Frontiers in Biomaterials

(Volume 4)

(Biomaterials for Tissue Engineering)

Edited by

Mehdi Razavi

Department of Radiology, School of Medicine, Stanford University, Palo Alto, California 94304, USA

General:

1. Any dispute or claim arising out of or in connection with this License Agreement or the Work (including non-contractual disputes or claims) will be governed by and construed in accordance with the laws of the U.A.E. as applied in the Emirate of Dubai. Each party agrees that the courts of the Emirate of Dubai shall have exclusive jurisdiction to settle any dispute or claim arising out of or in connection with this License Agreement or the Work (including non-contractual disputes or claims).
2. Your rights under this License Agreement will automatically terminate without notice and without the need for a court order if at any point you breach any terms of this License Agreement. In no event will any delay or failure by Bentham Science Publishers in enforcing your compliance with this License Agreement constitute a waiver of any of its rights.
3. You acknowledge that you have read this License Agreement, and agree to be bound by its terms and conditions. To the extent that any other terms and conditions presented on any website of Bentham Science Publishers conflict with, or are inconsistent with, the terms and conditions set out in this License Agreement, you acknowledge that the terms and conditions set out in this License Agreement shall prevail.

Bentham Science Publishers Ltd.
Executive Suite Y - 2
PO Box 7917, Saif Zone
Sharjah, U.A.E.
Email: subscriptions@benthamscience.org

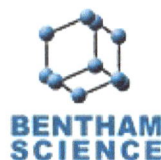

CONTENTS

FOREWORD

Biomaterials have come a long way since the first total joint replacements, which were introduced at a time when biomaterials were selected for their corrosion resistance. Orthopaedic surgeons initially selected materials which would stimulate the least reaction from the body. Materials used were "nearly inert" metal alloys and polymers. Total joint replacements revolutionised surgery and were life changing for patients. However, such materials are eventually rejected by the body, not in the same way as transplants, but because a thin layer of scar tissue forms around them, isolating them from the body, eventually causing the implant to be forced out of position. This became more problematic when clinicians attempted to repair or restore other parts of the skeleton or other tissues.

In 1969 (published in 1971), the invention of Bioglass® by Larry Hench, then at the University of Florida in Gainesville (USA), changed the face of orthopaedics. Bioglass was the first synthetic material that was found to bond with bone (no scar tissue). It is also biodegradable. However, it was not until the mid-1990s when the first Bioglass synthetic bone graft for bone regeneration reached the market. Now, it has been used in more than 1.5 million patients. Between the concept and clinical use of Bioglass, other bioactive ceramics reached clinicians first, such as synthetic hydroxyapatite, which is similar to bone mineral and also bonds with bone, albeit slower than Bioglass. This triggered the use of other calcium phosphate variants, such as tricalcium phosphate.

I mentioned that bioceramics can be biodegradable. This is possible by dissolution (also happens in water) or by cellular action (*e.g.* macrophages or osteoclasts). Hench termed the combination of biodegradation and bioactivity as 3rd Generation Biomaterials in a Science review in 2002.

Biomaterials are now being designed to deal with the body's own healing for many different clinical indications. To work well they must be used as temporary templates or scaffolding, specifically designed for the tissue that is being repaired. Scaffolds made of bioactive and biodegradable materials could present a 4th Generation if they are able to stimulate another course of action, *e.g.* blood vessel growth or bearing load. They can be labelled as 5th Generation, if they do both.

Remarkably, biomaterials have now gone beyond bone and orthopaedics. Almost every tissue in the body has received research attention, with clinical products at various stages of development. In this book, scaffolds for nerves, cardiovascular system, liver, kidney and skin applications are described in addition to bone, cartilage and dental. The translation of new devices from concept to clinic is a great challenge for biomaterials researchers, one that is certainly not lost on the authors of this book.

This book begins with important, and perhaps more conventional biodegradable materials, which are the biodegradable polymers that are used in sutures. Bioceramics are usually too brittle for load bearing structures that must take cyclic load, therefore, in this book they have been included within composites with polymers as the matrix. Metals are now also being made to be biodegradable.

Scaffolds are often designed to mimic the macrostructure of the host tissue, with blood vessels growing through the pore networks to feed the new tissue. Hydrogels are another important type of polymers which mimic the extracellular matrix of tissues. Hydrogels are particularly beneficial for cell types that exist in a 3D gel-like environment. Their unique property is their ability to transport nutrients through their watery networks to cells.

Scaffolds can be employed as an implant on their own, or can be seeded with cells (*e.g.* stem cells) *in vitro* prior to implantation, which is termed as tissue engineering.

The concept of bioactive, biodegradable and strong scaffolds is an important area in healthcare. The UK Government highlighted Eight Great Technologies in 2013, suggesting great need and opportunity for growth. Two of those are Advanced Materials and Regenerative Medicine. When new medical devices are created in the laboratory, they must be translated to clinic. In order to deliver these scaffolds, new manufacturing methods are also needed, such as Additive Manufacturing and 3D printing, which can create the required architectures and also promote reproducibility in large numbers.

Other aspects of technology transfer are the need to pass tests prescribed by regulatory bodies. The devices often highlight ambiguities in the tests, so new tests have to be developed. There is a large area of research in tests that can more closely assess the *in vivo* situation. While researchers often study how tissue specific cells respond to scaffolds, an important area often neglected is that how immune cells respond.

This new book provides a basic level of understanding of all of the above topics, starting from scaffold design; some key biomaterials; manufacturing techniques; to technology transfer aspects that include testing scaffolds both *in vivo* and *in vitro*. It provides the necessary foundation of science and technology. For the experienced researcher the book provides a comprehensive overview of the important current topics in the field. Happy reading.

Julian R. Jones
Department of Materials
Imperial College London
South Kensington Campus
London SW7 2AZ
UK
E-mail: julian.r.jones@imperial.ac.uk

PREFACE

Tissue engineering aims to regenerate damaged tissues by using a 3-dimensional bioscaffold, cells, biomolecules and growth factors. The success of this strategy depends on the biomaterials selection, design and development techniques of bioscaffolds and evaluation methods. Although, this field is new, upward advances are being made in order to be translated to patients. Therefore, it was found that an appropriate book which discusses the novel 3D bioscaffold designs and experimental procedures could be helpful for students and researchers. This book reviews the published resources and discusses the bioscaffolding materials, used techniques and presents the production parameters to clarify the evaluation protocols for analysis or testing. This book covers the chapters by leading bioengineers, biologists, dentists and clinicians. Therefore, the text has basic information that will be of use to bioengineers, clinicians and surgeons who deal with the tissue engineering strategies. This is a reference book for undergraduate and graduate courses and clinical laboratories. Finally, the editor thanks for the support of all the contributors and the publisher who made the publication of this book possible.

Mehdi Razavi
Department of Radiology, School of Medicine
Stanford University, Palo Alto, California 94304
USA
E-mail: mrazavi2659@gmail.com

List of Contributors

Amirsalar Khandan   Young Researchers and Elite Club, Khomeinishahr Branch, Islamic Azad University, Isfahan, Iran

Burak Ozdemir   Faculty of Chemistry and Metallurgical, Department of Bioengineering, Yildiz Technical University, Davutpasa St. No.127, 34210 Esenler, Istanbul, Turkey

Burcu Ozkan   Faculty of Chemistry and Metallurgical, Department of Bioengineering, Yildiz Technical University, Davutpasa St. No.127, 34210 Esenler, Istanbul, Turkey

Busra Ozkan   Faculty of Chemistry and Metallurgical, Department of Bioengineering, Yildiz Technical University, Davutpasa St. No.127, 34210 Esenler, Istanbul, Turkey

Drago Skrtic   Volpe Research Center, American Dental Association Foundation, Gaithersburg, Maryland, Unites States

Farnaz Naghizadeh   Biomedical Engineering Faculty, Amirkabir University of Technology (Tehran Polytechnic), Tehran, Iran

Hamidreza Mokhtari   Department of Materials Engineering, Isfahan University of Technology, Isfahan 84156-83111, Iran

Hossein Jazayeri   Marquette University, School of Dentistry, Milwaukee, WI 53233, USA

Ibrahim Isildak   Faculty of Chemistry and Metallurgical, Department of Bioengineering, Yildiz Technical University, Davutpasa St. No.127, 34210 Esenler, Istanbul, Turkey

Ilke Kurt   Faculty of Chemistry and Metallurgical, Department of Bioengineering, Yildiz Technical University, Davutpasa St. No.127, 34210 Esenler, Istanbul, Turkey

Joseph M. Antonucci   Biomaterials Group, Biosystems and Biomaterials Division, National Institute of Standards and Technology, Gaithersburg, Maryland, United States

Kubra Gozutok   Faculty of Chemistry and Metallurgical, Department of Bioengineering, Yildiz Technical University, Davutpasa St. No.127, 34210 Esenler, Istanbul, Turkey

Mahdis Hesami   Amirkabir University of Technology, Tehran, Iran

Mehdi Razavi   Department of Radiology, School of Medicine, Stanford University, Palo Alto, California 94304, USA

Mehtap Sert   Faculty of Chemistry and Metallurgical, Department of Bioengineering, Yildiz Technical University, Davutpasa St. No.127, 34210 Esenler, Istanbul, Turkey

Mina D. Fahmy   Marquette University, School of Dentistry, Milwaukee, WI 53233, USA

Nasim Kiaie   Department of Biomedical Engineering, Amirkabir University of Technology, Tehran, 15875, Iran

Nasrin Mokhtari   Department of Dentistry, Khorasgan University of Dentistry Sciences, Isfahan 81551-39998, Iran

Neslinur Ozcelik   Faculty of Chemistry and Metallurgical, Department of Bioengineering, Yildiz Technical University, Davutpasa St. No.127, 34210 Esenler, Istanbul, Turkey

Rabia Cakir-Koc   Faculty of Chemistry and Metallurgical, Department of Bioengineering, Yildiz Technical University, Davutpasa St. No.127, 34210 Esenler, Istanbul, Turkey

Yasemin Budama-Kilinc   Faculty of Chemistry and Metallurgical, Department of Bioengineering, Yildiz Technical University, Davutpasa St. No.127, 34210 Esenler, Istanbul, Turkey

Zeynep Kaya   Faculty of Chemistry and Metallurgical, Department of Bioengineering, Yildiz Technical University, Davutpasa St. No.127, 34210 Esenler, Istanbul, Turkey

CHAPTER 1

Synthetic Biopolymers

Mahdis Hesami[*]

Amirkabir University of Technology, Tehran, Iran

Abstract: The striking role of tissue engineering in saving people's life is inevitable. The number of patients waiting for an organ donor is increasing every minute. On the other hand, life expectancy has increased which results in a growing demand of scaffold production. The developed technology seeks for materials which target specific cells, proliferate, regenerate the targeted tissue and restores its function. To fulfill this, not only the material type but also the fabrication techniques should be engineered carefully. Among various materials, synthetic polymers have attracted more attention due to their tailorable properties. In this chapter an overview of various synthetic polymers, their degradation, application and their various blends is discussed. The polymeric nanocomposites used as scaffold have been introduced briefly and the future research in the material selection for porous scaffolds has been reviewed.

Keywords: Biocompatible, Biodegradable, Biomimetic, Polymer blend, Polymer physics, Porous scaffold, Synthetic polymer, Tissue engineering.

INTRODUCTION

Saving people's lives is an admirable goal throughout history. Various materials including metals, glasses and woods have been used in human body more than 2000 years ago. Romans, Chinese and Aztecs were the first who used gold in dentistry. During centuries, scientists and surgeons made lots of effort to treat patients who lost one of their organs. The first autografting was done in 17 century by a Dutch doctor with a piece of dog bone. Although the patient was excommunicated, the therapy worked well [1]. The next big jump toward implantations happened during world war II when the injured airplane pilots by shards of polymethyl methacrylate (PMMA) felt much better than those injured by standard glass [1]. Nowadays population is growing much faster than before while the life expectancy is growing even faster. According to world health organization (WHO) report, about 8.5 million people die every year as a result of

[*] **Corresponding author Mahdis Hesami:** Amirkabir University of Technology, Tehran, Iran; Tel: +49 6131 379-520; E-mail: mahdis.hesami@aut.ac.ir

Mehdi Razavi (Ed.)

injury. This number is 32% more than fatalities due to malaria, HIV and tuberculosis and highlights the necessity for a solution [2]. Organ transplantations including autografts and allografts have been regarded as an efficient therapy although they have disadvantages. In some cases the transplanted organ is rejected by the patient's body because of immunogenic responses. In many cases the shortage of donor organ leads to patient's death. Every 12 min, one name is added to the transplant waiting list while an average of 22 people die each day waiting for transplants [3]. Tissue engineering is a promising alternative which provides the potential for regenerating tissues and organs of the human body. Various materials have been employed for this purpose including: metals, ceramics, natural and synthetic polymers. Among them, synthetic polymers have attracted more attention due to their superior characteristics. Their Excellency is because of their tailorable properties, biodegradability, biocompatibility and mass production. Metals used as clinical sides are not bio-degradable which means they require a second surgery for removal [4]. On the other hand, bio activated ceramics confront similar problems. They may react with physiological fluids in the body and form unwanted bonds to hard or soft tissues. Consequently, their biocompatibility is not well guaranteed [5].

For tissue engineering purposes, the synthetic bio polymer must have tailorable chemical and mechanical properties as well as proper architecture and morphology [6]. This is specifically important in porous scaffolds where interconnected pore networks provide place for cell attachment and growth. Furthermore, synthetic bio polymers can be mass produced and have a long shelf time. Synthetic bio polymers offer distinct advantages of biological properties and versatility of chemistry which leads to produce scaffolds with predictable uniformity and free from immunogenicity concerns. However in order to achieve these goals some criteria should be considered for selecting the synthetic bio polymer used for scaffold applications. These include material chemistry, molecular weight, polymer architecture, solubility, hydrophilicity/hydrophobicity, lubricity, surface energy, water absorption, and erosion mechanism (bio-degradation mechanism where necessary) [5]. In this section, the effect of mentioned parameters will be explained. In section 2, different synthetic biopolymers used in porous scaffolds will be introduced. In section 3, the application of polymer nanocomposites in scaffolds will be discussed briefly and finally the future research trends in this field will be reviewed.

REQUIRED CHARACTERISTICS FOR A SCAFFOLD

• **Biocompatibility:** The scaffold applied inside the human body should be fabricated from biocompatible material in order not to cause an immunological reaction or foreign body attack [7]. This includes the blood compatibility as well. It means that the material should perform an appropriate host response and not cause toxic or injurious effects. Furthermore it should support the appropriate cellular activity such as facilitation of molecular signals [8].

- **Biodegradation:** The planted scaffold should be bio-adsorbed by the surrounding tissues in order to omit the necessity of a surgical removal. However to achieve this, two important issues should be considered. First, the degradation should not produce toxic and harmful byproducts. Second, the kinetic of degradation should be designed appropriately according to the final application. For example, in skeletal tissue engineering, bio-adsorption of the scaffold should be relatively slow, since the mechanical strength should be adequate until tissue regeneration is almost completed. However, for the skin scaffold, bio degradation rate should be relatively high. If the scaffold remains for a long time, the remaining material may retard the tissue regeneration rather than healing effect [9].

- **Processability:** In contrast to metals and ceramics which have poor processability, polymers can be processed easily [10]. There are plenty of methods for producing porous scaffolds based on synthetic biopolymers. The method selection depends on many parameters and should be engineered carefully. This issue will be discussed in another chapter.

- **Pore Density:** An important factor for a scaffold is porosity and adequate pore size. The mission of scaffolds is to provide an appropriate environment for attaching the cells and growing them. In order to fulfill this goal, interconnected micro pores with sufficient pore size are necessary. The cells can be seeded and grow on the micro pores which provide vascular formation as well as waste transport. For bone tissue engineering a minimum pore diameter of 150 μm is suggested while for soft tissue engineering a range of 200-250 μm is recommended [11].

- **Mechanical Properties:** Generally the mechanical properties of scaffold should be sufficient to shield cells from damaging under compressive or tensile forces [12]. However, in some applications mechanical properties play a striking role, *e.g.* in skeletal systems. Mechanical environments markedly affect the bone tissue scaffolds. The amount of load on the bone tissue engineering affects its reconstruction.

BIOPOLYMERS

Bio polymers can be divided into various classes regarding to synthesis, properties, biodegradability and application. The designed scaffold may be used as a 'soft' or 'hard' tissue; therefore the kind of material used differs. For soft tissues *e.g.* cardiovascular substitutes or skeletal muscle, generally a wide variety of polymers are employed. Hard tissues, *e.g.* bone substitutes, are usually fabricated from rigid polymers. In this section the synthetic polymers used as scaffold have been reviewed regardless their ways of categorizing. Their application, properties, synthesis and biodegradation mechanism have been scrutinized as well.

Polyesters (Poly (α-Hydroxy-Acid))

Among various synthetic bio polymers, poly (α-hydroxy-acid)s are very popular due to their distinct properties. The advantage of these poly esters is that their degradation rate is tailorable. Depending on the final application, their degradation period can be controlled from months to years [12]. This is the reason why these biopolymers are most common polymers for scaffold application. However just like a double edged sword, they also have disadvantages. Within degradation, poly (hydroxy acids) produce acidic species which may decrease the local pH and accelerate the degradation rate. This may cause inflammation for surrounding implant [13]. They also suffer from their hydrophobicity which hinders smooth cell seeding. To overcome these drawbacks, copolymers or blends can be used. The most applicable poly (hydroxy acids) include PLA, PCL and PGA.

Polycaprolactone

Polycaprolactone (PCL) is a semi-crystalline polymer with a glass transition temperature (Tg) of approximately –65°C and a melting point (Tm) of approximately 60 °C which is prepared by ring opening polymerization of ε-caprolactone. PCL imparts good biocompatibility, biodegradability and permeability and shows excellent cell attachment and growth. Scheme (**1**) shows its structure.

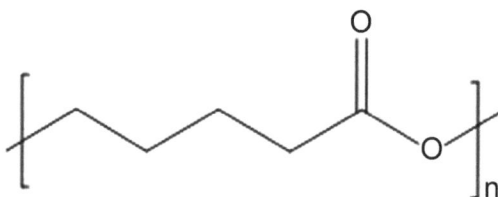

Scheme 1. Structure of polycaprolactone.

Biodegradation

The biodegradation of PCL takes place because of the ester linkages in the linear polyester which are susceptible to hydrolysis. In comparison to other aliphatic polyesters, degradation kinetics of PCL is slower because of its hydrophobic nature and high crystallinity. The products generated by biodegradation are either metabolized via the tricarboxylic acid (TCA) cycle or eliminated by direct renal secretion [14] Generally, degradation kinetics of poly(hydroxy acid) is affected by various factors including: degree of crystallinity, site of implantation [15] and molecular weight [16].

Scaffold Preparation Techniques

Polycaprolactone scaffolds can been constructed with a variety of solid free-form (SFF) techniques including fused deposition modeling (FDM) [17, 18], photo polymerization of a synthesized PCL macromere [14], shape deposition modeling [19], precision extruding deposition [20], low-temperature deposition [21] multi-nozzle free-form deposition [22] and selective laser sintering (SLS) [23]. The maximum porosity obtained by FDM technique was 80% while the non-woven method provides irregular porous structures with a pore size of 20-100 μm [23].

Direct solid free-form techniques provide porous scaffold with an appropriate control over porosity, pore size and interconnectivity. However they offer limited micro scale resolution and also require multifaceted manufacturing control. To overcome these problems and benefit the SFF technique, indirect SFF method has been employed [24]. Porogen-based SFF, a method of indirect SFF technique, has been recently applied for fabrication of PCL scaffolds as an alternative for bone tissue engineering. Employing this technique has resulted in scaffolds with a pore size of 200μm. Furthermore, the resolution of the 3D-SSF system was at least 2-fold as compared to directly built scaffolds [25].

In order to increase the surface area of PCL scaffolds, various methods have been employed *e.g.* fused deposition modeling [26]. Li *et al.* used needleless electro spinning for the first time to produce PCL 3D fibrous tissue engineering scaffolds. In comparison to the solvent casting method, needleless electrospun scaffolds showed higher porosity with higher surface-to-volume ratio which results in the enhancement of protein adsorption, cell attachment and proliferation. These scaffolds showed great potential in soft tissue engineering. With a 3D structure and larger pore size, fibroblasts were able to migrate up to 800 μm into the scaffolds [27].

Application

PCL is often used in bone tissue engineering and cartilage. In contrast to autogenic and allogenic grafts which suffer from various problems, bone tissues based on PCL have shown successful results. Disadvantages of grafting include organ rejection and donor site morbidity. On the other hand, metal implants used as bone tissues, can't perform healthy bone either. They are not bio-degradable so they require a second surgery for removal. Furthermore, they can't remodel during time and they may cause stress shielding. Another choice for bone tissue organs is bioceramic especially hydroxyapatite (HA) which is osteogenic.

However, HA is brittle and can't be processed into complex shapes [28]. PCL based scaffolds overcome these problems and recently they attracted much attention for bone repairment.

PCL-based scaffolds are also proper for skin replacement [29, 30] and nerve tissue engineering [31]. The application of PCL in tissue-engineered skin is because of its good mechanical properties as well as biocompatibility. Natural scaffolds such as collagen lattice used in skin tissue engineering suffer from shrinkage and interspecies pathogen transfer. Synthetic polymers also have shortcomings which must be considered. One of these shortcomings is low mechanical strength which can be compensated by producing biaxially stretched PCL. The results showed that cell attachment and proliferation of these stretched PCL was 20-40% better than that on polyurethane [29].

Another application of PCL-based scaffold is in nerve tissue engineering. In the case of nerve tissue engineering, electrical conductivity is vital. Consequently, applied scaffold should be prepared from conductive polymer or its blends. Since PCL is not conductive, its blends with a conductive polymer have been used for nerve tissue engineering which is explained in the following paragraphs.

Polycaprolactone Blends: PCL/ Hydrogels

Recently, the blends of PCL with natural hydrogels (gelatin, collagen, chitosan and alginate) have attracted much attention. Chitosan is a natural bio polymer which is extensively used for wound healing applications and for skin tissue engineering in combination with other biopolymers. Blending of two polymers is an appropriate method to bring desired physico-chemical characteristics of both polymers. Electrospun mats of chitosan/ PCL with a composition ratio of 1:5 were used for skin tissue engineering. In comparison to PCL alone, the blend showed enhanced cell adhesion, cell spreading and proliferation [32].

Introduction alginate to PCL can overcome the PCL deficiencies as well as alginate ones. PCL can produce acidic by-products during degradation, causing an inflammatory response. On the other hand, alginates have poor mechanical properties and limited 3D shape-ability due to their hydrophilic nature. Blending of these polymers can improve low mechanical strength and biocompatibility of alginate and PCL respectively. These nano fibrous scaffolds could be suitable for the regeneration of various hard tissues [33].

PCL/collagen composite scaffolds prepared by electrospinning have good mechanical properties as well as good cell adhesion and proliferation. They have been studied in various tissue engineering fields such as skin [34] and vascularization vessels [35].

PCL/ gelatin nano fibers were extensively studied by Ramakrishna *et al.* they used these scaffolds for dermal reconstitution [36] as well as neural tissue engineering. For this purpose C17.2 nerve stem cells were carried out. These cells can be used as neuron precursors since they are involved in the normal development of cerebellum, embryonic neocortex and other structures. In comparison to PCL, PCL/ gelatin nanofibers have promoted neurite extension [31].

Polycaprolactone Copolymers

In order to balance hydrophobicity and crystallinity of caprolactone, its copolymers with hydrophilic monomers has been prepared. Polyethylene glycols (PEGs) have been most commonly copolymerized with caprolactone to prepare hydrophilic, non-toxic, non-immunogenic and non-antigenic copolymers. Davaran *et al.* [37] synthesized triblock PCL-PEG-PCL copolymers by ring-opening polymerization of caprolactone in the presence of PEG and employed electrospinning to produce nano fibrous scaffolds. They studied the effect of composition and PEG molecular weight on morphology of nanofibers and concluded that, by increasing molecular weight of PEG, the fiber diameter decreased and the fiber morphology became finer. These results are of significant importance for design of scaffolds. By applying this method the favorable properties of PEG retains and the spin ability improves.

Polyglycolic Acid

Poly (glycolic acid) (PGA) -also called polyglycolide- is a rigid thermoplastic material with high crystallinity (46-50%). It can be prepared by polycondensation or ring-opening polymerization of glycolic acid. The glass transition temperature and melting point temperatures of PGA are 36°C and 225°C, respectively. According to some reports, PGA is not soluble in most organic solvents due to its high crystallinity; the exceptions are highly fluorinated organic solvents such as hexafluoro isopropanol [6]. Scheme (**2**) depicts the structure of PGA.

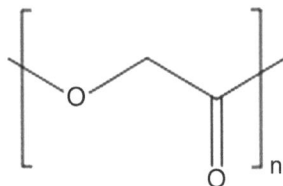

Scheme 2. structure of polyglycolic acid.

Biodegradation

Polyglycolic acid is a bulk degrading polymer, degrades by the non-specific scission of the ester backbone. The degradation process happens in two steps, first, diffusion of water molecules into the amorphous regions of the matrix and second, hydrolytic chain scission of the ester groups. Finally, the crystalline regions of the polymer will be triggered to degrade the polymer completely [6].

Application

Polyglycolic acid scaffolds have various applications including heart valve, myocardial tissue, esophagus, trachea [38] and wound dressing [39]. They are also served as the template for neocartilage formation. The grown neocartilage has stained positively for extracellular matrix structures found in native cartilage, such as sulfated glycosaminoglycan, collagen type II, and elastin [40].

Disadvantages of PCL include: high rate of degradation, acidic degradation products and low solubility. Therefore, several copolymers containing glycoside units are being developed to compensate the inherent shortages of polyglycolide [41]. The most common copolymer is poly (lactide-co-glycolide) which will be explained in the following paragraphs.

Polylactic Acid

Poly (lactic acid) –also called polylactide- is aliphatic polyester derived from renewable resources, such as corn starch, tapioca roots, chips or starch. It exist in three isomeric forms due to its monomer chirality: semi crystalline d(-), semi crystalline l(+) and racemic (d,l) which is amorphous [6]. Poly (L-lactide) (PLLA) is a semi crystalline polymer with 37% crystallinity. The degree of crystallinity depends on the molecular weight and polymer processing parameters. It has a glass transition temperature of 60–65°C and a melting temperature of approximately 175°C. PLLA has high tensile strength and modulus and therefore it is an ideal biomaterial for load bearing structures.

Poly (DL-lactide) (PDLLA) is an amorphous polymer due to the random distribution of L- and D-lactide units. It has a glass transition temperature of 55–60°C and a melting point of approximately 260°C. In comparison to PLLA, PDLLA shows much lower strength (1.9 GPa) which can be attributed to its amorphous nature. This polymer loses its strength within 1–2 months when hydrolyzed and undergoes a loss in mass within 12–16 months [41]. In Scheme (**3**) structure of PLA is shown.

Biodegradation

PLA degrades by bulk hydrolysis and produces lactic acid which exists in the human body. The body transports the produced L(+) lactic acid to the liver, converts it into pyruvic acid and upon entering the tricarboxylic acid cycle, secreting it as water and carbon dioxide and finally the carbon dioxide will excrete by the lungs [42]. However, some inflammatory responses have been reported since the produced lactic acid can lower the pH locally.

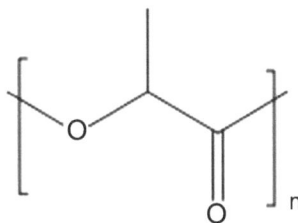

Scheme 3. Structure of polylactide.

The hydrolytic degradation of PLA is influenced by various factors including [43]:

- Water permeability, solubility (hydrophilicity/hydrophobicity).
- Additives presenting in the final scaffold (acidic, basic, monomers, solvents or even drugs): Basic compounds can catalyze ester linkage scission and thus accelerate polymer degradation on one hand and decelerate the degradation by absorbing the carboxylic acid sites on the other hand. The balancing between these two mechanisms determines the rate of degradation.
- Morphology of the PLA: (crystalline, amorphous and the degree of crystallinity), the higher the degree of crystallinity the lower rate of degradation.
- Porosity: by increasing the amount of porosity, the bio-degradation accelerates since the oligomers and low molecular weight produced during degradation can diffuse faster and expedite the degradation. These oligomeric chains are ended by carboxylic acid groups which may facilitate the autocatalytic degradation of the polymer.
- Glass transition temperature.
- Molecular weight and molecular weight distribution: wide molecular weight distribution means that the numbers of carboxylic end groups are higher compared to narrow molecular weight distribution which results in faster degradation rate.
- Sterilization: the types of materials used for sterilizations or the employed technique will affect the degradation.
- Site of implantation.

Scaffold Preparation Techniques

Porous scaffolds of PLA can be fabricated by different techniques including solvent casting [44], ice particle leaching method, gas foaming/ salt leaching method [45], freeze drying [46] and thermally induced phase separation. For producing fibrous scaffolds, electrospinning [47] or wet spinning can be also employed.

Application

Polylactic acid (PLA), and their copolymers have different applications in three dimensional culture and transplantation of articular, auricular, nasal, costochondral, tracheal, chondrocytes and intervertebral disk [48]. several cell types were successfully grown on the surface of PLA scaffolds including MC3T3-E1 osteoprogenitor cells [49], osteoblasts [50] chondrocyte [51], keratinocytes [52], hepatocytes [53], Bone marrow-derived mesenchymal stem cells (BMSCs) (cardiovascular applications such as tissue-engineered heart valves) [54], pneumocytes [55], Hep G2 cells [56] and neural stem cells [57].

Polylactide Copolymers and Composites; Poly(lactic-glycolic Acid)

PLGA is a linear copolymer with a Tg around 37°C that can be prepared at different ratios between its constituent monomers, lactic (LA) and glycolic acid (GA). It is preferred for the fabrication of bone substitute because of its superior control over degradation rates, crystallization and physico-chemical properties such as hydrophobicity/hydrophilicity balance. PLGA can be synthesized via different synthesis processes including solution poly-condensation, melt/solid polycondensation process and ring opening polymerization. In spite of the molecular weight of the monomers and their ratio, tacticity (stereochemistry) of the copolymer also influences dramatically the ultimate properties. By increasing the molecular weight, the degradation rate decreases. Also if the ratio of LA to GA enhances the degradation rate decreases because LA component is less hydrophilic compared to GA. PLGA degrades by hydrolysis of its ester linkages and converts into LA and GA byproducts [58].

PLGA materials have been used extensively to fabricate scaffolds for engineering musculoskeletal tissue. These include scaffolds for bone [59] cartilage and meniscus. PLGA scaffolds showed acceptable results by culturing various cells including 3T3 fibroblasts [60], osteoblasts [50, 61, 62], chondrocytes [63], keratinocytes [52], Bone marrow-derived mesenchymal stem cells (BMSCs) [54, 64], Primary neonatal Schwann cells [65] and Adipose tissue [66].

In order to produce porous scaffold out of PLGA, various techniques have been employed including phase separation [67], gas forming [68], porogen leaching [44] and solid free form techniques [69]. Porogen leaching method has been widely used by different researchers however this technique suffers from some serious problems such as incomplete solvent removal and restricted thickness. Some improvements are exerted by combining two methods *e.g.* gas forming and particulate leaching which omits the need of solvent and combination of the porogen leaching and melt-molding. Nowadays, selective laser sintering is used as a useful technique for producing scaffolds of PLGA [58]. Scheme (**4**) depicts the structure of PLGA.

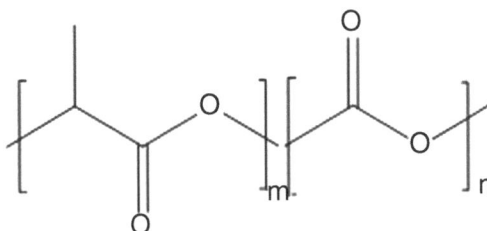

Scheme 4. Structure of poly (lactide-co-glycolide).

Polylactide/ Poly(lactic-glycolic Acid) (PLA/PLGA) Blends

An important issue in polymer blends is their miscibility which determines the physicochemical and final properties of the blend. In tissue engineering field, this aspect is of great importance because tailoring the ultimate properties is influenced by the blend characteristics. The miscibility of blends can be investigated by various method such as thermal (detecting the Tg), rheological methods and microscopic methods.

The researches have shown that blends of PLLA and PLGA (LA: GA=50:50) are immiscible and create a biphasic morphology (matrix-droplet). However in some compositions (75/25 PLA/PLGA) a certain degree of compatibility has been observed. In addition to blend composition, other factors also affect the miscibility including lactic to glycolic ratio in PLGA, blending method and molecular weight of each component [70, 71].

Addition of PLGA to PLLA has some benefits: the *in vitro* degradation of the blend has accelerated compared to its component. Furthermore, presence of PLGA can reduce the inflammatory reaction at the site of implantation.

Polylactide/ Polycaprolactone (PLA/PCL)

In order to overcome the brittleness of PLA, blending with a tough bio-polymer has been suggested. PCL is a bio degradable polymer which also improves the fracture toughness of PLA. Blends of PLLA and PCL form immiscible phases, with the PCL phases finely dispersed in the PLLA-rich matrix phase [72]. The presence of PCL in PLLA/PCL blends reduces the crystallinity of PLA. As a consequence, elongation at break increases and ductility improves. These blends have been used for bone regeneration and their efficacy tested using bovine periosteal tissues. The addition of PCL decreased the brittleness of PLLA membranes and at 50% PCL content, the elongation was also improved without decreasing the porosity on the membrane surface which is important for tissue adherence [73].

Polylactide/ Polyethylene Glycole (PLA/PEG)

The high hydrophobicity of PLA restricts its applications in some certain fields of tissue engineering. Therefore copolymerization with a hydrophilic bio-polymer such as PEG has been considered. Another way is blending of PLA with PEG which results in a partial miscible blend. Introduction of PEG to PLA also increases the biodegradation rate due to the enhancement of the surface hydrophilicity. These scaffolds can be used both in bone and skin tissue engineering. The result of dermal fibroblast cell culturing has proved the cellular interaction with nanofibrous mats. Cultivation of osteoblasts-like MG-63 cells also showed the adherence and proliferation of cells in the scaffold [74, 75].

In addition to electrospinning and freeze drying methods, gas forming technique has also been employed for preparation of PLA/PEG scaffolds. In this technique porosity is created by dispersing gas bubbles inside a viscous polymer solution. The gas bubbles can be formed by a blowing agent *via* chemical reactions. Dehghani *et al.* used this method for preparation of PLA/PEG scaffolds by tailoring the porosity. According to their results, mechanical properties of PLA/PEG blends with less than 30wt% PEG were suitable for the fabrication of porous scaffolds. However, increasing the concentration of PEG to above 50% resulted in blends that were brittle and had low mechanical integrity [76].

Introduction of PEG to PLA not only improves the hydrophilicity of PLA but also increases the porosity. In comparison to PLA, blends of PLA/PEG have a higher porosity. The porous films of PLA/PEG can be used for wound dressing. The enhanced porosity and hydrophilicity result in a higher water vapor transmission rate and higher oxygen permeability which are essential parameters for healing a wound. In order to prepare antimicrobial wound dressings, antibiotic drugs can be loaded on these porous matrix films. The results published by Phaechamud *et al.* confirm that these drug-loaded porous films, will efficiently inhibit the bacterial growth so they can be used as an effective dressing for treatment or prevention of bacterial wound infection [77].

Polylactide/ Polyhydroxybutyratevalerate (PLA/ PHBV)

Despite of suitable properties of PLA, it exhibits some drawbacks such as high brittleness and low heat resistance. These drawbacks need to be addressed in order to widen its range of applications in tissue engineering. Polyhydroxy-butyratevalerate (PHBV) is a copolymer of PHB with randomly arranged 3-

hydroxybutyrate (HB) groups and 3-hydroxyvalarate (HV) groups which exhibits high stiffness and crystallinity. This polymer is a good candidate for blending with PLA to improve its brittleness. Peng *et al.* [78] studied the effect of the PLA/PHBV blend composition on the morphology as well as thermal and mechanical properties of microcellular PLA/PHBV injection molded component. According to their results, PLA/PHBV blends containing less than 30% PHBV were miscible. It was proved that addition of PHBV to PLA improves the strain-at-break significantly.

The capability of cell adhesion and growth on PLA/PHBV substrates was studied by Stantos *et al.* They used Vero cells (a fibroblastic cell line established from the kidney of the African green monkey) for this case and studied various blend compositions. They concluded that (60/40) and (50/50) PLA/PHBV blends had the best cell adhesion among other compositions [79].

Hybrid of Poly (Hydroxyl Acids) with Collagen

As mentioned before, poly (hydroxy acids) suffer from their hydrophobic property which results in lack cell-recognition signals and hinders smooth cell seeding. In contrast, naturally derived collagen has the potential advantages of specific cell interactions and hydrophilicity, but collagen based scaffolds have poor mechanical strength. In order to benefit the properties of each polymer, hybridization of collagen and polyesters have been employed. Chen *et al.* produced PLGA-collagen hybrids by combining porogen leaching and freeze-drying techniques. By applying this method pore structures of the polymer sponges could be manipulated. These hybrids benefit both the synthetic polymers and collagens [80].

Polyhydroxyalkonates

Polyhydroxyalkonates (PHA) are aliphatic polyesters which are produced by microorganisms under unbalanced growth conditions. PHAs are generally biodegradable and have good biocompatibility therefore, they have been regarded as good candidates for tissue engineering biomaterials. Today, there are more than 100 known PHAs which have different structures and various physical-mechanical properties [81]. The most applicable PHA in tissue engineering include poly 3-hydroxybutyrate (PHB), 3-hydroxyvalerate (PHBV), poly 4-hydroxybutyrate (P4HB), hydroxyhexanoate (PHBHHx) and poly 3-hydroxyoctanoate (PHO). PHB is the most common member of the PHA family which has good biocompatibility for adrenocortical cells, osteoblasts, epithelial cells, fibroblasts, endothelium cells, and isolated hepatocytes [82]. Scheme (**5**) shows the general structure of polyhydroxyalkonates.

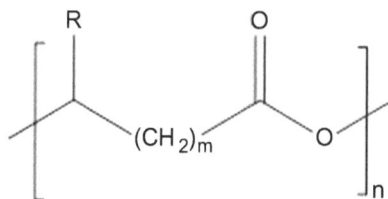

Scheme 5. Structure of polyhydroxyalkonate: *m=1, R=CH3*, the monomer structure is 3-hydroxybutyrate; *m=1, R=C3H7* monomer is hydroxyhexanoate.

Biodegradation

Another superiority of PHB among various PHAs is its existence in blood. Low molecular weight PHB is widely distributed in biological cells, being found in representative organism of nearly all phyla [83]. However the toxicological properties of other PHAs should be checked before use. For example hydroxyvalerate may be cytotoxic and may cause inflammatory effects. In general, various parameters affect biodegradation of PHAs including: composition of the material, methods of processing, crystallinity and molecular weight [81].

Scaffold Preparation Techniques

There are currently several methods available for fabrication of PHA scaffolds, including solution casting, electrospinning, phase separation, solvent casting, fiber bonding and particulate leaching, solid freeform fabrication, and particle sintering [84].

Application

The main application of PHAs is in the bone tissue engineering. Application of PHB as bone tissue showed no evidence of an undesirable chronic inflammatory [85]. Poly(3-hydroxybutyrate-co-3-hydroxyhexanoate) PHBHHx scaffolds have been applied for tendon repairing. In order to evaluate their facilitation of tendon movement recovery and complete restoration of load bearing and function, rats marrow recipient were employed [86].

Another application of PHAs is in neuro tissue engineering. PHA scaffolds can be used for cultivation of neural stem cells which may be useful for repairing central nervous system injury [84]. An example is PHBHHx which promotes neural stem cells differentiation into neurons. Nanofiber scaffolds prepared from PHBHHx, are good candidates for treating central nervous system defects [84].

Blends of (Polyhydroxy Alkonate) PHAs: Poly 3-hydroxybutyrate/ Polyethylene Glycol (PHB/PEG)

A drawback of PHB is its poor hydrophilicity. In order to improve the hydrophilicity, it would be practical to blend it with a hydrophilic polymer such as PEG. Cheng *et al.* [87] produced PHB/PEG blends for blood vessel. Their results showed that PEG played an important role in resisting platelet adhesion. Furthermore, by increasing the PEG loading, the number of live cells increased which is an evidence for the suitability of the blend for blood vessel.

Recently, Karahaliloglu *et al.* [88] used plasma polymerization to graft PEG on the surface of PHB nanofibers. In order to improve the drawbacks of PHB, they used surface modification. At first nanofibers of PHB were produced by electrospinning then PEG was grafted on its surface. L-929 cells were used to test the proliferation. The results proved that surface modification has improved the proliferation.

Poly 3-hydroxybutyrate/Poly (lactic-co-caprolactone)(PHB/PLCL)

Punyodom *et al.* [89] produced a blend of PLCL, PHB by electrospinning. They observed that by increasing PLCL loading in PHB blends, the average fiber diameters and the distribution of diameters in the electrospun scaffolds decreases significantly. Furthermore, PLCL has improved the brittleness of PHB. On the other hand presence of PHB improved cell adhesion and growth of PLCL.

Poly 3-hydroxybutyrate /Poly (3-hydroxyvalerate) (PHB/PHBV)

PHB is known as a rigid and highly crystalline polymer with slow degradation rate that results in a poor processing window. In contrast, PHBV has lower glass transition and melting temperatures and therefore it is more flexible and easier to process. Blending of PHB with PHBV will decrease the melting temperature, leading to the possibility to process the materials at lower temperature. Blends of PHB/PHBV have been studied in various compositions. PHB/PHBV 50/50 scaffolds have been used in bone tissue engineering [90] and PHB/PHBV 30/70 have been used as scaffold for human adipose tissue-derived stem cells [91]. Recently, Morshed *et al.* [92] prepared random and aligned PHB/PHBV nanofibers by electrospinning and evaluated the Schwann cells (SCs) effect on them. They observed that aligned nanofibrous scaffolds showed higher SCs proliferation after 14 days compared to random nanofibers. These results confirm the suitability of the scaffolds for using in nerve tissue engineering.

Poly (Propylene Fumarate)

Poly (propylene fumarate) (PPF) is a linear polyester polymerized of fumaric acid. The fumarate double bonds are reactive and crosslink at low temperatures, making it valuable as an in situ polymerizable biomaterial especially for orthopedic applications. Although crosslinked networks may be formed from PPF alone, a variety of crosslinking agents have been explored in combination with PPF for the formation of crosslinked, degradable polymer networks with tunable material properties. For example, crosslinked networks of PPF with *N*-vinyl pyrrolidinone, poly(ethylene glycol)-dimethacrylate, PPF-diacrylate and diethyl fumarate have been developed [93]. In Scheme (**6**), the structure of poly (propylene fumarate) has been shown.

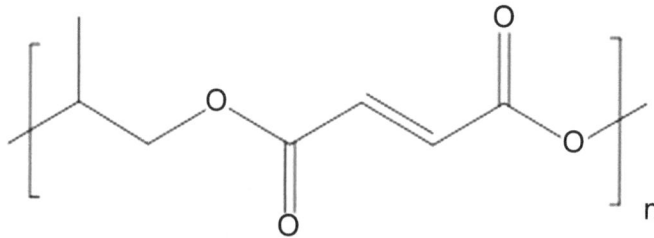

Scheme 6. Structure of poly (propylene fumarate).

Biodegradation

Degradation of PPF starts by hydrolysis of the ester bonds (as shown in Scheme **6**) and results into fumaric acid and propylene glycol which are biocompatible and insoluble in water [94].

Application

The double bonds in PPF allow the linear polymer to be crosslinked into a solid, polymeric network which makes it appropriate for bone tissue engineering scaffolds. This polymer was either used as an injectable in situ curing material or as preformed scaffold [95]. The PPF scaffolds were used for large cranial defects in a rabbit model. The scaffolds were photo crosslinked by UV laser and produced with various porosities. The results showed that bone ingrowth in PPF scaffolds implanted into cranial defects was <3% of the defect area which confirms their suitability as platform for bone tissue engineering [96].

Although PPF has good mechanical properties, for bone tissue application it must mimic the bone extracellular matrix. Bone is a structure composed of hydroxyapatite crystals deposited within an organic matrix consisting of □95% type I collagen. Therefore, hydroxyapatite and other calcium phosphate have been introduced to PPF to improve bone regeneration capacity. The results revealed that scaffolds with each of the calcium phosphate coatings were capable of sustaining recombinant human bone morphogenetic protein-2 (rhBMP-2) release and retained an open porous structure [97].

Polyanhydride

Polyanhydrides are a class of biodegradable and biocompatible polymers which degrade by surface erosion. Generally, they are polymerized by polycondensation method through dehydration of the diacid or a mixture of diacids [98].The dicarboxylic acid monomers are converted to the mixed anhydride of acetic acid by reflux in excess acetic anhydride. High molecular weight polymers are prepared by melt-polycondensation of pre polymer in vacuum under nitrogen sweep [6].

Polyanhydrides are chemically reactive which has both advantage and disadvantage. Their advantage is their degradation by surface erosion without the need of incorporation various catalysts or excipients. However because of high reactivity, polyanhydrides may react with compounds containing free amino groups or other nucleo polyanhydrides [99]. Another drawback of polyanhydrides is their limited mechanical properties which restrict their use in load–bearing applications such as orthopedics. For orthopedic means they are blended or copolymerized with other polymers [6].

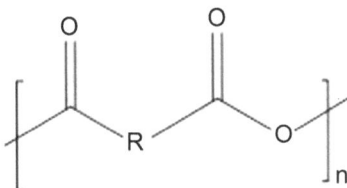

Scheme 7. Structure of polyanhydride.

Biodegradation

Polyanhydrides are surface eroding polymers which do not allow water to penetrate into the material and erode layer by layer. Their degradation proceeds by hydrolysis of the anhydride linkage. By choosing appropriate diacid monomers, the hydrolytic degradation rates can be manipulated. Poly (sebacic acid) degrades quickly (about 54 days in saline), while poly (1,6-bis(-*p*-carboxyphenoxy) hexane degrade much more slowly (estimated 1 year). In order to control degradation rate for a specific application, different amounts of these monomers can be combined in polymer [100].

Application

Polyanhydrides may have an orthopedic application but their Young's Modulus should be improved by formation of cross-linked networks. Two various strategies have been employed to improve mechanical properties of polyanhydrides: copolymerization and photo polymerization.

Incorporation of aromatic imide groups to anhydride monomers can increase the thermal and mechanical properties of the copolymers. Langer *et al.* [101] first, synthesized a series of poly(anhydride- co-imides) containing pyromellitic acid derivatives for potential use as degradable, high compressive strength materials. Their results proved that the mechanical and thermal stability of the materials are increased by the incorporation of imide groups in the polymer backbone.

To produce photopolymerizable polyanhydride, cross linkable methacrylate groups were introduced to polyanhydride chains which results in controlled degradation and improves mechanical properties. In general, the core of the molecule consists of hydrophobic repeating units, such as sebacic acid, carboxyphenoxy propane, or carboxyphenoxy hexane but other anhydride monomers, including methacrylated tricarballylic acid (MTCA, trimethacrylated) and methacrylated pyromellitylimidoalanine (MPMA-ala, amino-acid containing) have been synthesized to impart greater crosslinking density and a biologically recognized component, respectively [102].

Photo crosslinkable polyanhydrides have been employed for several applications. Because they are injectable, they can be formed directly in a bone defect through a photo initiated polymerization. When new bone fills the defect, the injected polymer will degrade [103].

Polyurethane

Polyurethanes can be tailored to have a broad range of properties, from soft to hard tissue applications [6, 104] In contrast to aliphatic linear polyesters that are more appropriate for hard tissue engineering due to their high glass transition temperature and high modulus, polyurethanes can be used as soft tissue scaffolds as well. They exhibit a wide range of properties through variability of the hard segment (diisocyanate), the soft segment (polyethers or polyesters), the chain extenders, and the ratios in which they are reacted [105]. Scheme (**8**) shows a general structure of polyurethanes.

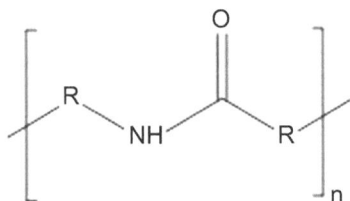

Scheme 8. Structure of polyurethane.

Biodegradation and Biocompatibility

An important issue in polyurethanes is the toxicity of their degradation product which limits their usage as bio materials. Recently polyurethanes with non-toxic degradation products have been developed. Guan *et al.* [106] synthesized polyurethanes from polycaprolactone (PCL) and 1,4-diisocyanatobutane (BDI) with putrescine used as a chain extender. The hard segments of polyurethane were built by BDI and the soft segments were prepared by polyethylene glycol (PEG) which also increases the hydrophilicity of the scaffold. Putrescine, as a polyamine can improve cell growth and differentiation, following complete degradation. This group also studied the degradation of the polyurethanes. According to their results, there was no evidence of an autocatalytic effect during the degradation process. Furthermore, degradation behavior is different from that of poly (α-hydroxyester) such as poly (L-lactide) and poly (lactide-*co*-glycolide). In contrast to polyhydroxy esters, the pH will not decrease during degradation. In addition, the use of BDI as a hard segment with chain extension by putrescine would be expected to ultimately yield a hard segment degradation product of putrescine, which is already present in the body and has been implicated as an important mediator of cellular growth and differentiation in response to growth factors [107, 108].

Scaffold Preparation Techniques

Methods used for preparing polyurethane porous scaffolds include electrospinning [109, 110], solvent casting/salt leaching [111], phase inversion [112], laser excimer [113] and thermally induced phase separation [114]. Electrospun polyurethanes are elastomeric, have small diameter, high porosity and controlled degradation rate. Although these properties aid the development of soft tissue scaffolds, it is difficult to make a scaffold with large pore sizes [110]. In the case of solvent casting/salt leaching method, pore size can be controlled by manipulating the size of the salt particulate. However, the resulting scaffold may have limited interconnectivity, which would adversely influence cell seeding and ingrowth [111]. Phase inversion method results in scaffolds with low interconnectivity and week control over pore size [112]. Scaffolds prepared by laser excimer method exhibit straight pores but achieving connectivity is still a challenge [113]. In the case of thermally induced phase separation method, pore size and pore structure can be controlled by varying the preparation conditions [114].

Application

Polyurethanes have a vast majority of applications including hard and soft tissues. However, the diversity of soft-tissue applications is far greater. These include endothelium, cardiovascular [107, 111], epithelial, cartilage skin related tissue [114] and bladder muscle reconstruction.

For endothelium reconstruction, the surface of polyurethane is usually amino modified. The introduced amino groups provide the opportunity to immobilize bio macromolecules such as gelatin, chitosan or collagen onto PU scaffold surface which in return enhance cell–material interaction and accelerate the endothelium regeneration [115].

In order to reduce the toxicity of the degraded products of conventional polyurethanes, (lysine diisocyanate) LDI–glucose polyurethanes can be employed. In this kind of polyurethanes, LDI is the hard segment and glucose is the hydroxyl donor. These scaffolds are biocompatible because their major degradation products are lysine and glucose which convert to CO_2 and ethanol. These scaffolds allow cell attachment and support cell growth of bone marrow stromal cells (BMSCs) which favors them as osteoblast precursor [108].

Polyphosphazenes

Polyphosphazenes are inorganic-organic polymers with a number of different skeletal architectures. Due to their flexible linkage (P=N) and versatile compositions, they have various application both in soft and hard tissue engineering. The general structure for polyphosphazenes is shown in Scheme (**9**) where R can be an alkoxy, aryloxy, or amino acid group or a combination of different functional groups. Because of various structures, polyphosphazenes have different physicochemical properties.

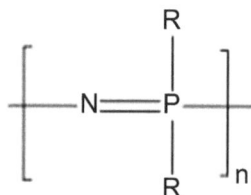

Scheme 9. Structure of polyphosphazene.

Some researchers categorize polyphosphazenes into nonionic and ionic hydrogels. Polyphosphazene gels containing water-soluble compounds such as glucosyl or glyceryl side groups are classified as nonionic while those containing divalent ions or 60Co gamma irradiation are classified as ionic polyphosphazenes [116].

Biodegradation

Replacing the chlorine atoms of polydichlorophosphazene by groups such as imidazolyl, amino acid esters, glyceryl, glycosyl, and lactic or glycolic acid esters will result into biodegradable polyphosphazenes. Incorporation of these groups to the polymer backbone will accelerate the hydrolytic degradation. Furthermore polyphosphazenes can degrade by both surface and bulk erosion. The degradation rate depends on several factors including hydrophilicity (water adsorption will influence the hydrolysis), pH, lability of the bond and solubility of the degradation products [117].

Two mechanistic pathways have been proposed for the hydrolytic instability of aminophosphazenes. The degradation of these compounds can be initiated by the protonation of atoms either in the skeleton or in the side groups. If skeletal protonation happens, nitrogen would lead directly to ring cleavage which leads to the conversion of the compound to ammonium ion, phosphoric acid and the free amine salt. When the side group nitrogen is protonated, nucleophilic attack by water at phosphorus will take place, yielding a monohydroxycyclophosphazene, which, on further hydrolysis, would undergo ring cleavage and eventual degradation [118].

Application

Polyphosphazenes can be used in bone tissue engineering [119], as wound dressing scaffold, nerve generation scaffolds and also periodontal cavity [48]. For bone tissue scaffolds, the polymer must have sufficient mechanical strength to support bone growth as well as the ability to degrade into non-toxic product. As mentioned before, PLGA is an excellent choice for this purpose however it produces acidic byproducts during hydrolysis which may cause inflammations. Polyphosphazenes as another candidate are good alternatives which are tailorable due to their side groups [120].

Polyorthoesters

Polyorthoesters (POE) are heterocycle rings created by reacting ketene acetals with diols. They have been under development since 1970 and four generations (I-IV) of these polymers have been developed which are shown in Scheme (**10**). The application of the first generation (POE I) has been limited due to its low glass transition temperature and autocatalytic hydrolysis [121]. Their hydrophobic nature allows them to undergo surface degradation rather than bulk degradation [48].

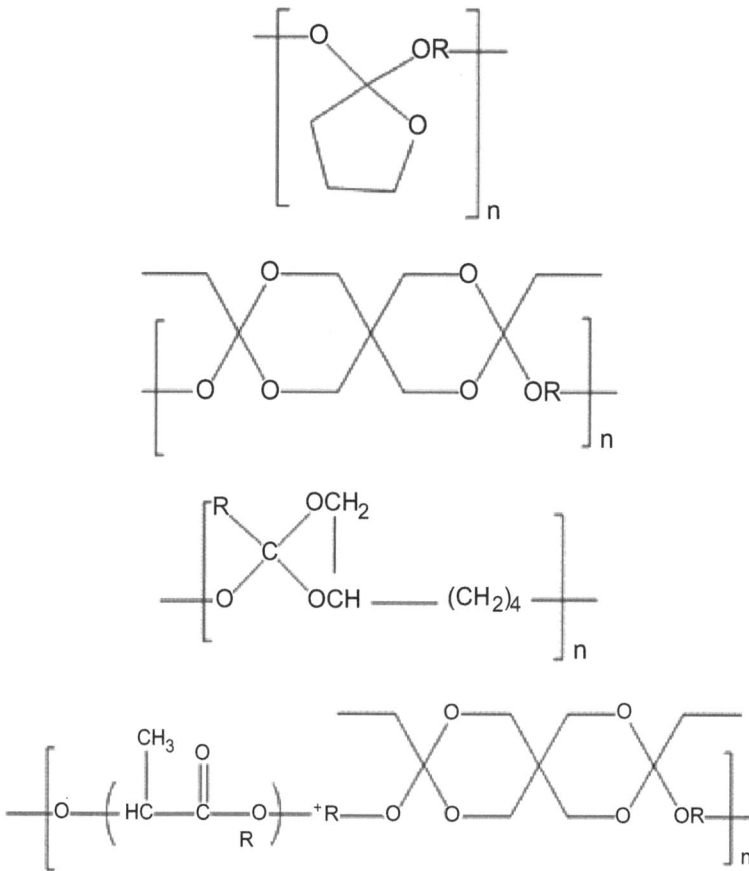

Scheme 10. Structure of various polyorthoesters (from top to down: POE I, POE II, POE III and POE IV).

Biodegradation

The degradation mechanism for each generation differs from the other one. However, they all have some similarities. The dominant mechanism is hydrolysis of the ester linkage in the backbone of the polymer. The hydrophobic nature of polyorthoesters surface allows this polymer to undergo surface degradation and bulk of material remains structurally intact. By incorporating short acid groups, such as glycolic acid or lactic, degradation rate can be controlled. Since the last generations of POE (POE IV) are more popular, their degradation mechanism will be explained here. The hydrolysis proceeds in three consecutive steps. In the first step, the lactic acid or glycolic acid groups in the polymer backbone hydrolyze to generate a polymer fragment containing a carboxylic acid end-group. A second cleavage produces free α-hydroxy acid that also catalyzes hydrolysis of the ortho ester link. Further hydrolysis proceeds and generates mixture of diols and carboxylic acids [121].

Application

Polyorthoesters have application in bone and cartilage tissues [122]. However their mechanical properties are week compared to other bio-polymers such as PLA, PCL and PLGA. Currently, polyorthoesters have generated little interest in orthopedic applications. Their main application is in drug delivery systems because of their superior properties like surface degradation and structure control [42].

Conductive Polymers: Polypyrrole

Polypyrrole (PPy) is a conductive synthetic polymer formed by polymerization of pyrrole. PPy is a potential vehicle for drug delivery while the polymer matrix serves as a container for proteins. Another advantage of polypyrrole, is its ability to be easily doped so that properties such as wettability and charge density can be varied to best mimic neural structure [123]. Due to the high degree of conjugation in the molecular backbone, this polymer is very rigid and almost insoluble in common solvents. In order to optimize the advantages of PPy electrical conductivity for biomedical, and particularly tissue engineering applications, it must be transformed into a mechanically manageable and processable form [124]. The structure of polypyrrole is shown in Scheme (**11**).

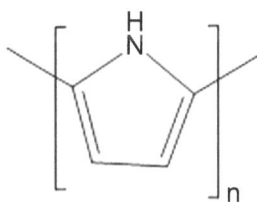

Scheme 11. Structure of polypyrrole.

The biocompatibility of PPy has been proved by several researchers [125, 126] [127, 128]. The biocompatibility was confirmed *in vivo* and *in vitro* with fibroblast (L929), neuroblastoma (neuro2a) [125] cells and also spinal cord tissue [128].

Scaffold Preparation Techniques

Electrochemical polymerization is the most widely used method for preparation of PPy. In this method, PPy is polymerized in situ on the surface of an electrode. The technique is desirable because of polymerization on complex surface geometries but, large amount production of PPy at one time is impossible due to restricted surface area of electrodes. Furthermore preparing PPy/polymer composite is difficult because most synthetic polymers are insulators which cannot be used as electrodes [124].

Application

Polypyrroles are well known for their conductivity and since electronic interaction is an important factor for neuronal tissue regeneration, they are mostly used in neuronal tissue regeneration. Schmidt and her coworkers were the first who employed PPy for tissue engineering purposes, demonstrating that electrical stimulation enhanced nerve growth factor induced neuronal differentiation of PC 12 cells [129].

As mentioned before, PPy can be easily doped to mimic the neural structure. George *et al.* doped PPy with polystyrene sulfonate or sodium dodecyl benzenesulfonate to examine their efficiency for neural networks. Neural networks have grown on the PPy surfaces and were surgically implanted in the cerebral cortex of the rat. The results were compared to stab wounds and Teflon implants (currently a gold standard for neural implants) of the same size and proved that, these doped scaffolds can be beneficial in disease states where neuronal replacement is required, such as in stroke or in Parkinson's disease [123].

Polypyrorrole/ Polylactide (PPy/PLA)

Electrically conductive polymeric scaffolds regulate cellular activities by providing an electrical way. These scaffolds can be used alone for cell cultures which are based on salt bridges [130], or on metallic or indium-tin oxide (ITO)-coated or conductive polymer-coated electrodes [131]. The electrode method has some limitations *e.g.* difficult to confine and uniformly distribute in a defined volume of tissue or body fluid with a complex geometry. Polymer blending was employed as an efficient method to apply electrical simulating only to the cells cultured on a scaffold [132]. Shi *et al.* have developed a biodegradable conductor made of 5% PPy and 95% polylactide (PLA) [133]. Compared to electrodes, a conductor has several advantages: (i) the electro simulation is spatially localized on the surface and within the conductor (scaffold); (ii) by changing the conductor resistivity, the electrical potential gradient can be controlled (iii) conductors can be bio activated to provide a multifunctional surface for cell growth; and (iv) conductors can be easily prepared as 3-D microporous structures, such as conductive nerve guidance channels [132].

As mentioned before polypyrroles suffer from their week process ability. In order to improve process ability as well as biodegradability of PPy, blends of PPy with biodegradable PDLLA have been employed. Since PPy is considered non-biodegradable, its content should be reduced as low as possible. To fulfill this goal, emulsion polymerization can be employed which results PPy nanoparticles in PDLLA substrate. Fibroblasts were cultured on these composite membranes and were stimulated with various DC currents. The PPy nanoparticles inside the PDLLA substrate, formed aggregations, micro domains and networks. In comparison to traditional electrical stimulation with electrodes, the electrical stimulation applied through a scaffold made of conductive polymer is confined in the boundary of the scaffold, therefore can be much more precisely controlled [124].

Polypyrrol/ Polycaprolactone (PPy/PCL)

In order to benefit both electrical properties of PPy and biodegradability of PCL, polymer blending was introduced. Xie *et al.* present a new type of scaffold, comprised of conductive core-sheath nanofibers prepared *via in situ* polymerization of pyrrole on electrospun PCL nanofibers. In their research, PCL was chosen as the core materials due to its biocompatibility, slow degradation rate and good processability. PPy was also chosen for the sheath because of its high electrical conductivity. Since PPy is considered as a non-biodegradable polymer and might remain in tissue for a relatively long period of time, it was used as a thin coating on biodegradable nanofibers, in order to reduce its amount. The scaffold was used for neural tissue [134].

Polyaniline

Polyaniline (shown in Scheme (**12**)) is an electrically conducting stimulus-responsive polymer, which can be synthesized to form a biomaterial. Conductive polymers, which are versatile and dynamic (the physical characteristics of the material are not set at the time of synthesis), have advantages over conventional nonconductive biomaterials. For example, they are sensitive to numerous stimuli and can be made to respond to those stimuli. They can also store information and energy and are capable of performing numerous intelligent functions [135].

In vitro and *in vivo* biocompatibility of PANI in long-term animal studies was demonstrated by Mattioli-Belmonte *et al.* [136]. In order to improve biocompatibility of PANI, various methods have been employed: (i) covalently grafting various adhesive peptides onto the surface of prefabricated conducting polymer films or into the polymer structures during the synthesis, (ii) co-electrospinning or blending with natural proteins to form conducting nanofibers or films, and (iii) preparing conducting polymers using biopolymers, such as collagen, as templates [137].

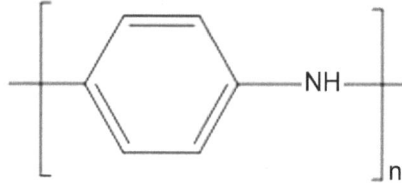

Scheme 12. Structure of polyaniline.

Application

Electroactive PANI scaffolds have applications in neuronal and cardiac tissue engineering [137]. To alleviate neurodegenerative injuries or damage to the brain, usually, transplantation of different kinds of cell suspensions into neural lesions is employed. This method leads to replacing dead or dysfunctional cells with transplanted cells via an appropriate scaffold [138]. Electroactive polymers such as PANI are a good choice for this purpose. These kind of polymers assist the bio functionality of neurite and axonal outgrowth. For such nerve regeneration not only mechanical support for neural cell growth and prevention of fibrous scar tissue ingrowth is required, but also chemical and electrical signals to direct the neurites and axonal growth to the distal stump is significant. Electroactive polymer scaffolds could be used either *in vitro* or *in vivo* to promote the growth of neuronal cells [139]. However, PANI is brittle and rigid, and therefore it is difficult to use it alone [138].

Blends of Polyaniline: PANI/ Poly (Hydroxyesters)

Shin *et al.* [140] have recently developed blends of poly[(L-lactide)-co-(caprolactone)] (PLCL) and PANI for regeneration of muscle tissue. This nano-/microfibrous structure has a high specific surface area that provides more substrate for cell attachment [141]. They showed that myogenic differentiation of myoblasts cultured on these electrically conductive electrospun fibers can be significantly enhanced as compared to pure PLCL fibers without external electrical stimulation.

Polyaniline/Gelatin

Gelatin is a frequently used biomaterial for tissue engineering application, especially in cardiac tissue engineering [142] while PANI is an electroactive polymer. Combining these biomaterials together leads to a blend with desired properties of each component. Lee *et al.* prepare homogeneous electrospun fibers of PANI and gelatin and studied the effect of PANI concentration on the fiber size and mechanical properties of scaffolds. According to their report, by increasing PANI concentration, size of nanofibers has reduced from approximately 800nm to less than 100nm and the tensile modulus of scaffolds has increased. Furthermore the conductivity of electrospun PANI-gelatin blends has enhanced by increasing the amount of PANI. They also cultured H9c2 rat cardiac myoblast cells on these fibrous substrates, in order to generate scaffolds for engineering cardiac tissues *in vivo*. They observed that cardiac myoblast cells proliferate similarly on all substrates since the fibrous substrates, being rougher, provide more surfaces for the cells to grow [143].

Polyaniline/Poly (hydroxybutyrate) (PANI/PHB)

Poly (hydroxybutyrate) is an attractive alternative for scaffolds, as it is totally bioresorbable. The biocompatibility of PHB was confirmed in case of variable cells and tissues [144]. On the other hand, in some tissue engineering applications, electrical stimulation of the tissue growing process is advantageous. Polyaniline as a proper candidate is chemically and thermally stable in a wide range of parameters. To benefit both characteristics of these two polymers, Fryczkowski *et al.* prepared electrospun fibers of PANI/PHB with an optimize composition. According to their results, the solvent should be chosen properly in order to obtain the uniform spinning solution. The non-woven scaffolds are applicable for tissue engineering [145].

Hydrogels

Hydrogels are attractive candidates in bio material applications. They can fill irregularly shaped defects and incorporate cells and other bioactive materials. Since they have structural similarity to the macromolecular-based components in the body, they are considered as biocompatible [30]. However they are often applied as space filling agents but, they also have other applications such as delivery vehicles for bioactive molecules, and also three-dimensional structures that organize cells and provide stimuli to create a desired tissue. In addition, bioactive molecules are delivered from hydrogel scaffolds in a variety of applications including promotion of angiogenesis and encapsulation of secretory cells. Hydrogel scaffolds are being applied to transplant cells and to engineer nearly every tissue in the body, including cartilage, bone, smooth muscle, urinary incontinence treatment [146] and vesicoureteral reflux [147]. They are also utilized to stabilize and deliver bioactive molecules and encapsulate secretory cells. This group of bio materials can also provide chemical signals to the cells through the incorporation of growth factors and mechanical signals by manipulation of the mechanical properties of the material [148].

Biodegradation of Hydrogels

Hydrogels can be degraded in four different mechanisms: solubilization, chemical hydrolysis, enzyme-induced degradation and other mechanisms such as ion-exchange. These degradations result in soluble or bio-absorbable moieties. Hydrogels such as PVA and PEO which are water soluble, degrade simply due to their ability to absorb water. The water diffuses into the hydrophilic polymer leading to the formation of a swollen system which ultimately dissolves. This mechanism depends on various factors such as hydrophilicity of polymer, pH, ionic strength and temperature. Chemical hydrolysis which is also common in other bio-polymers, takes place by the hydrolysis of ester linkages leading to the formation of a carboxylic acid and alcohol. Crystallinity, hydrophilicity and molecular weight affect the hydrolysis. Enzymatic hydrolysis of hydrogels takes place due to the presence of hydrolases, glycosidases or other bacterial enzymes. Some hydrogels are able to be degraded by enzymes; these include: gelatin, collagen, albumin and also synthetic hydrogels such as PVA and polydiols. In order to control the degree of degradation, specific sites which accelerate enzymatic degradation are introduced to the substrate of hydrogel [149].

The degradation behavior of hydrogels generally depends on the cross-linking density. Degradation rate and mechanical properties of cross-linked gels are typically coupled to each other. However, sometimes those properties can be decoupled by intentionally introducing network defects, resulting in the formation of soft hydrogels with longer degradation times than stiffer, more crosslinked gels. For example hydrogels with many dangling single-end molecules have showed a retarded degradation behavior irrespective of their low initial modulus and low degree of cross-linking density [150].

Application

The structure of hydrogels is similar to cartilage, which is a highly hydrated tissue composed of chondrocytes embedded in type II collagen and glycosaminoglycans. Thus, hydrogel scaffolds can be efficiently utilized in cartilage tissue. They are also being widely used in the area of non-load bearing bone tissue engineering. Generally, hydrogels do not exhibit sufficient mechanical strength to be used in load bearing applications, but they can be placed into critical defects to promote regeneration. Hydrogels can also be used for vascular smooth muscles. Photo crosslinked PEG scaffolds incorporating adhesion proteins, enzymatic degradation sites, and/or growth factors have been employed to increase collagen production by smooth muscle cells [151].

Both natural and synthetic polymers can be used for preparation of hydrogels. The most important natural hydrogels include collagen, hyaluronate, fibrin, agarose, alginate and chitosan which will not be discussed here. There are also versatile synthetic hydrogels which are explained in the following:

Poly (Acrylic Acid)

Various poly (acrylic acids) have been used in tissue engineering field. The most important ones are poly (2-hydroxyethyl methacrylate) (HEMA) and poly (*N*-isopropylacrylamide) (PNIPAAm). Poly(2 hydroxyethyl methacrylate) is often used for cartilage replacement [152]. In order to make this polymer degradable, dextran-modified poly (HEMA) gels have been synthesized. This copolymer is able to be degraded by enzymes [153]. Scheme (**13**) shows structures of poly (HEMA) and PNIPAAm.

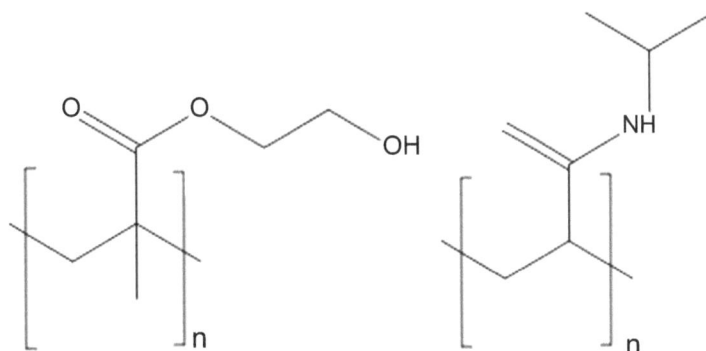

Scheme 13. Structure of various poly (acrylic acid) (left: poly (2-hydroxymethyl methacrylate), right: poly (*N*-isopropylacrylamide)).

Poly(*N*-isopropylacrylamide) (PNIPAAm) is an injectable delivery vehicle for cartilage and pancreas engineering [154]. Since this polymer has a lower critical solution temperature of approximately 32°C (body temperature), it can be easily prepared by a mixed solution of cells and the polymer at room temperature and be injected into the desired site of body. However this polymer has also limitations due to its non-degradability. In order to overcome this problem, Huh *et al.* synthesized dextran-grafted PNIPAAm copolymers which are enzymatic degradable [155].

Poly (Ethylene Oxide)

PEO (Scheme **14**) is a hydrophilic polymer which can be synthesized by anionic or cationic polymerization of ethylene oxide. PEO gels can be prepared by UV photo polymerization of the precursor that consists of PEO with acrylate termini at each end in the presence of R-hydroxy acid.

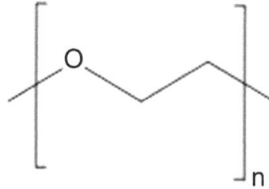

Scheme 14. Structure of poly (ethylene oxide).

Hydrogels are well known because of their high water content, which facilitates transport of nutrients, and tissue-like elastic properties. Among various hydrogels, PEO have shown success in encapsulating chondrocytes. Elisseeff *et al.* [156] were the first who provided successful investigation of transdermally photo polymerizing chondrocytes into athymic mice for cartilage tissue engineering. The photo polymerization has various advantages including: ability to convert rapidly a liquid monomer or macromere to a gel at physiological temperatures, temporal and spatial control during polymerization and formation of complex three-dimensional architectures *in vivo* with controlled mechanics.

In another attempt Anseth *et al.* [157] encapsulated chondrocytes in poly(ethylene oxide) hydrogels and used photo polymerization technology to produce cartilaginous tissue for partial and full thickness defects. According to their results, under *in vitro* conditions, photo crosslinked hydrogels can be used to encapsulate chondrocytes and regenerate cartilaginous tissue in scaffolds. They have shown that chondrocytes encapsulated in an 8mm thick photo crosslinked hydrogel and cultured *in vitro* for 6 weeks produced cartilaginous tissue throughout the construct.

Alginate/ Polyethylenoxide

Sodium alginate is a linear anionic polysaccharide which has been studied extensively in tissue engineering, including the regeneration of skin, cartilage, bone, liver and cardiac tissues. However it can't be electrospun from an aqueous solution lonely because of its electrical conductivity and surface tension. Addition of an electrospinable polymer such as PEO (which is also water soluble) can solve this problem since it provides molecular entanglement which is necessary for electrospinning [158, 159]. Core-shell structured nanofibers can be produced by electrospinning of the PEO/alginate solution. In order to improve the anti-water property of the electrospun membranes, cross-linking with Ca^{2+} can be employed which facilitates practical tissue engineering applications. These produced membranes can promote fibroblasts cells attachment and proliferation [159].

Poly (Vinyl Alcohol)

Poly (vinyl alcohol) (PVA) (Scheme **15**) is prepared by alcoholysis, hydrolysis, or aminolysis of poly (vinyl acetate). By controlling the extent of hydrolysis and molecular weight, hydrophilicity and solubility of PVA can be controlled. PVA can be regarded as hydrogels, by chemical cross-linking with glutaraldehyde or epichlorohydrin. Recently, freezing/thawing method, or electron beam has been applied to form PVA hydrogels. These methods prevail over the chemical crosslinking techniques since the toxicity and leaching problems of chemical cross-linking agents have been cancelled [116]. The gels formed by the repeated freezing/thawing method were stable at room temperature, and highly elastic. However, these gelling methods lead to two series of problems: first, they are not appropriate inside the body in situ, and second, PVA is not degradable in most physiological situations. Therefore, these gels are most likely to be useful as a long-term or permanent scaffold. PVA hydrogels have been utilized in tissue engineering for regeneration of artificial articular cartilage [160 - 162] and hybrid-type artificial pancreas [163].

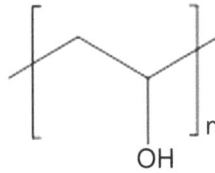

Scheme 15. Structure of poly (vinyl alcohol).

Poly(vinyl alcohol)PVA Blends: PVA/Chitosan

Electrospun polyvinyl alcohol (PVA)/chitosan nanofibrous scaffolds are a proper choice for nervous tissue engineering and repair. The PVA scaffolds containing 10wt% chitosan were used for *in vitro* cell culture in contact with PC12 nerve cells, and they were found to exhibit the most balanced properties to meet the basic required specifications for nerve cells. According to the researches, addition of a small amount of chitosan to the PVA scaffolds enhances viability and proliferation of nerve cells and is useful for neural-friendly applications [164].

Poly(vinyl alcohol)/Hydroxyapatite (PVA/HA)

Poly(vinyl alcohols) are good candidates for cartilage tissues. Since hydroxyapatite (HA) is the main mineral component of bone, its combination with PVA seems to be profitable. Wang *et al.* synthesized PVA mixed with HA and gelatin by emulsification technique. They employed the composite to create a cartilage scaffold for tissue engineering and studied the performance by implanting it subcutaneously in the dorsal region of rats for 12 weeks. The results indicated that the composite scaffold HA/PVA/gelatin is biocompatible and may serve as a cartilage scaffold for tissue engineering applications [162].

NANOCOMPOSITES

Incorporation of nanofillers to polymeric materials exhibited improvement in ultimate properties of the nanocomposite including gas barrier properties, flame retardancy [165], and other loadbearing applications. Recently, biopolymer-based nanocomposites are considered to be a 'stepping stone toward a greener and sustainable environment [166]. Various nano fillers have been added to biopolymers. However not all of them are suitable for tissue engineering purposes. In the following the nanofillers used in tissue engineering polymers are discussed.

Hydroxyapatite is a naturally occurring mineral form of calcium apatite with the formula $Ca_5 (PO4)_3(OH)$. Since 65wt% of bone is made of HA, it promotes bone ingrowth. HA improves the osteoconductivity of the bone tissue. The nano-sized HA may have even better properties due to its small size and huge surface to volume area. Webster *et al.* observed an increase in protein adsorption and osteoblast adhesion on the nanosized ceramic materials [167]. Nano hydroxyapatite (nHA) has been used in polymers which are almost for bone tissues like PCL [168] and PLA [169]. By incorporation of synthesized nHA to PLA, higher mechanical strength and more regular microarchitecture has been observed. This can be attributed to the higher surface area, surface reactivity and ultra-fine structure [169].

Carbon nanotubes (CNTs) have been used in biomedical applications due to their honeycomb-like structure, electrical conductivity and reinforcing ability. However they have a drawback which is their non-biodegradability. Bizios *et al.* prepared PLA/ CNT nanocomposites to deliver electrical stimulation to osteoblasts. According to their results, this electrical stimulation promotes various important osteoblast functions, such as cell proliferation, expression of genes for collagenous and non-collagenous proteins, and calcium deposition in the extracellular matrix. The prepared scaffolds are useful in bone repair, healing and regeneration [170].

In vitro work revealed that several different cells types have been successfully grown on carbon nanotubes or its nanocomposites. For example, nanocomposites based on single wall carbon nanotube (SWCNT) with collagen support smooth muscle cell growth. L929 mouse fibroblasts have been successfully grown on carbon nanotube scaffolds. Because multi wall carbon nanotubes (MWCNTs) have diameters approximately 100 nm, they can possibly be used to mimic neural fibers for neuronal growth. It has been shown that hippocampal neurons from 0- to 2-day-old Sprague-Dawley rats were able to grow on carbon nanotubes coated with 4-hydroxynonenal [171]. Despite of the desired properties of CNT nanocomposites, their dispersion in polymeric matrix is still a challenge [172]. Furthermore, their cytotoxicity is under debate therefore they should be employed carefully.

Nano diamonds (NDs) synthesized by detonation are one of the most promising materials for use in biomedical applications. Zhou *et al.* prepared PLLA and octadecylamine functionalized ND for using in bone scaffolds. According to their results strain to failure and fracture energy improved dramatically which are desirable in bone tissue scaffolds [173].

CONCLUDING REMARKS

As discussed before various materials including metals, ceramics and polymers can be used to produce scaffolds. Metals are not biodegradable and do not provide a biomimetic matrix for cell growth and tissue formation and ceramics have also limited biodegradability and are not suitable for preparing highly porous structures. In contrast, bio-polymers have biodegradability, can mimic the cell matrix and have the flexibility to produce various porous shapes. In the first part of this chapter, various synthetic polymers have been introduced and their application, bio-degradation and alternative forms have been discussed. However synthetic polymers are preferred to metals and ceramics but, they also require improvements and therefore there are still unsolved problems in this field. The most important features for producing a synthetic polymer available in scaffolds have been reviewed in the following.

FUTURE RESEARCH

Functionalization and Surface Modification

In order to expand the application of a certain scaffold, it would be desirable to incorporate biologically active moieties onto the scaffolding surface. Since the cells are often acting on the surface rather than the bulk, surface modification is preferred. Furthermore, bulk modifications often alter the mechanical and processing properties of the scaffold. The mechanisms in which functionalized scaffolds influence cell differentiation, proliferation, and morphology is still an unsolved problem [174].

Tailoring the Properties of Synthetic Polymer, Importance of Polymer Physics

In 2005, Hollister *et al.* stated that "The art of scaffolding is where to put the holes and the bio factors" [175]. In other words, precise control over pore size, pore distribution, permeability, and stiffness is necessary for scaffold design. Control over these characteristics may enhance cell infiltration and mass transport of nutrients and metabolic waste throughout the scaffold. Computational topology design and solid free form fabrication methods can be used for designing the architecture of porous scaffold. However it should be mentioned that focusing on fabrication method is not enough. Selecting of an appropriate bio-polymer for a specific application is significant. Tailoring the properties of material is only feasible when the chemistry and physics of the polymeric chains are well understood. In the past decades, the chemical aspects were mostly considered but nowadays the physics of polymer has been regarded as well.

Blending and Thermodynamic Aspects

The number of papers regarding the properties of newly developed materials based on the polymer blends, is increasing dramatically. However, many research results are far from commercialization. Therefore it can be concluded that in the near future a huge interest in the production of new products should arise based on the blends [176]. For various polymer blends there are discrepancies between research groups on the miscibility. For example Kumar *et al.* [177] showed, that chitosan and PVA were miscible in both diluted solution as well as in solid state. However, Lewandowska reported that chitosan and PVA are poorly miscible in the solid state [178]. In our group, phase behavior of blends based on polylactide is studied using various methods including rheological, thermal and microscopic methods.

The thermodynamic aspects are not only crucial for polymer blends but also significant in homopolymers *e.g.* in hydrogels. As discussed before, gelling is inevitable for hydrogels. Ionic crosslinking with multivalent counter ions is a simple way to form hydrogels. However, in this method the original properties of hydrogels is out of control because the ions could be exchanged with other ionic molecules in aqueous environments. Another alternative which can control the cross-linking density precisely is covalent cross-linking but its toxicity must be considered. Non-degradable cross-link formation may be harmful in most tissue engineering applications. Recently, the utilization of the phase transition behavior of certain polymers has been employed to form hydrogels. For example, a very small change of temperature near the lower critical solution temperature (LCST) can trigger the phase transition of a polymer solution to a gel, and significant research has been performed to control the LCST (*e.g.*, design it to be close to body temperature) [116]. Thermodynamic and phase behavior is an appropriate tool to engineer effective hydrogels.

Soft Nanoparticles

Towards the end of the last century, it was commonly thought that the term "nanotechnology" was coined exclusively for "hard materials" but this has changed as polymeric materials became more common ingredients in nanometric systems [179]. Among the first nanotechnology drug delivery systems were lipid vesicles (liposomes) which were described in the mid1960s. Their drawback was their rapid degradation due to the macrophage phagocyte system which leads to the inability to achieve sustained drug delivery over a prolonged period of time. In order to overcome this problem poly (ethylene glycol) (PEG) has been incorporated to them. The resulted material called Stealth liposome is the most commonly used soft nanoparticles for clinical applications. Apart from liposomes, polymer-based nano formulations constitute the majority of the nanoparticle therapeutic agents available for clinical use [180].

Biodegradable polymeric micelles with a size of 10–200nm have attracted considerable attention as drug delivery nanocarriers. There are various polymer based soft nanoparticles but hydrogels are the most important ones. So far, soft nanoparticles have been used in drug delivery systems. Their application in tissue scaffolds have not been reported yet. However, in 1980s, soft nanoparticles have been used for gene therapy [181].

Polymer based soft nanoparticles are a new class of materials which can also be used to regenerate the tissues. They can be designed as stimuli-responsive material which are smart and can react differently depending on their stimulus (temperature, electric and magnetic field, light intensity, pressure, pH, ionic strength). The selection of the polymer and also its synthesis techniques are challenges to the researchers.

Biomimetic Strategies

Mimicking biology or nature has attracted a great interest during last few years. The field of biomimetics is highly interdisciplinary. It involves the understanding of biological functions, structures, and principles of various objects found in nature by biologists, physicists, chemists, and material scientists and the design and fabrication of various materials and devices of commercial interest by engineers, material scientists, chemists, and others [182]. Scaffold tissues are the most important materials which need to mimic the structure and action of the actual tissue.

Despite the recent advances toward the development of biomimetic materials for tissue engineering applications, several challenges still remain including cell–biomaterial interactions, the design of adhesion molecules for specific cell types as needed for guided tissue regeneration and the synthesis of materials exhibiting the mechanical responsiveness of living tissues [183, 184].

CONFLICT OF INTEREST

The author declares no conflict of interest, financial or otherwise.

ACKNOWLEDGEMENTS

First and foremost, I would like to thank my husband for standing beside me throughout writing this book chapter. He always motivated me for continuing research and admired me to write a book. I also thank my wonderful parents who were always like a rock for me. They taught me how to think, move and achieve my goals. I appreciate my parents because they were not only good teachers for me but also good parents for students whom they devote their lives.

REFERENCES

[1]   http://www.infusebonegraft.com/healthcare-providers/bone-grafting-options/history-of-bone-grafting/index.htm

[2]   http://www.who.int/violence_injury_prevention/en/

[3]   http://www.organdonor.gov/about/data.html

[4]   Ambrose CG, Clanton TO. Bioabsorbable implants: review of clinical experience in orthopedic surgery. Ann Biomed Eng 2004; 32(1): 171-7.
       [http://dx.doi.org/10.1023/B:ABME.0000007802.59936.fc] [PMID: 14964733]

[5]   Dhandayuthapani B, Yoshida Y, Maekawa T, Kumar DS. Polymeric scaffolds in tissue engineering application: a review. Int J Polymer Sci 2011; 2011: Article ID 290602.
       [http://dx.doi.org/10.1155/2011/290602]

[6]   Gunatillake PA, Adhikari R. Biodegradable synthetic polymers for tissue engineering. Eur Cell Mater 2003; 5(1): 1-16.
       [http://dx.doi.org/10.22203/eCM.v005a01] [PMID: 14562275]

[7]   Hutmacher DW. Scaffolds in tissue engineering bone and cartilage. Biomaterials 2000; 21(24): 2529-43.
       [http://dx.doi.org/10.1016/S0142-9612(00)00121-6] [PMID: 11071603]

[8]   Williams DF. On the mechanisms of biocompatibility. Biomaterials 2008; 29(20): 2941-53.
       [http://dx.doi.org/10.1016/j.biomaterials.2008.04.023] [PMID: 18440630]

[9]   Ikada Y. Challenges in tissue engineering. J R Soc Interface 2006; 3(10): 589-601.
       [http://dx.doi.org/10.1098/rsif.2006.0124] [PMID: 16971328]

[10]   Chen G, Ushida T, Tateishi T. Scaffold Design for Tissue Engineering. Macromol Biosci 2002; 2(2): 67-77.
       [http://dx.doi.org/10.1002/1616-5195(20020201)2:2<67::AID-MABI67>3.0.CO;2-F]

[11]   Cooper JA, Lu HH, Ko FK, Freeman JW, Laurencin CT. Fiber-based tissue-engineered scaffold for ligament replacement: design considerations and *in vitro* evaluation. Biomaterials 2005; 26(13): 1523-

32.
[http://dx.doi.org/10.1016/j.biomaterials.2004.05.014] [PMID: 15522754]

[12]   Sokolsky-Papkov M, Agashi K, Olaye A, Shakesheff K, Domb AJ. Polymer carriers for drug delivery in tissue engineering. Adv Drug Deliv Rev 2007; 59(4-5): 187-206.
[http://dx.doi.org/10.1016/j.addr.2007.04.001] [PMID: 17540473]

[13]   Fu K, Pack DW, Klibanov AM, Langer R. Visual evidence of acidic environment within degrading poly(lactic-co-glycolic acid) (PLGA) microspheres. Pharm Res 2000; 17(1): 100-6.
[http://dx.doi.org/10.1023/A:1007582911958] [PMID: 10714616]

[14]   Kweon H, Yoo MK, Park IK, *et al.* A novel degradable polycaprolactone networks for tissue engineering. Biomaterials 2003; 24(5): 801-8.
[http://dx.doi.org/10.1016/S0142-9612(02)00370-8] [PMID: 12485798]

[15]   Matsusue Y, Yamamuro T, Oka M, Shikinami Y, Hyon SH, Ikada Y. *In vitro* and *in vivo* studies on bioabsorbable ultra-high-strength poly(L-lactide) rods. J Biomed Mater Res 1992; 26(12): 1553-67.
[http://dx.doi.org/10.1002/jbm.820261203] [PMID: 1484062]

[16]   Li S, Garreau H, Vert M. Structure-property relationships in the case of the degradation of massive poly (α-hydroxy acids) in aqueous media. J Mater Sci Mater Med 1990; 1(4): 198-206.
[http://dx.doi.org/10.1007/BF00701077]

[17]   Rohner D, Hutmacher DW, Cheng TK, Oberholzer M, Hammer B. *In vivo* efficacy of bone-marro--coated polycaprolactone scaffolds for the reconstruction of orbital defects in the pig. J Biomed Mater Res B Appl Biomater 2003; 66(2): 574-80.
[http://dx.doi.org/10.1002/jbm.b.10037] [PMID: 12861610]

[18]   Hutmacher DW. Scaffold design and fabrication technologies for engineering tissues--state of the art and future perspectives. J Biomater Sci Polym Ed 2001; 12(1): 107-24.
[http://dx.doi.org/10.1163/156856201744489] [PMID: 11334185]

[19]   Marra KG, Szem JW, Kumta PN, DiMilla PA, Weiss LE. *In vitro* analysis of biodegradable polymer blend/hydroxyapatite composites for bone tissue engineering. J Biomed Mater Res 1999; 47(3): 324-35.
[http://dx.doi.org/10.1002/(SICI)1097-4636(19991205)47:3<324::AID-JBM6>3.0.CO;2-Y]   [PMID: 10487883]

[20]   Wang F, Shor L, Darling A, *et al.* Precision extruding deposition and characterization of cellular poly-ε-caprolactone tissue scaffolds. Rapid Prototyping J 2004; 10(1): 42-9.
[http://dx.doi.org/10.1108/13552540410512525]

[21]   Xiong Z, Yan Y, Wang S, Zhang R, Zhang C. Fabrication of porous scaffolds for bone tissue engineering *via* low-temperature deposition. Scr Mater 2002; 46(11): 771-6.
[http://dx.doi.org/10.1016/S1359-6462(02)00071-4]

[22]   Sun W, Darling A, Starly B, Nam J. Computer-aided tissue engineering: overview, scope and challenges. Biotechnol Appl Biochem 2004; 39(Pt 1): 29-47.
[http://dx.doi.org/10.1042/BA20030108] [PMID: 14563211]

[23]   Williams JM, Adewunmi A, Schek RM, *et al.* Bone tissue engineering using polycaprolactone scaffolds fabricated *via* selective laser sintering. Biomaterials 2005; 26(23): 4817-27.
[http://dx.doi.org/10.1016/j.biomaterials.2004.11.057] [PMID: 15763261]

[24]   Taboas JM, Maddox RD, Krebsbach PH, Hollister SJ. Indirect solid free form fabrication of local and global porous, biomimetic and composite 3D polymer-ceramic scaffolds. Biomaterials 2003; 24(1): 181-94.
[http://dx.doi.org/10.1016/S0142-9612(02)00276-4] [PMID: 12417192]

[25]   Mondrinos MJ, Dembzynski R, Lu L, *et al.* Porogen-based solid freeform fabrication of polycaprolactone-calcium phosphate scaffolds for tissue engineering. Biomaterials 2006; 27(25): 4399-408.

[http://dx.doi.org/10.1016/j.biomaterials.2006.03.049] [PMID: 16678255]

[26]   Christensen BB, Foldager CB, Hansen OM, *et al.* A novel nano-structured porous polycaprolactone scaffold improves hyaline cartilage repair in a rabbit model compared to a collagen type I/III scaffold: *in vitro* and *in vivo* studies. Knee Surg Sports Traumatol Arthrosc 2012; 20(6): 1192-204.
[http://dx.doi.org/10.1007/s00167-011-1692-9] [PMID: 21971941]

[27]   Kim MS, Kim G. Three-dimensional electrospun polycaprolactone (PCL)/alginate hybrid composite scaffolds. Carbohydr Polym 2014; 114: 213-21.
[http://dx.doi.org/10.1016/j.carbpol.2014.08.008] [PMID: 25263884]

[28]   Lieb E. Bone tissue engineering from marrow stromal cells: Universität Regensburg. 2003.

[29]   Ng KW, Hutmacher DW, Schantz J-T, *et al.* Evaluation of ultra-thin poly(ε-caprolactone) films for tissue-engineered skin. Tissue Eng 2001; 7(4): 441-55.
[http://dx.doi.org/10.1089/10763270152436490] [PMID: 11506733]

[30]   Ungaro F, Biondi M, Indolfi L, *et al.* Bioactivated polymer scaffolds for tissue engineering. Topics in Tissue engineering. 2005; 2.

[31]   Ghasemi-Mobarakeh L, Prabhakaran MP, Morshed M, Nasr-Esfahani M-H, Ramakrishna S. Electrospun poly(epsilon-caprolactone)/gelatin nanofibrous scaffolds for nerve tissue engineering. Biomaterials 2008; 29(34): 4532-9.
[http://dx.doi.org/10.1016/j.biomaterials.2008.08.007] [PMID: 18757094]

[32]   Prasad T, Shabeena EA, Vinod D, Kumary TV, Anil Kumar PR. Characterization and *in vitro* evaluation of electrospun chitosan/polycaprolactone blend fibrous mat for skin tissue engineering. J Mater Sci Mater Med 2015; 26(1): 5352.
[http://dx.doi.org/10.1007/s10856-014-5352-8] [PMID: 25578706]

[33]   Li D, Wu T, He N, *et al.* Three-dimensional polycaprolactone scaffold *via* needleless electrospinning promotes cell proliferation and infiltration. Colloids Surf B Biointerfaces 2014; 121: 432-43.
[http://dx.doi.org/10.1016/j.colsurfb.2014.06.034] [PMID: 24996758]

[34]   Klumpp D, Rudisile M, Kühnle RI, *et al.* Three-dimensional vascularization of electrospun PCL/collagen-blend nanofibrous scaffolds *in vivo.* J Biomed Mater Res A 2012; 100(9): 2302-11.
[PMID: 22508579]

[35]   Zhang YZ, Venugopal J, Huang Z-M, Lim CT, Ramakrishna S. Characterization of the surface biocompatibility of the electrospun PCL-collagen nanofibers using fibroblasts. Biomacromolecules 2005; 6(5): 2583-9.
[http://dx.doi.org/10.1021/bm050314k] [PMID: 16153095]

[36]   Chong EJ, Phan TT, Lim IJ, *et al.* Evaluation of electrospun PCL/gelatin nanofibrous scaffold for wound healing and layered dermal reconstitution. Acta Biomater 2007; 3(3): 321-30.
[http://dx.doi.org/10.1016/j.actbio.2007.01.002] [PMID: 17321811]

[37]   Valizadeh A, Bakhtiary M, Akbarzadeh A, Salehi R, Frakhani SM, Ebrahimi O, *et al.* Preparation and characterization of novel electrospun poly (ε-caprolactone)-based nanofibrous scaffolds. Artif Cells Nanomed Biotechnol 2014; (0): 1-6.
[PMID: 25307268]

[38]   Fuchs JR, Nasseri BA, Vacanti JP. Tissue engineering: a 21st century solution to surgical reconstruction. Ann Thorac Surg 2001; 72(2): 577-91.
[http://dx.doi.org/10.1016/S0003-4975(01)02820-X] [PMID: 11515900]

[39]   Yonezawa H, Yamada S, Yanamoto S, Yoshitomi I, Kawasaki G, Umeda M. Effect of polyglycolic acid sheets with fibrin glue (MCFP technique) on the healing of wounds after partial resection of the border of the tongue in rabbits: a preliminary study. Br J Oral Maxillofac Surg 2012; 50(5): 459-63.
[http://dx.doi.org/10.1016/j.bjoms.2011.07.012] [PMID: 21820772]

[40]   Homicz MR, Chia SH, Schumacher BL, *et al.* Human septal chondrocyte redifferentiation in alginate, polyglycolic acid scaffold, and monolayer culture. Laryngoscope 2003; 113(1): 25-32.

[http://dx.doi.org/10.1097/00005537-200301000-00005] [PMID: 12514377]

[41] Nair LS, Laurencin CT. Biodegradable polymers as biomaterials. Prog Polym Sci 2007; 32(8): 762-98.
[http://dx.doi.org/10.1016/j.progpolymsci.2007.05.017]

[42] Agrawal CM, Ray RB. Biodegradable polymeric scaffolds for musculoskeletal tissue engineering. J Biomed Mater Res 2001; 55(2): 141-50.
[http://dx.doi.org/10.1002/1097-4636(200105)55:2<141::AID-JBM1000>3.0.CO;2-J] [PMID: 11255165]

[43] Anderson JM, Shive MS. Biodegradation and biocompatibility of PLA and PLGA microspheres. Adv Drug Deliv Rev 2012; 64: 72-82.
[http://dx.doi.org/10.1016/j.addr.2012.09.004]

[44] Mikos AG, Thorsen AJ, Czerwonka LA, Bao Y, Langer R, Winslow DN, *et al.* Preparation and characterization of poly (L-lactic acid) foams. Polymer (Guildf) 1994; 35(5): 1068-77.
[http://dx.doi.org/10.1016/0032-3861(94)90953-9]

[45] Yoon JJ, Park TG. Degradation behaviors of biodegradable macroporous scaffolds prepared by gas foaming of effervescent salts. J Biomed Mater Res 2001; 55(3): 401-8.
[http://dx.doi.org/10.1002/1097-4636(20010605)55:3<401::AID-JBM1029>3.0.CO;2-H] [PMID: 11255194]

[46] Woo BH, Kostanski JW, Gebrekidan S, Dani BA, Thanoo BC, DeLuca PP. Preparation, characterization and *in vivo* evaluation of 120-day poly(D,L-lactide) leuprolide microspheres. J Control Release 2001; 75(3): 307-15.
[http://dx.doi.org/10.1016/S0168-3659(01)00403-5] [PMID: 11489318]

[47] Doshi J, Reneker DH. Electrospinning process and applications of electrospun fibers. Industry Applications Society Annual Meeting, 1993, Conference Record of the 1993 IEEE; 1993: IEEE.
[http://dx.doi.org/10.1109/IAS.1993.299067]

[48] Patel H, Bonde M, Srinivasan G. Biodegradable polymer scaffold for tissue engineering. Trends Biomater Artif Organs 2011; 25(1): 20-9.

[49] Badami AS, Kreke MR, Thompson MS, Riffle JS, Goldstein AS. Effect of fiber diameter on spreading, proliferation, and differentiation of osteoblastic cells on electrospun poly(lactic acid) substrates. Biomaterials 2006; 27(4): 596-606.
[http://dx.doi.org/10.1016/j.biomaterials.2005.05.084] [PMID: 16023716]

[50] El-Amin SF, Botchwey E, Tuli R, *et al.* Human osteoblast cells: isolation, characterization, and growth on polymers for musculoskeletal tissue engineering. J Biomed Mater Res A 2006; 76(3): 439-49.
[http://dx.doi.org/10.1002/jbm.a.30411] [PMID: 16541483]

[51] Yang H-S, Park K-D, Ahn K-D, Kim B-S, Han D-K. Optimal hydrophilization and chondrocyte adhesion of PLLA films and scaffolds by plasma treatment and acrylic acid grafting. Polymer Korea 2006; 30(2): 168-74.

[52] Beckstead BL, Pan S, Bhrany AD, Bratt-Leal AM, Ratner BD, Giachelli CM. Esophageal epithelial cell interaction with synthetic and natural scaffolds for tissue engineering. Biomaterials 2005; 26(31): 6217-28.
[http://dx.doi.org/10.1016/j.biomaterials.2005.04.010] [PMID: 15913763]

[53] Török E, Vogel C, Lütgehetmann M, *et al.* Morphological and functional analysis of rat hepatocyte spheroids generated on poly(L-lactic acid) polymer in a pulsatile flow bioreactor. Tissue Eng 2006; 12(7): 1881-90.
[http://dx.doi.org/10.1089/ten.2006.12.1881] [PMID: 16889518]

[54] Engelmayr GC Jr, Sales VL, Mayer JE Jr, Sacks MS. Cyclic flexure and laminar flow synergistically accelerate mesenchymal stem cell-mediated engineered tissue formation: Implications for engineered heart valve tissues. Biomaterials 2006; 27(36): 6083-95.
[http://dx.doi.org/10.1016/j.biomaterials.2006.07.045] [PMID: 16930686]

[55] Lin YM, Boccaccini AR, Polak JM, Bishop AE, Maquet V. Biocompatibility of poly-DL-lactic acid (PDLLA) for lung tissue engineering. J Biomater Appl 2006; 21(2): 109-18.
[http://dx.doi.org/10.1177/0885328206057952] [PMID: 16443629]

[56] Sakai Y, Otsuka M, Hanada S, Nishiyama Y, Konishi Y, Yamashita A. A novel poly-L-lactic acid scaffold that possesses a macroporous structure and a branching/joining three-dimensional flow channel network: its fabrication and application to perfusion culture of human hepatoma Hep G2 cells. Mater Sci Eng C 2004; 24(3): 379-86.
[http://dx.doi.org/10.1016/j.msec.2003.12.007]

[57] Yang F, Xu CY, Kotaki M, Wang S, Ramakrishna S. Characterization of neural stem cells on electrospun poly(L-lactic acid) nanofibrous scaffold. J Biomater Sci Polym Ed 2004; 15(12): 1483-97.
[http://dx.doi.org/10.1163/1568562042459733] [PMID: 15696794]

[58] Gentile P, Chiono V, Carmagnola I, Hatton PV. An overview of poly(lactic-co-glycolic) acid (PLGA)-based biomaterials for bone tissue engineering. Int J Mol Sci 2014; 15(3): 3640-59.
[http://dx.doi.org/10.3390/ijms15033640] [PMID: 24590126]

[59] Félix Lanao RP, Jonker AM, Wolke JG, Jansen JA, van Hest JC, Leeuwenburgh SC. Physicochemical properties and applications of poly(lactic-co-glycolic acid) for use in bone regeneration. Tissue Eng Part B Rev 2013; 19(4): 380-90.
[http://dx.doi.org/10.1089/ten.teb.2012.0443] [PMID: 23350707]

[60] Yang W-S, Roh H-W, Lee WK, Ryu GH. Evaluation of functions and tissue compatibility of poly (D,L-lactic-co-glycolic acid) seeded with human dermal fibroblasts. J Biomater Sci Polym Ed 2006; 17(1-2): 151-62.
[http://dx.doi.org/10.1163/156856206774879108] [PMID: 16411605]

[61] Ishaug-Riley SL, Crane GM, Gurlek A, et al. Ectopic bone formation by marrow stromal osteoblast transplantation using poly(DL-lactic-co-glycolic acid) foams implanted into the rat mesentery. J Biomed Mater Res 1997; 36(1): 1-8.
[http://dx.doi.org/10.1002/(SICI)1097-4636(199707)36:1<1::AID-JBM1>3.0.CO;2-P] [PMID: 9212383]

[62] Kim S-S, Sun Park M, Jeon O, Yong Choi C, Kim B-S. Poly(lactide-co-glycolide)/hydroxyapatite composite scaffolds for bone tissue engineering. Biomaterials 2006; 27(8): 1399-409.
[http://dx.doi.org/10.1016/j.biomaterials.2005.08.016] [PMID: 16169074]

[63] Shin HJ, Lee CH, Cho IH, et al. Electrospun PLGA nanofiber scaffolds for articular cartilage reconstruction: mechanical stability, degradation and cellular responses under mechanical stimulation in vitro. J Biomater Sci Polym Ed 2006; 17(1-2): 103-19.
[http://dx.doi.org/10.1163/156856206774879126] [PMID: 16411602]

[64] Uematsu K, Hattori K, Ishimoto Y, et al. Cartilage regeneration using mesenchymal stem cells and a three-dimensional poly-lactic-glycolic acid (PLGA) scaffold. Biomaterials 2005; 26(20): 4273-9.
[http://dx.doi.org/10.1016/j.biomaterials.2004.10.037] [PMID: 15683651]

[65] Moore MJ, Friedman JA, Lewellyn EB, et al. Multiple-channel scaffolds to promote spinal cord axon regeneration. Biomaterials 2006; 27(3): 419-29.
[http://dx.doi.org/10.1016/j.biomaterials.2005.07.045] [PMID: 16137759]

[66] Patrick CW Jr, Chauvin PB, Hobley J, Reece GP. Preadipocyte seeded PLGA scaffolds for adipose tissue engineering. Tissue Eng 1999; 5(2): 139-51.
[http://dx.doi.org/10.1089/ten.1999.5.139] [PMID: 10358221]

[67] Zhang R, Ma PX. Poly (α-hydroxyl acids)/hydroxyapatite porous composites for bone-tissue engineering. I Preparation and morphology 1999.

[68] Harris LD, Kim B-S, Mooney DJ. Open pore biodegradable matrices formed with gas foaming. 1998.

[69] Zein I, Hutmacher DW, Tan KC, Teoh SH. Fused deposition modeling of novel scaffold architectures for tissue engineering applications. Biomaterials 2002; 23(4): 1169-85.

[http://dx.doi.org/10.1016/S0142-9612(01)00232-0] [PMID: 11791921]

[70]   Carmagnola I, Nardo T, Gentile P, Tonda-Turo C, Mattu C, Cabodi S, *et al.* Poly (Lactic acid)-based blends with tailored physicochemical properties for tissue engineering applications: A case study. International Journal of Polymeric Materials and Polymeric Biomaterials 2015; 64(2): 90-8.
[http://dx.doi.org/10.1080/00914037.2014.886247]

[71]   Goonoo N, Bhaw-Luximon A, Jhurry D. Biodegradable polymer blends: miscibility, physico-chemical properties and biological response of scaffolds. Polym Int 2015.
[http://dx.doi.org/10.1002/pi.4937]

[72]   Vilay V, Mariatti M, Ahmad Z, Pasomsouk K, Todo M. Characterization of the mechanical and thermal properties and morphological behavior of biodegradable poly (L-lactide)/poly (ε-caprolactone) and poly (L-lactide)/poly (butylene succinate-co-L-lactate) polymeric blends. J Appl Polym Sci 2009; 114(3): 1784-92.
[http://dx.doi.org/10.1002/app.30683]

[73]   Kouya T, Tada S-i, Minbu H, *et al.* Microporous membranes of PLLA/PCL blends for periosteal tissue scaffold. Mater Lett 2013; 95: 103-6.
[http://dx.doi.org/10.1016/j.matlet.2012.12.076]

[74]   Ni P, Fu S, Fan M, *et al.* Preparation of poly(ethylene glycol)/polylactide hybrid fibrous scaffolds for bone tissue engineering. Int J Nanomedicine 2011; 6: 3065-75.
[PMID: 22163160]

[75]   Spasova M, Stoilova O, Manolova N, Rashkov I, Altankov G. Preparation of PLLA/PEG nanofibers by electrospinning and potential applications. J Bioact Compat Polym 2007; 22(1): 62-76.
[http://dx.doi.org/10.1177/0883911506073570]

[76]   Ji C, Annabi N, Hosseinkhani M, Sivaloganathan S, Dehghani F. Fabrication of poly-D--lactide/polyethylene glycol scaffolds using the gas foaming technique. Acta Biomater 2012; 8(2): 570-8.
[http://dx.doi.org/10.1016/j.actbio.2011.09.028] [PMID: 21996623]

[77]   Chitrattha S, Phaechamud T. Porous poly(DL-lactic acid) matrix film with antimicrobial activities for wound dressing application. Mater Sci Eng C 2016; 58: 1122-30.
[http://dx.doi.org/10.1016/j.msec.2015.09.083] [PMID: 26478412]

[78]   Zhao H, Cui Z, Sun X, Turng L-S, Peng X. Morphology and properties of injection molded solid and microcellular polylactic acid/polyhydroxybutyrate-valerate (PLA/PHBV) blends. Ind Eng Chem Res 2013; 52(7): 2569-81.
[http://dx.doi.org/10.1021/ie301573y]

[79]   Santos AR Jr, Ferreira BM, Duek EA, Dolder H, Wada RS, Wada ML. Differentiation pattern of Vero cells cultured on poly(L-lactic acid)/poly(hydroxybutyrate-co-hydroxyvalerate) blends. Artif Organs 2004; 28(4): 381-9.
[http://dx.doi.org/10.1111/j.1525-1594.2004.47199.x] [PMID: 15084200]

[80]   Chen G, Ushida T, Tateishi T. Development of biodegradable porous scaffolds for tissue engineering. Mater Sci Eng C 2001; 17(1): 63-9.
[http://dx.doi.org/10.1016/S0928-4931(01)00338-1]

[81]   Shishatskaya EI, Volova TG. A comparative investigation of biodegradable polyhydroxyalkanoate films as matrices for *in vitro* cell cultures. J Mater Sci Mater Med 2004; 15(8): 915-23.
[http://dx.doi.org/10.1023/B:JMSM.0000036280.98763.c1] [PMID: 15477744]

[82]   Chang HM, Wang ZH, Luo HN, *et al.* Poly(3-hydroxybutyrate-co-3-hydroxyhexanoate)-based scaffolds for tissue engineering. Braz J Med Biol Res 2014; 47(7): 533-9.
[http://dx.doi.org/10.1590/1414-431X20143930] [PMID: 25003631]

[83]   Reusch RN. Low molecular weight complexed poly(3-hydroxybutyrate): a dynamic and versatile molecule *in vivo*. Can J Microbiol 1995; 41(13) (Suppl. 1): 50-4.

[http://dx.doi.org/10.1139/m95-167] [PMID: 7606668]

[84] Xu X-Y, Li X-T, Peng S-W, *et al.* The behaviour of neural stem cells on polyhydroxyalkanoate nanofiber scaffolds. Biomaterials 2010; 31(14): 3967-75.
[http://dx.doi.org/10.1016/j.biomaterials.2010.01.132] [PMID: 20153524]

[85] Doyle C, Tanner ET, Bonfield W. *In vitro* and *in vivo* evaluation of polyhydroxybutyrate and of polyhydroxybutyrate reinforced with hydroxyapatite. Biomaterials 1991; 12(9): 841-7.
[http://dx.doi.org/10.1016/0142-9612(91)90072-I] [PMID: 1764555]

[86] Webb WR, Dale TP, Lomas AJ, *et al.* The application of poly(3-hydroxybutyrate-c--3-hydroxyhexanoate) scaffolds for tendon repair in the rat model. Biomaterials 2013; 34(28): 6683-94.
[http://dx.doi.org/10.1016/j.biomaterials.2013.05.041] [PMID: 23768899]

[87] Cheng G, Cai Z, Wang L. Biocompatibility and biodegradation of poly(hydroxybutyrate)/poly(ethylene glycol) blend films. J Mater Sci Mater Med 2003; 14(12): 1073-8.
[http://dx.doi.org/10.1023/B:JMSM.0000004004.37103.f4] [PMID: 15348500]

[88] Karahaliloğlu Z, Demirbilek M, Şam M, Erol-Demirbilek M, Sağlam N, Denkbaş EB. Plasma polymerization-modified bacterial polyhydroxybutyrate nanofibrillar scaffolds. J Appl Polym Sci 2013; 128(3): 1904-12.

[89] Daranarong D, Chan RTH, Wanandy NS, Molloy R, Punyodom W, Foster LJR. Electrospun polyhydroxybutyrate and poly(L-lactide-co-ε-caprolactone) composites as nanofibrous scaffolds. BioMed Research International 2014; 2014: 12.

[90] Sombatmankhong K, Sanchavanakit N, Pavasant P, Supaphol P. Bone scaffolds from electrospun fiber mats of poly (3-hydroxybutyrate), poly (3-hydroxybutyrate-co-3-hydroxyvalerate) and their blend. Polymer (Guildf) 2007; 48(5): 1419-27.
[http://dx.doi.org/10.1016/j.polymer.2007.01.014]

[91] Zonari A, Novikoff S, Electo NR, *et al.* Endothelial differentiation of human stem cells seeded onto electrospun polyhydroxybutyrate/polyhydroxybutyrate-co-hydroxyvalerate fiber mesh. 2012.

[92] Masaeli E, Morshed M, Nasr-Esfahani MH, *et al.* Fabrication, characterization and cellular compatibility of poly(hydroxy alkanoate) composite nanofibrous scaffolds for nerve tissue engineering. PLoS One 2013; 8(2): e57157.
[http://dx.doi.org/10.1371/journal.pone.0057157] [PMID: 23468923]

[93] Kasper FK, Tanahashi K, Fisher JP, Mikos AG. Synthesis of poly(propylene fumarate). Nat Protoc 2009; 4(4): 518-25.
[http://dx.doi.org/10.1038/nprot.2009.24] [PMID: 19325548]

[94] He S, Timmer M, Yaszemski M, Yasko A, Engel P, Mikos A. Synthesis of biodegradable poly (propylene fumarate) networks with poly (propylene fumarate)–diacrylate macromers as crosslinking agents and characterization of their degradation products. Polymer (Guildf) 2001; 42(3): 1251-60.
[http://dx.doi.org/10.1016/S0032-3861(00)00479-1]

[95] Lee K-W, Wang S, Dadsetan M, Yaszemski MJ, Lu L. Enhanced cell ingrowth and proliferation through three-dimensional nanocomposite scaffolds with controlled pore structures. Biomacromolecules 2010; 11(3): 682-9.
[http://dx.doi.org/10.1021/bm901260y] [PMID: 20112899]

[96] Fisher JP, Vehof JW, Dean D, *et al.* Soft and hard tissue response to photocrosslinked poly(propylene fumarate) scaffolds in a rabbit model. J Biomed Mater Res 2002; 59(3): 547-56.
[http://dx.doi.org/10.1002/jbm.1268] [PMID: 11774313]

[97] Dadsetan M, Guda T, Runge MB, *et al.* Effect of calcium phosphate coating and rhBMP-2 on bone regeneration in rabbit calvaria using poly(propylene fumarate) scaffolds. Acta Biomater 2015; 18: 9-20.

[http://dx.doi.org/10.1016/j.actbio.2014.12.024] [PMID: 25575855]

[98]   Domb A, Langer R, Polyanhydrides I. Preparation of high molecular weight polyanhydrides. J Polym Sci A Polym Chem 1987; 25(12): 3373-86.
[http://dx.doi.org/10.1002/pola.1987.080251217]

[99]   Ranter B, Hofman A, Schoen F, Lemon J. Biomateria science an introduction to materials in medecine. Press A, editor 1996.

[100] Mikos AG, Temenoff JS. Formation of highly porous biodegradable scaffolds for tissue engineering. Electron J Biotechnol 2000; 3(2): 23-4.
[http://dx.doi.org/10.2225/vol3-issue2-fulltext-5]

[101] Uhrich KE, Gupta A, Thomas TT, Laurencin CT, Langer R. Synthesis and characterization of degradable poly (anhydride-co-imides). Macromolecules 1995; 28(7): 2184-93.
[http://dx.doi.org/10.1021/ma00111a012]

[102] Young JS, Gonzales KD, Anseth KS. Photopolymers in orthopedics: characterization of novel crosslinked polyanhydrides. Biomaterials 2000; 21(11): 1181-8.
[http://dx.doi.org/10.1016/S0142-9612(00)00018-1] [PMID: 10817271]

[103] Ifkovits JL, Burdick JA. Review: photopolymerizable and degradable biomaterials for tissue engineering applications. Tissue Eng 2007; 13(10): 2369-85.
[http://dx.doi.org/10.1089/ten.2007.0093] [PMID: 17658993]

[104] Pinchuk L. A review of the biostability and carcinogenicity of polyurethanes in medicine and the new generation of 'biostable' polyurethanes. J Biomater Sci Polym Ed 1994; 6(3): 225-67.
[http://dx.doi.org/10.1163/156856294X00347] [PMID: 7986779]

[105] Martina M, Hutmacher DW. Biodegradable polymers applied in tissue engineering research: a review. Polym Int 2007; 56(2): 145-57.
[http://dx.doi.org/10.1002/pi.2108]

[106] Guan J, Sacks MS, Beckman EJ, Wagner WR. Synthesis, characterization, and cytocompatibility of elastomeric, biodegradable poly(ester-urethane)ureas based on poly(caprolactone) and putrescine. J Biomed Mater Res 2002; 61(3): 493-503.
[http://dx.doi.org/10.1002/jbm.10204] [PMID: 12115475]

[107] Guan J, Fujimoto KL, Sacks MS, Wagner WR. Preparation and characterization of highly porous, biodegradable polyurethane scaffolds for soft tissue applications. Biomaterials 2005; 26(18): 3961-71.
[http://dx.doi.org/10.1016/j.biomaterials.2004.10.018] [PMID: 15626443]

[108] Zhang J-Y, Beckman EJ, Hu J, Yang G-G, Agarwal S, Hollinger JO. Synthesis, biodegradability, and biocompatibility of lysine diisocyanate-glucose polymers. Tissue Eng 2002; 8(5): 771-85.
[http://dx.doi.org/10.1089/10763270260424132] [PMID: 12459056]

[109] Lee KH, Kim HY, Ryu YJ, Kim KW, Choi SW. Mechanical behavior of electrospun fiber mats of poly (vinyl chloride)/polyurethane polyblends. J Polym Sci, B, Polym Phys 2003; 41(11): 1256-62.
[http://dx.doi.org/10.1002/polb.10482]

[110] Demir MM, Yilgor I, Yilgor E, Erman B. Electrospinning of polyurethane fibers. Polymer (Guildf) 2002; 43(11): 3303-9.
[http://dx.doi.org/10.1016/S0032-3861(02)00136-2]

[111] Fujimoto K, Minato M, Miyamoto S, *et al.* Porous polyurethane tubes as vascular graft. J Appl Biomater 1993; 4(4): 347-54.
[http://dx.doi.org/10.1002/jab.770040409] [PMID: 10146534]

[112] Kowligi RR, von Maltzahn WW, Eberhart RC. Fabrication and characterization of small-diameter vascular prostheses. J Biomed Mater Res 1988; 22(3) (Suppl.): 245-56.
[http://dx.doi.org/10.1002/jbm.820221405] [PMID: 3235462]

[113] Doi K, Nakayama Y, Matsuda T. Novel compliant and tissue-permeable microporous polyurethane

vascular prosthesis fabricated using an excimer laser ablation technique. J Biomed Mater Res 1996; 31(1): 27-33.
[http://dx.doi.org/10.1002/(SICI)1097-4636(199605)31:1<27::AID-JBM4>3.0.CO;2-S]   [PMID: 8731146]

[114] Saad B, Matter S, Ciardelli G, *et al.* Interactions of osteoblasts and macrophages with biodegradable and highly porous polyesterurethane foam and its degradation products. J Biomed Mater Res 1996; 32(3): 355-66.
[http://dx.doi.org/10.1002/(SICI)1097-4636(199611)32:3<355::AID-JBM8>3.0.CO;2-R]   [PMID: 8897140]

[115] Zhu Y, Gao C, He T, Shen J. Endothelium regeneration on luminal surface of polyurethane vascular scaffold modified with diamine and covalently grafted with gelatin. Biomaterials 2004; 25(3): 423-30.
[http://dx.doi.org/10.1016/S0142-9612(03)00549-0] [PMID: 14585690]

[116] Lee KY, Mooney DJ. Hydrogels for tissue engineering. Chem Rev 2001; 101(7): 1869-79.
[http://dx.doi.org/10.1021/cr000108x] [PMID: 11710233]

[117] Lakshmi S, Katti DS, Laurencin CT. Biodegradable polyphosphazenes for drug delivery applications. Adv Drug Deliv Rev 2003; 55(4): 467-82.
[http://dx.doi.org/10.1016/S0169-409X(03)00039-5] [PMID: 12706046]

[118] Allcock H, Fuller T, Matsumura K. Hydrolysis pathways for aminophosphazenes. Inorg Chem 1982; 21(2): 515-21.
[http://dx.doi.org/10.1021/ic00132a009]

[119] Laurencin CT, Morris CD, Pierre-Jacques H, Schwartz ER, Keaton AR, Zou L. Osteoblast culture on bioerodible polymers: studies of initial cell adhesion and spread. Polym Adv Technol 1992; 3(6): 359-64.
[http://dx.doi.org/10.1002/pat.1992.220030612]

[120] Deng M, Kumbar SG, Wan Y, Toti US, Allcock HR, Laurencin CT. Polyphosphazene polymers for tissue engineering: an analysis of material synthesis, characterization and applications. Soft Matter 2010; 6(14): 3119-32.
[http://dx.doi.org/10.1039/b926402g]

[121] Heller J, Barr J, Ng SY, Abdellauoi KS, Gurny R. Poly(ortho esters): synthesis, characterization, properties and uses. Adv Drug Deliv Rev 2002; 54(7): 1015-39.
[http://dx.doi.org/10.1016/S0169-409X(02)00055-8] [PMID: 12384319]

[122] Andriano KP, Tabata Y, Ikada Y, Heller J. *In vitro* and *in vivo* comparison of bulk and surface hydrolysis in absorbable polymer scaffolds for tissue engineering. J Biomed Mater Res 1999; 48(5): 602-12.
[http://dx.doi.org/10.1002/(SICI)1097-4636(1999)48:5<602::AID-JBM3>3.0.CO;2-6]   [PMID: 10490673]

[123] George PM, Lyckman AW, LaVan DA, *et al.* Fabrication and biocompatibility of polypyrrole implants suitable for neural prosthetics. Biomaterials 2005; 26(17): 3511-9.
[http://dx.doi.org/10.1016/j.biomaterials.2004.09.037] [PMID: 15621241]

[124] Shi G, Rouabhia M, Wang Z, Dao LH, Zhang Z. A novel electrically conductive and biodegradable composite made of polypyrrole nanoparticles and polylactide. Biomaterials 2004; 25(13): 2477-88.
[http://dx.doi.org/10.1016/j.biomaterials.2003.09.032] [PMID: 14751732]

[125] Wang X, Gu X, Yuan C, *et al.* Evaluation of biocompatibility of polypyrrole *in vitro* and *in vivo*. J Biomed Mater Res A 2004; 68(3): 411-22.
[http://dx.doi.org/10.1002/jbm.a.20065] [PMID: 14762920]

[126] Jiang X, Marois Y, Traoré A, *et al.* Tissue reaction to polypyrrole-coated polyester fabrics: an *in vivo* study in rats. Tissue Eng 2002; 8(4): 635-47.
[http://dx.doi.org/10.1089/107632702760240553] [PMID: 12202003]

[127]   Williams R, Doherty P. A preliminary assessment of poly (pyrrole) in nerve guide studies. J Mater Sci Mater Med 1994; 5(6-7): 429-33.
[http://dx.doi.org/10.1007/BF00058978]

[128]   Olayo R, Ríos C, Salgado-Ceballos H, *et al.* Tissue spinal cord response in rats after implants of polypyrrole and polyethylene glycol obtained by plasma. J Mater Sci Mater Med 2008; 19(2): 817-26.
[http://dx.doi.org/10.1007/s10856-007-3080-z] [PMID: 17665119]

[129]   Kotwal A, Schmidt CE. Electrical stimulation alters protein adsorption and nerve cell interactions with electrically conducting biomaterials. Biomaterials 2001; 22(10): 1055-64.
[http://dx.doi.org/10.1016/S0142-9612(00)00344-6] [PMID: 11352099]

[130]   McCaig CD, Rajnicek AM, Song B, Zhao M. Controlling cell behavior electrically: current views and future potential. Physiol Rev 2005; 85(3): 943-78.
[http://dx.doi.org/10.1152/physrev.00020.2004] [PMID: 15987799]

[131]   Kimura K, Yanagida Y, Haruyama T, Kobatake E, Aizawa M. Gene expression in the electrically stimulated differentiation of PC12 cells. J Biotechnol 1998; 63(1): 55-65.
[http://dx.doi.org/10.1016/S0168-1656(98)00075-3] [PMID: 9764482]

[132]   Shi G, Zhang Z, Rouabhia M. The regulation of cell functions electrically using biodegradable polypyrrole-polylactide conductors. Biomaterials 2008; 29(28): 3792-8.
[http://dx.doi.org/10.1016/j.biomaterials.2008.06.010] [PMID: 18602689]

[133]   Shi G, Rouabhia M, Meng S, Zhang Z. Electrical stimulation enhances viability of human cutaneous fibroblasts on conductive biodegradable substrates. J Biomed Mater Res A 2008; 84(4): 1026-37.
[http://dx.doi.org/10.1002/jbm.a.31337] [PMID: 17668861]

[134]   Xie J, Macewan MR, Willerth SM, *et al.* Conductive core-sheath nanofibers and their potential application in neural tissue engineering. Adv Funct Mater 2009; 19(14): 2312-8.
[http://dx.doi.org/10.1002/adfm.200801904] [PMID: 19830261]

[135]   Garner B, Georgevich A, Hodgson AJ, Liu L, Wallace GG. Polypyrrole-heparin composites as stimulus-responsive substrates for endothelial cell growth. J Biomed Mater Res 1999; 44(2): 121-9.
[http://dx.doi.org/10.1002/(SICI)1097-4636(199902)44:2<121::AID-JBM1>3.0.CO;2-A]   [PMID: 10397912]

[136]   Mattioli-Belmonte M, Giavaresi G, Biagini G, *et al.* Tailoring biomaterial compatibility: *in vivo* tissue response *versus in vitro* cell behavior. Int J Artif Organs 2003; 26(12): 1077-85.
[PMID: 14738191]

[137]   Li M-y, Bidez P, Guterman-Tretter E, Guo Y, MacDiarmid AG, Lelkes PI, *et al.* Electroactive and nanostructured polymers as scaffold materials for neuronal and cardiac tissue engineering. Chin J Polym Sci 2007; 25(04): 331-9.
[http://dx.doi.org/10.1142/S0256767907002199]

[138]   Bhang SH, Jeong SI, Lee TJ, *et al.* Electroactive electrospun polyaniline/poly[(L-lactide)-co-(ε-caprolactone)] fibers for control of neural cell function. Macromol Biosci 2012; 12(3): 402-11.
[http://dx.doi.org/10.1002/mabi.201100333] [PMID: 22213547]

[139]   Whitehead MA, Fan D, Akkaraju GR, Canham LT, Coffer JL. Accelerated calcification in electrically conductive polymer composites comprised of poly(ε-caprolactone), polyaniline, and bioactive mesoporous silicon. J Biomed Mater Res A 2007; 83(1): 225-34.
[http://dx.doi.org/10.1002/jbm.a.31547] [PMID: 17647228]

[140]   Jun I, Jeong S, Shin H. The stimulation of myoblast differentiation by electrically conductive sub-micron fibers. Biomaterials 2009; 30(11): 2038-47.
[http://dx.doi.org/10.1016/j.biomaterials.2008.12.063] [PMID: 19147222]

[141]   Rosso F, Giordano A, Barbarisi M, Barbarisi A. From cell-ECM interactions to tissue engineering. J Cell Physiol 2004; 199(2): 174-80.
[http://dx.doi.org/10.1002/jcp.10471] [PMID: 15039999]

[142] Zimmermann W-H, Eschenhagen T. Cardiac tissue engineering for replacement therapy. Heart Fail Rev 2003; 8(3): 259-69.
[http://dx.doi.org/10.1023/A:1024725818835] [PMID: 12878835]

[143] Li M, Guo Y, Wei Y, MacDiarmid AG, Lelkes PI. Electrospinning polyaniline-contained gelatin nanofibers for tissue engineering applications. Biomaterials 2006; 27(13): 2705-15.
[http://dx.doi.org/10.1016/j.biomaterials.2005.11.037] [PMID: 16352335]

[144] Cheng S, Chen G-Q, Leski M, Zou B, Wang Y, Wu Q. The effect of D,L-β-hydroxybutyric acid on cell death and proliferation in L929 cells. Biomaterials 2006; 27(20): 3758-65.
[http://dx.doi.org/10.1016/j.biomaterials.2006.02.046] [PMID: 16549197]

[145] Fryczkowski R, Kowalczyk T. Nanofibres from polyaniline/polyhydroxybutyrate blends. Synth Met 2009; 159(21): 2266-8.
[http://dx.doi.org/10.1016/j.synthmet.2009.09.008]

[146] Dmochowski RR, Appell RA. Injectable agents in the treatment of stress urinary incontinence in women: where are we now? Urology 2000; 56(6) (Suppl. 1): 32-40.
[http://dx.doi.org/10.1016/S0090-4295(00)01019-0] [PMID: 11114561]

[147] Läckgren G, Wåhlin N, Sköldenberg E, Stenberg A. Long-term followup of children treated with dextranomer/hyaluronic acid copolymer for vesicoureteral reflux. J Urol 2001; 166(5): 1887-92.
[http://dx.doi.org/10.1016/S0022-5347(05)65713-8] [PMID: 11586255]

[148] Drury JL, Mooney DJ. Hydrogels for tissue engineering: scaffold design variables and applications. Biomaterials 2003; 24(24): 4337-51.
[http://dx.doi.org/10.1016/S0142-9612(03)00340-5] [PMID: 12922147]

[149] Kamath KR, Park K. Biodegradable hydrogels in drug delivery. Adv Drug Deliv Rev 1993; 11(1): 59-84.
[http://dx.doi.org/10.1016/0169-409X(93)90027-2]

[150] Lee KY, Bouhadir KH, Mooney DJ. Degradation behavior of covalently cross-linked poly (aldehyde guluronate) hydrogels. Macromolecules 2000; 33(1): 97-101.
[http://dx.doi.org/10.1021/ma991286z]

[151] Mann BK, Schmedlen RH, West JL. Tethered-TGF-β increases extracellular matrix production of vascular smooth muscle cells. Biomaterials 2001; 22(5): 439-44.
[http://dx.doi.org/10.1016/S0142-9612(00)00196-4] [PMID: 11214754]

[152] Oxley HR, Corkhill PH, Fitton JH, Tighe BJ. Macroporous hydrogels for biomedical applications: methodology and morphology. Biomaterials 1993; 14(14): 1064-72.
[http://dx.doi.org/10.1016/0142-9612(93)90207-I] [PMID: 8312461]

[153] Meyvis T, De Smedt S, Demeester J, Hennink W. Influence of the degradation mechanism of hydrogels on their elastic and swelling properties during degradation. Macromolecules 2000; 33(13): 4717-25.
[http://dx.doi.org/10.1021/ma992131u]

[154] Stile RA, Burghardt WR, Healy KE. Synthesis and characterization of injectable poly (N-isopropylacrylamide)-based hydrogels that support tissue formation *in vitro*. Macromolecules 1999; 32(22): 7370-9.
[http://dx.doi.org/10.1021/ma990130w]

[155] Huh KM, Hashi J, Ooya T, Yui N. Synthesis and characterization of dextran grafted with poly (N□isopropylacrylamide□co□N, N□dimethyl□acrylamide). Macromol Chem Phys 2000; 201(5): 613-9.
[http://dx.doi.org/10.1002/(SICI)1521-3935(20000301)201:5<613::AID-MACP613>3.0.CO;2-I]

[156] Elisseeff J, Anseth K, Sims D, McIntosh W, Randolph M, Langer R. Transdermal photopolymerization for minimally invasive implantation. Proc Natl Acad Sci USA 1999; 96(6): 3104-7.

[http://dx.doi.org/10.1073/pnas.96.6.3104] [PMID: 10077644]

[157] Bryant SJ, Anseth KS. The effects of scaffold thickness on tissue engineered cartilage in photocrosslinked poly(ethylene oxide) hydrogels. Biomaterials 2001; 22(6): 619-26.
[http://dx.doi.org/10.1016/S0142-9612(00)00225-8] [PMID: 11219727]

[158] Saquing CD, Tang C, Monian B, *et al.* Alginate–Polyethylene Oxide Blend Nanofibers and the Role of the Carrier Polymer in Electrospinning. Ind Eng Chem Res 2013; 52(26): 8692-704.
[http://dx.doi.org/10.1021/ie302385b]

[159] Ma G, Fang D, Liu Y, Zhu X, Nie J. Electrospun sodium alginate/poly (ethylene oxide) core–shell nanofibers scaffolds potential for tissue engineering applications. Carbohydr Polym 2012; 87(1): 737-43.
[http://dx.doi.org/10.1016/j.carbpol.2011.08.055]

[160] Noguchi T, Yamamuro T, Oka M, *et al.* Poly(vinyl alcohol) hydrogel as an artificial articular cartilage: evaluation of biocompatibility. J Appl Biomater 1991; 2(2): 101-7.
[http://dx.doi.org/10.1002/jab.770020205] [PMID: 10171121]

[161] Kobayashi M, Toguchida J, Oka M. Preliminary study of polyvinyl alcohol-hydrogel (PVA-H) artificial meniscus. Biomaterials 2003; 24(4): 639-47.
[http://dx.doi.org/10.1016/S0142-9612(02)00378-2] [PMID: 12437958]

[162] Baker MI, Walsh SP, Schwartz Z, Boyan BD. A review of polyvinyl alcohol and its uses in cartilage and orthopedic applications. J Biomed Mater Res B Appl Biomater 2012; 100(5): 1451-7.
[http://dx.doi.org/10.1002/jbm.b.32694] [PMID: 22514196]

[163] Young T-H, Chuang W-Y, Hsieh M-Y, Chen L-W, Hsu J-P. Assessment and modeling of poly(vinyl alcohol) bioartificial pancreas *in vivo*. Biomaterials 2002; 23(16): 3495-501.
[http://dx.doi.org/10.1016/S0142-9612(02)00075-3] [PMID: 12099294]

[164] Alhosseini SN, Moztarzadeh F, Mozafari M, *et al.* Synthesis and characterization of electrospun polyvinyl alcohol nanofibrous scaffolds modified by blending with chitosan for neural tissue engineering. Int J Nanomedicine 2012; 7: 25-34.
[PMID: 22275820]

[165] Hesami M, Bagheri R, Masoomi M. Combination effects of carbon nanotubes, MMT and phosphorus flame retardant on fire and thermal resistance of fiber-reinforced epoxy composites. Iran Polym J 2014; 23(6): 469-76.
[http://dx.doi.org/10.1007/s13726-014-0241-z]

[166] Okamoto M, John B. Synthetic biopolymer nanocomposites for tissue engineering scaffolds. Prog Polym Sci 2013; 38(10): 1487-503.
[http://dx.doi.org/10.1016/j.progpolymsci.2013.06.001]

[167] Webster TJ, Ergun C, Doremus RH, Siegel RW, Bizios R. Enhanced functions of osteoblasts on nanophase ceramics. Biomaterials 2000; 21(17): 1803-10.
[http://dx.doi.org/10.1016/S0142-9612(00)00075-2] [PMID: 10905463]

[168] Bianco A, Di Federico E, Moscatelli I, *et al.* Electrospun poly(ε-caprolactone)/Ca-deficient hydroxyapatite nanohybrids: Microstructure, mechanical properties and cell response by murine embryonic stem cells. Mater Sci Eng C 2009; 29(6): 2063-71.
[http://dx.doi.org/10.1016/j.msec.2009.04.004]

[169] Nejati E, Mirzadeh H, Zandi M. Synthesis and characterization of nano-hydroxyapatite rods/poly(l-lactide acid) composite scaffolds for bone tissue engineering. Compos, Part A Appl Sci Manuf 2008; 39(10): 1589-96.
[http://dx.doi.org/10.1016/j.compositesa.2008.05.018]

[170] Supronowicz PR, Ajayan PM, Ullmann KR, Arulanandam BP, Metzger DW, Bizios R. Novel current-conducting composite substrates for exposing osteoblasts to alternating current stimulation. J Biomed Mater Res 2002; 59(3): 499-506.

[http://dx.doi.org/10.1002/jbm.10015] [PMID: 11774308]

[171] Harrison BS, Atala A. Carbon nanotube applications for tissue engineering. Biomaterials 2007; 28(2): 344-53.
[http://dx.doi.org/10.1016/j.biomaterials.2006.07.044] [PMID: 16934866]

[172] Hesami M, Bagheri R, Masoomi M. Flammability and thermal properties of epoxy/glass/MWNT Composites. J Appl Polymer Sci 2014; 131(4)

[173] Zhang Q, Mochalin VN, Neitzel I, *et al.* Mechanical properties and biomineralization of multifunctional nanodiamond-PLLA composites for bone tissue engineering. Biomaterials 2012; 33(20): 5067-75.
[http://dx.doi.org/10.1016/j.biomaterials.2012.03.063] [PMID: 22494891]

[174] Liu X, Holzwarth JM, Ma PX. Functionalized synthetic biodegradable polymer scaffolds for tissue engineering. Macromol Biosci 2012; 12(7): 911-9.
[http://dx.doi.org/10.1002/mabi.201100466] [PMID: 22396193]

[175] Hollister SJ. Porous scaffold design for tissue engineering. Nat Mater 2005; 4(7): 518-24.
[http://dx.doi.org/10.1038/nmat1421] [PMID: 16003400]

[176] Sionkowska A. Current research on the blends of natural and synthetic polymers as new biomaterials. Prog Polym Sci 2011; 36(9): 1254-76. [Review].
[http://dx.doi.org/10.1016/j.progpolymsci.2011.05.003]

[177] Kumar HN, Prabhakar M, Prasad CV, *et al.* Compatibility studies of chitosan/PVA blend in 2% aqueous acetic acid solution at 30 C. Carbohydr Polym 2010; 82(2): 251-5.
[http://dx.doi.org/10.1016/j.carbpol.2010.04.021]

[178] Lewandowska K. Miscibility and thermal stability of poly (vinyl alcohol)/chitosan mixtures. Thermochim Acta 2009; 493(1): 42-8.
[http://dx.doi.org/10.1016/j.tca.2009.04.003]

[179] Nayak S, Lyon LA. Soft nanotechnology with soft nanoparticles. Angew Chem Int Ed Engl 2005; 44(47): 7686-708.
[http://dx.doi.org/10.1002/anie.200501321] [PMID: 16283684]

[180] Estelrich J, Quesada-Pérez M, Forcada J, Callejas-Fernández J. Introductory Aspects of Soft Nanoparticles. 2014.

[181] Marshall E. Gene therapy death prompts review of adenovirus vector. Science 1999; 286(5448): 2244-5.
[http://dx.doi.org/10.1126/science.286.5448.2244] [PMID: 10636774]

[182] Nosonovsky M, Bhushan B. Green Tribology. Springer 2012.
[http://dx.doi.org/10.1007/978-3-642-23681-5]

[183] Pina S, Oliveira JM, Reis RL. Biomimetic strategies to engineer mineralised human tissues. 2015.
[http://dx.doi.org/10.1007/978-3-319-09230-0_25-1]

[184] Shin H, Jo S, Mikos AG. Biomimetic materials for tissue engineering. Biomaterials 2003; 24(24): 4353-64.
[http://dx.doi.org/10.1016/S0142-9612(03)00339-9] [PMID: 12922148]

CHAPTER 2

Polymer-Based Biocomposites

Yasemin Budama-Kilinc[*], Rabia Cakir-Koc, Ilke Kurt, Kubra Gozutok, Busra Ozkan, Burcu Ozkan and Ibrahim Isildak

Faculty of Chemistry and Metallurgical Engineering, Department of Bioengineering, Yildiz Technical University, Davutpasa St., 34210 Esenler, Istanbul, Turkey

Abstract: Polymer-based biocomposites consist of two or more different polymers that exhibit superior and unique properties when bound together. Currently, a large variety of composites are being produced in order to meet the requirements of numerous biomedical applications. This chapter focuses on synthetic polymer science, which aids in the design of novel materials for biomedical and pharmaceutical applications. In terms of current biomedical technology, many rapid developments in modern medicine have been influenced by the utilization of synthetic polymeric biocomposites (SPBc). This chapter will illuminate the advantages, specific mechanical properties, manufacturing methods, and wide range of applications (*i.e.* dental, orthopedic and cardiovascular applications, drug delivery systems, artificial skin, artificial cornea, surgical sutures, and biosensors) of SPBc.

Keywords: Artificial Cornea, Artificial Skin, Artificial Tendons, Biocomposite, Biocomposite Production, Biomaterial, Biosensor, Dental, Drug Delivery, Implant, Ligament, Orthopedic, Polymer.

INTRODUCTION

Since the middle of the 20[th]century, researchers have focused on using synthetic polymeric biocomposite (SPBc) materials in numerous different application areas. The term 'biocomposite material' generally refers to materials with different chemical structures, compositions, and morphologies, which have been bound together in order to obtain particular chemical, physical, and mechanical properties by preserving the boundaries and features of the original materials [1 - 7]. Therefore, the composite material has properties that its constituent components could not have by themselves [6, 7]. In other words, such materials include different types of materials or phases that were combined to reduce the

[*] **Corresponding author Yasemin Budama Kılınc:** Faculty of Chemistry and Metallurgical Engineering, Department of Bioengineering, Yildiz Technical University, İstanbul, Turkey; Tel: +90 (212) 383 4647; Fax: +90 (212) 383 4625; E-mail: yaseminbudama@gmail.com

Mehdi Razavi (Ed.)

weaknesses of each individual material and to provide superior properties to the biocomposites [8, 9].

The main goal of preparing a biocomposite material is to combine the best properties of various different materials in order to form a homogeneous appearance in a single material [10, 11].

Components involved in the effective formation of structures in biocomposite materials must be inert and insoluble in each other [12]. Biocomposites should ideally include one or more components that stimulate the healing process as well as non-toxic components that can interact well with the human body *in vivo* [13, 14].

Synthetic polymeric biocomposites that used in various application fields must be selected specifically and for this reason response of organs and tissues against synthetic polymeric biocomposites should be well understood [15]. Organs and tissues are generally classified into two classes including hard and soft tissues. Bones and tooth are the examples of hard tissues and organs; whereas heart, blood vessels, tendons, skin and cornea are the examples of soft tissues and organs [2]. Bone is a fragile structure such as ceramics that composed of hydroxyapatite, collagen and soft polimeric protein tissue [16]. In addition the enamel enamel on the teeth is the hardest tissue in the body. There are large apatite crystals and 97% calcium phosphate salt in its structure [17]. When considered in terms of structural compatibility metals or ceramics are suitable for hard tissue applications and the synthetic polymeric biocomposites can be used for soft tissue applications [18, 19]. One of the most common problems in hard tissue applications is elastic modulus which is one of the mechanical properties of the metal or ceramic material used that is not the same as the elastic modulus of the bones and teeth. This causes deformation of the bone [20, 21]. Cardiovascular devices provide therapeutic support for the heart and vessels. Thrombus formation is the most critical issue for materials that are placed in contact with blood and depends on firmly surface properties, implant site and implant time [22]. When heart, bone, skin and cornea are considered to the design of synthetic polymeric biocomposites for tissue regeneration and other medical applications; special attention is paid to features such as vascularization rate and nutrients/waste permeability for heart; surface topography for bone; oxygen and nutrient/waste permeability for skin and cornea [23]. Also, material that is used in the body must be corrosion resistant and biocompatible, doesn't cause allergic reactions in the tissues and considering body weight its tensile strength must be sufficient to carry the load transmitted by the body [21, 24]. Biocomposites with the desired morphological structure that allowing the growth of tissues or cells and having properties such as biocompatible and biodegradable can be produced and their tensile strengths can be adjusted. All of these structures and properties taken into account; synthetic polymeric biocomposites have the advantage of use compared to other materials [23].

A biocomposite structure is formed from both a continuous phase and a discontinuous phase. The continuous phase is known as the matrix, while the discontinuous phase can be either reinforcing agents or fillers. Additives (*i.e.* heat and light stabilizers, plasticizers, pigments) are often added to provide specific properties. The species and reinforcing geometry incorporate strength into the matrix and ensure that the obtained composite possess the best possible features (high specific strength, hardness, rigidity, *etc.*) [4, 5, 25]. Today, synthetic fossil-based polymers are generally preferred to other sources, and recyclable or raw thermoplastics (polyethylene, polypropylene, polystyrene, and polyvinyl chloride), raw thermosets (unsaturated polyesters, phenol formaldehyde, isocyanate, and epoxy) or both can be used [15]. This chapter briefly introduces the concept of synthetic polymeric biocomposite (SPBc) materials. The effect of both structural and chemical characteristics of SPBc on cell behaviors such as adhesion, proliferation, migration and differentiation are also evaluated. The most frequently used synthetic derived polymeric biocomposite materials and various fabrication technologies for SPBc are elaborated.

IMPORTANCE OF SYNTHETIC POLYMERIC BIOCOMPOSITES (SPBC)

Nowadays, biocomposite materials are used in various applications due to the many benefits and diverse properties that they offer. Studies on methods to strengthen plastic material characterized by low hardness and durable properties were accelerated, and in the 1950s polymer-based composites were developed. There are several other reasons behind the preference for using polymer in the construction of biocomposites, including straight forward production methods, less parts required for design, and ease of transport *etc.* Polymer-based biocomposites also have a low cost when compared to other materials [26]. Most biocomposites aim to improve the mechanical properties of the matrix such as hardness and durability. Hence, researchers also focus on erosion resistance, transport properties (electrical or thermal), radiopacity, and other properties such as density or biodegradability [13, 27, 28].

Synthetic polymeric biocomposites are produced in controlled conditions. Therefore, such biocomposites exhibit predictable behaviors and standard physical-mechanical properties such as degradation rate, tensile strength, and elastic modulus. Furthermore, any impurities of synthetic polymeric biocomposites can be controlled [7, 29]. Polymers are different from steel and other conventional materials because of their construction. Their usage is expanding due to increased realization of the advantageous aspects of polymers. Being at least as strong as a steel material, weightless, resistant to high temperatures, and economical are the main goals of polymer-polymer biocomposites.

Researchers have investigated several synthetic biocomposites for biomedical applications [1, 30, 31]. Biocomposites can be used in various fields of application (*i.e.* wound dressing materials, drug delivery systems) because they can be synthesized with the desired degradation rate and mechanical durability, and due to the non-toxic effect of their decomposition byproducts and their biocompatibility [3, 7]. Further, biocomposites can be used in applications such as artificial tissues and organs because of their compatibility with human tissues and the ease of adjusting their degree of hardness, as well as other properties like mechanical durability and lightness [11]. In biomedical applications, the mechanical and biological characteristics of biocomposites are the most significant issues that must be considered when choosing an application area.

SPECIFIC MECHANICAL AND BIOLOGICAL PROPERTIES OF SPBC

The mechanical and biological properties of biocomposites are greatly influenced by monomer-polymer conversion. Furthermore, the mechanical and biological properties of each polymer involved in the biocomposite are different. Also, the mechanical properties of biocomposites vary according to the biocomposites' production method and the proportion of the reinforcement. Some of the polymers most commonly used in the design of biocomposites are listed in Table **1**.

Table 1. Mechanical properties of polymers used in biocomposites.

Material	Modulus (GPa)	Tensile Strength (MPa)	Reference
Ultra-high-molecular-weight polyethylene (UHMWPE)	4-12	>35	[32]
Polypropylene	1.1-1.55	28-36	[32]
Polytetrafluoroethylene (PTFE)	0.5	27.5	[32, 33]
Polymethylmethacrylate (PMMA)	2.55	59	[32, 33]
Polyethylene terephthalate (PET)	2.85	61	[32, 33]
Polysulfone (PS)	2.65	75	[33]
Polyetheretherketone (PEEK)	8.3	139	[33]
Polyacetal (PA)	2.1	67	[33]
Poly(glycolic acid) (PGA)	7.0	60.8 to 71.8	[34, 35]

(Table 1) contd.....

Material	Modulus (GPa)	Tensile Strength (MPa)	Reference
Poly(l-lactic acid) (PLLA)	2.7	50 to 70	[36]
Poly(d,l-lactic acid) (PDLLA)	1.9	40 to 53	[36]
Poly(d,l-lactic-co-glycolic acid) (85/15)	2.0	87.6	[37, 38]
Polycaprolactone (PCL)	0.4	10.5 to 16.1	[39]
Polyanhydrides	45	4 to 19	[40, 41]
Poly(ortho esters) (POE)	20	20	[42, 43]
Poly(propylene fumarate) (PPF)	2 to 30	61 to 70	[44]

The mechanical performance of the biocomposite structure depends on the filler-matrix interface, which affects its long-term success and stability in the biological environment. Therefore, the applications of biocomposites vary according to differences in their performance. The main characteristics of some common biocomposite materials are briefly described in the following subsections.

Poly(dimethyl siloxane)/Poly(N-isopropylacrylamide)(PDMS/PNIPAAM)

Poly(N-isopropylacrylamide) (PNIPAAM) is one of the most commonly used polymers for controlled drug release applications because of its lower critical solution temperature (LCST), biocompatibility, and hydrophilic structure [45].

The PDMS/PNIPAAM copolymer was produced to provide a biocomposite with better wettability and mechanical strength than the PDMS and PNIPAAM homopolymers. It is also used to form biocomposites that are able to permeate oxygen and glucose. Further, PDMS/PNIPAAM IPNs (PDMS-V and PDMS-OH IPNs, respectively), which terminated with hydroxyl and transparent vinyl, were obtained [46, 47].

PDMS-based biocomposites are widely used in ophthalmic applications and microfluidic-based biosensor devices because of their properties such as biocompatibility, inert nature, easy fabrication ability, non-toxicity, *etc* [48 - 50].

Poly(ethylene glycol)/Poly(butylene terephthalate) (PEG/PBT)

PEG/PBT biocomposites are synthesized using hydrophobic PBT and hydrophilic PEG segments, and their structure includes a series of segmented block copolymers. The proper combination of the two polymer segments can regulate the copolymer matrix properties (*i.e.* degradation, rate of controlled release, strength, and swelling).The tensile strength rates can change between8 and 23 MPa, while water uptake can also have a changeable range from 4% to 210% [51, 52].

The hydrophilic PEG segments determine the water uptake capability of PEG/PBT copolymers. The copolymers enforce a swelling pressure on tissues, while mechanical restrictions from tissues in contact with the biocomposite prevent the swelling of the copolymer in fluid. For example, when generating a strong interface bond between PEG/PBT and bone, the most significant factor is the swelling pressure applied by drypress-fit implanted PEG/PBT biocomposites [53, 54].

For the development of biocomposites as a bone graft, PEG, PBT and its derivatives are used [55]. Besides that, PEG/PBT biocomposites are utilized for dentistry [56, 57].

Poly(ethylene oxide)/Poly(butylene terephthalate)(PEO/PBT)

Commercially available poly(ethylene oxide) (PEO) and poly(butylene terephthalate) (PBT) are approved by the FDA and are commonly used in biomedical engineering. Their mechanical and degradation properties, structures, and combination rates can feature diverse settings. Also, polymer sequences that have a variety of mechanical and degradation properties can be obtained by shifting the PEO feed rate (to 1,4-butanediol and the M_w of the PEO). A high PEO content leads to faster degradation of the PEO/PBT copolymer [58]. The tensile strengths vary between 8 and 23 MPa [59, 60].

In biosensor applications, polyethylene oxide (PEO) and its copolymers are used [61].

Poly(lactic acid)/Poly(glycolic acid) (PLA/PGA)

Poly(glycolic acid) (PGA), poly(lactic acid) (PLA), and their copolymers have been utilized more than any other kind of biodegradable polymers for many applications. The PLA/PGA copolymer is considered safe, non-toxic, and biocompatible by regulatory agencies in all of the developed countries. PLA and PGA are biodegradable polyesters, and the ester bonds in their structures can degrade to harmless and non-toxic compounds in the body through a simple hydrolysis [29, 62]. The glass transition temperature of the PLA-PGA copolymer varies between 37°C and 55°C [43, 63].

PLA/PGA biocomposites have favorable properties such as non-toxicity and no tissue reaction for applications of intracutaneous closures, abdominal and thoracic surgeries, and also vascular grafts [64 - 66], cardiovascular [67, 68] spine cage, plate, rods, screws, disc, finger joint, intramedullary nails, abdominal wall prosthesis [69, 70], drug delivery [67], surgical sutures [57].

Poly(tetrafluoroethylene)/Poly(urethane)(PTFE/PU)

A PTFE-PU structure is used because the PTFE surface has an appropriate amount of surface roughness, which will allow binding to a thin layer of PU. Thus, surface defects (*i.e.* leakage) cannot occur. The PTFE/PU membrane shows better elastic recovery in the presence of PU [71].

An additional membrane made of PU is used to protect the PTFE surface so that the PTFE membrane is not contaminated and it is possible to obtain the desired performance. PU membranes can be modified to be hydrophilic because they do not allow water passage in [72].

PTFE/PU biocomposites are used for joint replacements [73, 74] and vascular applications due to its electronegative luminar surface and improving the antithrombotic effects of the vascular grafts and this biocomposite is used in bypass grafts [2, 75, 76].

Bisphenol A glycidyl methacrylate/Tri(ethylene glycol) dimethacrylate (BisGMA/TEGDMA)

To increase the viscosity of Bis-GMA, a diluent monomer such as tri(ethylene glycol) dimethacrylate (TEGDMA) is added due to its highly viscous structure [77, 78]. Dental composites that consist of a polymeric resin matrix and inorganic fillers have been available for decades. Such composites exhibit better aesthetic and safety features than dental amalgams, and they give reasonably satisfactory clinical results [79].

Bis-GMA/TEGDMA-based dental composites have a bending strength of between 100 and 140 MPa and so can fulfill minor repair needs, although they are insufficient for repairs that carry a lot of stress. Also, the strength of dental composites is significantly reduced following long-term water aging. The average life of a dental composite is less than five years [80, 81].

Poly(ethylene oxide)/Poly(propylene oxide) (PEO/PPO)

Different molar ratios of poly(ethylene oxide)-co-poly(propylene oxide)-co-poly(ethylene oxide) (PEO-PPO-PEO) block copolymers were examined to analyze the effect of formed morphologies, as well as the interactions between components, on the mechanical properties of the mixture. Morphological, dynamic, and mechanical analyses indicated that the observed increase in the flexural modulus may be related to the decrease in the free volume [82, 83]. In general, tissues are classified into soft and hard tissues. Cartilage, skin, tendon, ligaments and blood vessels are described as soft tissues; tooth and bone are described as hard tissues. Generally, the hard tissues are harder (tensile strength) and stiffer (flexural modulus) than the soft tissues. Soft tissues have considerably lower Young's modulus (stiffness) and they are usually weaker (with lower tensile strength) as compared with hard tissues. One of the main reasons for usage of biomaterials is to change hard and soft tissues that have damaged or destroyed [84].

The final morphology and the mechanical properties are controlled by various parameters (*i.e.* degree of thermoset polymerization, volume ratio of each block, composition of the mixture, and interaction between the epoxy resin and the block) [85, 86].

In the case of block copolymers, PEO and PPO blocks have similar Tg values. Thus, all of the block copolymers show a single Tg degree of around -73°C, which is similar to the Tg of PPO, regardless of the content of each block and the PEO:PPO ratio. Different final morphologies can be obtained as a function of the copolymer content and cure cycle [86].

Water-soluble copolymers of polyethylene oxide and polypropylene oxide (PEOn–PPOm) are used in drug delivery [56] and biosensor enzyme immobilization applications [87].

Poly(Vinyl Alcohol)/Poly(Vinyl Pyrrolidone) (PVA/PVP)

PVP has good characteristics in terms of its outstanding absorption and ability for complex formation [88]. At the same time, PVA exhibits significant features such as high hydrophilicity, known biodegradability, biocompatibility, electro-chemical stability, non-toxicity, and good film-forming ability [89]. In addition, these synthetic polymers are water-soluble [90]. PVP shows greater hydrophilic property than PVA [90 - 92]. The degree of swelling is higher for PVA/PVP mixtures than for PVA alone. This situation can be explained by reducing the crystallinity of the PVP mixture. Implants that are useful in the medium- or long-term can be produced with the appropriate combinations of polymer and additives that can modify the mechanical properties [93].

PVA-based biocomposites are used for artificial cornea and skin applications [94 - 96].

MANUFACTURING METHODS FOR SPBC

Many methods have been developed for the manufacture of SPBc. The most commonly used of these manufacturing methods are injection molding, compression molding, filament winding, and the pultrusion method.

Injection Molding

The polymer injection procedure is characterized by a fast production speed, low cost, and variable strength (low to medium). The procedure allows the manufacture of polymers with a small size and a complex shape [26, 97, 98] as shown in Fig. (**1**).

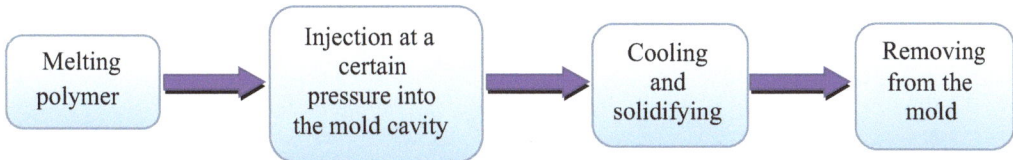

Fig. (1). Injection molding process.

Scaffolds have been widely fabricated by using injection molding method. Reignier used PCL with polyethylene oxide (PEO) to produce a scaffold that has porous and interconnected channels. In this application, injection molding method has been used due to its advantage of fabrication of scaffolds that have the same geometry as the mold cavity. Teng *et al.* produced L-shaped nasal scaffolds and Ghosh *et al.* created a PLLA/PEO porous scaffold by using this method [99].

In addition to this method, Turng and Kramschuster used microcellular injection molding to fabricate scaffold with polylactide (PLA) with water-soluble polyvinyl alcohol (PVOH) and sodium chloride (NaCl) [100].

Compression Molding

Compression molding results in medium strength, variable size (small to medium), and changeable shape (simple to complex) when compared to injection molding [46]. Manufacturing procedure is shown as in Fig. (**2**).

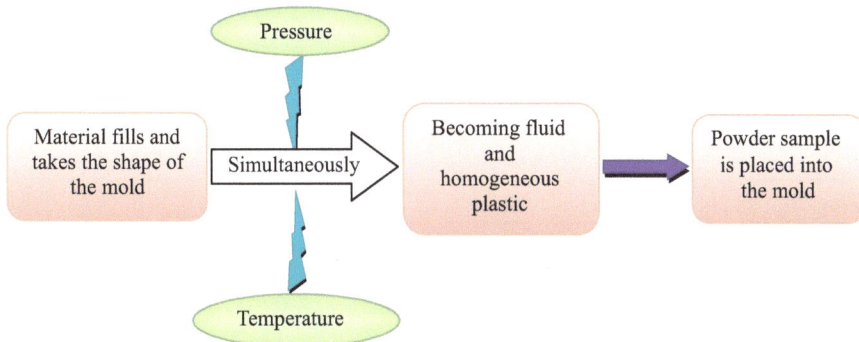

Fig. (2). Compression Molding Process.

Filament Winding

Filament winding is utilized when there is a need for a fast production speed, variable cost (low to high), high strength, changeable size (small to large), and different shape characteristics (cylindrical and axisymmetric). However, filament winding is only applicable for certain product shapes such as cylindrical and axisymmetric [46, 101, 102]. Manufacturing process is shown in Fig. (**3**).

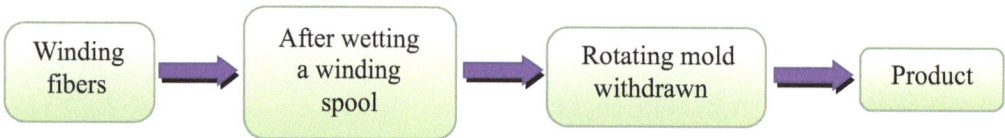

Fig. (3). Filament winding process.

Pultrusion

The pultrusion method involves a fast production speed, variable cost (low to medium), high strength (along the longitudinal axis), small to medium size cross-section (without restriction on length), and constant cross-section shape [46, 67, 97]. The manufacturing procedure is shown in Fig. (**4**).

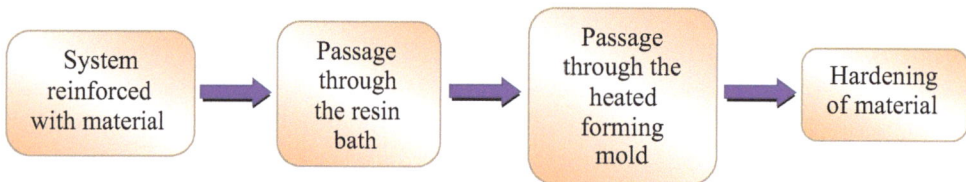

Fig. (4). Pultrusion process.

APPLICATION OF SPBC'S

SPBc which are widely used in the following important applications are shown in Table **2**.

Table 2. Applications of biocomposites used in the human body.

Applications	Types of Materials	References
Dentistry	UHMWPE/PMMA, BisGMA/ TEDGMA, PEGT-HA/PBT, PEG/PBT	[56, 57]
Cardiovascular	PU/PU-PELA, PGA/PLA, PLLA/PLGA, PLLA/P4HB, PLLA/PCL	[56, 68]

(Table 2) contd.....

Applications	Types of Materials	References
Joint Replacements	PET/PHEMA, PET/PU, PTFE/PU, UHMWPE/UHMWPE	[73, 74]
Bone Replacement Materials	HA/PHB, HA/PEG-PHB, PET/PU, HA/HDPE, HA/PE, HA/PLA, UHMWPE/UHMWPE	[56, 103]
Spine Cage, Plate, Rods, Screws, Disc, Finger Joint, Intramedullary Nails, Abdominal Wall Prosthesis	PET/PU, PLLA/HA, PGA/PLA	[69, 70]
Drug Delivery	PLA/PGA, PEG/PLGA, PEO/PPO	[56]
Surgical Sutures	PP/PA, PTMC/P3HB, PGA/PLA	[57]
Artificial Skin	PLLA/PU, PLGA/PVA	[104]
Bone Cement	UHMWPE/PMMA, HA/PMMA	[2]
Biosensors	PEG/PEO, PEO/PPO	[105, 106]

Dental Applications

Composite materials such as metals and ceramics are used for repairing anterior and posterior teeth in clinical applications. However, the SPBc structures are superior to the ceramic and metal alloys due to a number of key properties, including having a low elastic module, resembling the natural tooth structure, and minimizing both the stress field and tissue response [2, 22, 107, 108]. Polymer matrix composites are used for replacing missing teeth, repairing broken teeth, and filling gaps in restorative dentistry (Fig. **5**). In most applications, dental composites consist of acrylic or methacrylic polymeric matrices that are reinforced with ceramic particles. The long-term performance of dental composites depends on the dimensional stability, polymerization tensile tracking, corrosion resistance, and mechanical properties [2, 109, 110]. Corrosion and the mechanical properties strongly depend on the filler-matrix adhesion. Polymeric matrices are based on bisphenol-A-glycidyl dimethacrylate (Bis-GMA), although tri (ethylene glycol) dimethacrylate (TEGDMA) is added to reduce viscosity [2, 22, 111 - 113].

The amount of extracted TEGDMA is occasionally seen to be higher than the acceptable cytotoxic limit [2, 114]. Meanwhile, matrix shrinkage can be reduced by the addition of inorganic filler particles, while matrix shrinkage and water uptake increase as a result of the decomposition of mechanical properties caused by TEGDMA. This increase can be one reason behind the dilution of monomers and, consequently, the decrease in the molecular volume of Bis-GMA [22, 115]. Dimensional stability and the mechanical properties of Bis-GMA can be improved by using monomers with a greater molar volume [112, 116].

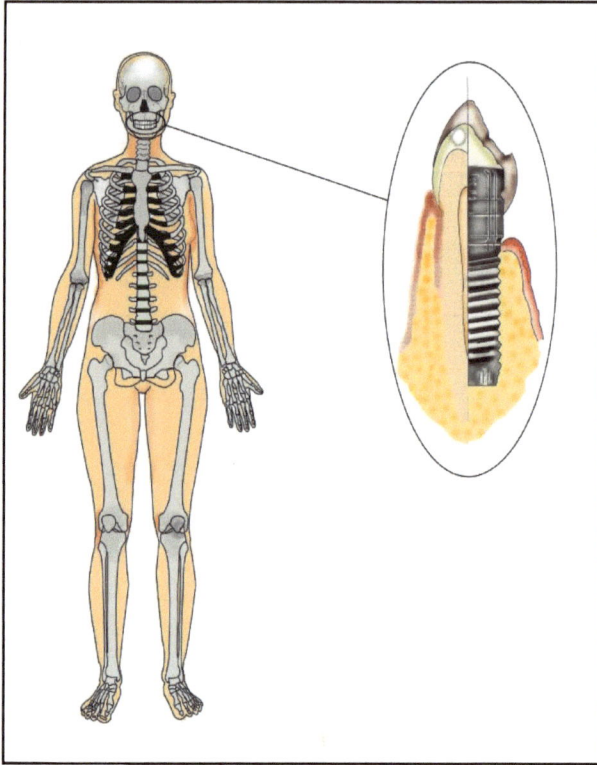

Fig. (5). Dental applications: UHMWPE/PMMA, BisGMA/TEDGMA, PEGT-HA/PBT, PEG/PBT are the polymeric biocomposites that used in dental applications.

Orthopedic Applications

Bone is complex, intelligent and includes multiple phases due to both its composite structure and its self-renewal ability [117]. The human body contains 206 bones, each of which has different elastic properties. The bone tissue changes constantly and it shows regeneration after injury according to the applied stress. However, the use of bone grafts is appropriate in several cases: (i) if injuries are serious; (ii) if the loss in bone volume is quite significant; and (iii) if the fibrous tissue cannot regenerate its mechanical properties [117, 118].

Orthopedics is a highly advanced field of medicine in terms of both the commercial and the research areas of biomaterial applications. The improvement of prosthesis materials available for the human body is arguably one of the most interesting research areas of biomaterial science.

Incompatibility between the hardness of the implant and the bone is one of the major problems encountered in orthopedic surgery [2, 22]. The modulated elasticity of SPBc allows the production of biocomposite implants that have different elasticities for several parts of the human body. The use of SPBc in orthopedics thus provides the opportunity to tailor the individual properties of the device and to vary new implant designs [64, 119].

Composite materials are produced in order to ensure continued long-term stability by increasing the femoral stem performance of bone cement, changing the cartilage structure, remodeling tendons and ligaments, and also reconstructing the bone grafts. The other significant advantages of SPBc in orthopedic applications when compared to metal-based composites are [119 - 122]:

• No requirement for a second surgical operation.
• Reduces the tendency to break the broken bone again after removal of the bone implant.
• Allows the applied load to be transferred in a stepwise manner from the implant to the recovering bone at the same time as providing a degradation of the mechanism at a particular speed.
• Metals exposed to abrasion in a physiological environment can be toxic.

Due to their many advantages, SPBc are most commonly used in the following areas of orthopedic application:

Bone Grafts

Bone grafting, also known as bone tissue transplantation, is a beneficial surgical procedure used for replacing new bone or bone fragments in order to repair injured or broken bones, provide bone union, and support bone healing around surgically implanted devices (Fig. **6**). Bone graft sources can be autologous, allografts or synthetic so long as they have similar mechanical properties to the bone [2, 22].

PEG, PBT, PLLA, PHB, and its derivatives are used to develop partially absorbable biocomposites. The foam form of the poly(glycolic acid) (PGA) and poly(lactic acid) (PLA) copolymer, biodegradable biocomposite PLGA that is reinforced with a short fiber structure of HA, are used in the field of bone regeneration [55, 119, 123]. In order to enhance the mechanical and osteoconductive properties of PLGA scaffolds; Laurencin *et al.* combined PLGA and HAP polymers. The cell adhesion, function and mineral generation were observed in osteoblast cell culture of the PLGA/HAP composite matrix within 21 days. Kim created a nanocomposite that contain HA and PCL by using oleic acid as a surfactant, thus the HA nanoparticles were dispersed homogeneously within the PCL matrix. When compared with conventional nanocomposite and pure PCL this nanocomposite has considerably higher mechanical strength (22 MPa). In addition the nanocomposites exhibit higher development of osteoblastic cell proliferation than conventional nanocomposites [124]. This nanocomposite can be beneficial in bone tissue regeneration. Novel scaffold that consists of PLGA microspheres, n-HA and BMP-2, is developed by Jeon *et al.* for bone regeneration. The determination of the proliferation and osteogenic differentiation of human adipose-derived stem cells inside the HA/BMP-2/PLGA microspheres; the dynamic 3D cell culture system was used. According to the results; immobilized surface of the PP-n-HA enhanced the cell attachment, osteoconduction and proliferation. Also, the BMP-2 promoted the bone tissue regenerative activity of the porous microspheres in terms of osteoinductive property [125].

The use of materials that are produced by the combination of high density polyethylene (HDPE) and HA particles standout in bone prosthesis applications. Interaction between the blood plasma and the bone-like HA-reinforced polymeric surface coating easily induces the growth of osteoblast cells [2, 123].

Good osteoblast cell adhesion to the HA surface particles and growth in the osteoblast cells were observed with the increase of the HA content. However, having the low mechanical properties of composites in this structure limit the use of these materials in load endurable applications (*i.e.* craniofacial repair) as a bone graft [55].

Bone Plates, Screws and Fixation Devices

Fixation devices are implanted into the body temporarily in order to keep the bone pieces together and to speed up the healing process.

An ideal SPBc fixation device should have high mechanical strength so as to avoid fractures as well as having hardness and elastic properties close to those of natural bone tissue [126, 127]. A fixation device that consists of a thermoset polymer-based composite structure is not preferred because it may lead to toxic reactions that result in the release of unreacted monomers [120]. That is why scientists have turned their attention to developing thermoplastic composites such as carbon fiber-reinforced PMMA, polysulfone, PP, PA, PBT, and polyetheretherketone (PEEK) [22].

Entirely bioresorbable internal fixation materials are made from reinforced PLLA polymer with raw ultra-HA particles. The obtained biocomposite structure has an ultra-high strength, excellent processability, and elasticity close to that of natural bone structure [128 - 130].

Metal plates and screws are used frequently in treatment that requires surgery to repair the broken bone. Bone plates formed of reinforced SPBc are successful in decreasing the stress shielding phenomenon. In the use of SPBc as bone plates, PLA supplementation increases the resorbability. However, this feature improves degradation and reduces the mechanical properties [119, 121, 131].

Osteosynthesis plates, screws, and even spine implants are the most popular orthopedic applications of biocomposites. Biocomposites reinforced with PEEK are used in the most demanding applications, such as hip and knee arthroplasty [132].

Bone Cement

Bone cements are used to fill any gaps between the implant and the host bone tissue, thereby preventing the loosening of the bond between the bone and the implant by increasing adhesion and improving the shear strength (Fig. **6**). UHMWPE fibers increase the fatigue life and reduce the crack deformation when added to the PMMA matrix [133 - 135]. The reason that PMMA causes bone necrosis, mechanical damage, and instability is because it has non-reactive cytotoxic monomers. The addition of HA in the fillers that form HA and PMMA provides direct bone fusion and osteoblast bonding [136, 137]. The PMMA and HA filler have a low rate of flexibility, compressibility, and tensile strength, which are a key disadvantages of this filler [2, 113].

Total Hip Prosthesis (Femoral Stem-Acetabular Cup)

Total hip replacement is a surgical procedure involving replacing the hip joint with a prosthetic implant (Fig. **6**). This process is most commonly used in the treatment of joint failure caused by diseases such as osteoarthritis, rheumatoid arthritis, hip fractures, *etc.* The aims of the procedure are to eliminate the pain and improve hip function [118, 122, 138, 139].

A hip joint prosthesis consists of three main parts:

- A metal femoral stem fixed to the endoprosthesis femur bone.
- An acetabular cup, usually consisting of ceramic or polyethylene, placed in the pelvis.
- A head part made of metal or ceramics, performing function with the acetabular cup and friction.

A total hip joint prosthesis is an endoprosthesis process and its life time ranges from 10 to 15 years. Adverse effects of endoprosthesis such as toxic, immunogenic and mutagenic effects that occur after corrosion, osteolysis activity occurring around the implant, and the difficulty of repeated surgical implantation procedures are the most important risk parameters encountered in materials produced for endoprosthesis applications.

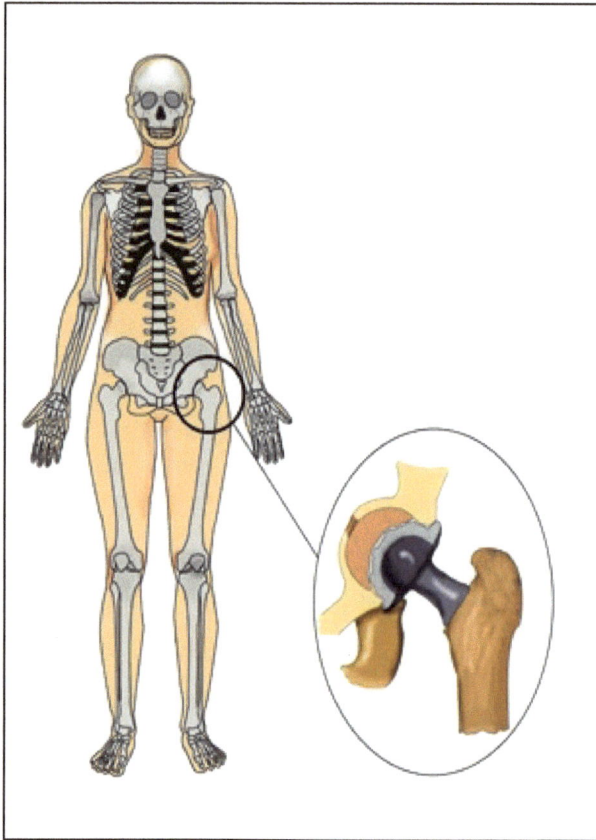

Fig. (6). Orthopedic applications: HDPE/HA for bone graft, UHMWPE/ PMMA and HA/PMMA for cement, UHMWPE/UHMWPE for acetabular prothesis are the polymeric biocomposites that used in orthopedic applications.

The acetabular cup is the component that is placed into the acetabulum. PTFE is preferred in acetabular cup applications owing to its hydrophobic structure, stable chemical environment, low friction coefficient of the inert structure, solidity within the body, and high thermal stability properties. However, the tissue reaction that is caused by corrosion in clinical trials can be a reason behind granuloma formation [2].

Due to the negative effects of PTFE, UHMWPE is now used instead of PTFE. Yet, unfortunately, UHMWPE is seen as the weakest link in the hip prosthesis due to reasons such as corrosion, erosion, crack deformation, and plastic distortion in long-term use. UHMWPE forms SPBc with carbon fiber or a strengthening polymer material to resolve the negative consequences resulting from long-term use of UHMWPE and improve the performance [140].

Carbon fiber-reinforced PEEK SPBc contain high levels of fiber structure. This structure results in a decrease in the corrosion rate and also shows good dimensional stability properties. For this reason, carbon fiber-reinforced PEEK biocomposite structures offer a better alternative in acetabular cup applications when compared with UHMWPE/UHMWPE, metal/ceramic composite components or the usual UHMWPE [22, 113].

The femoral stem is the component of a total hip prosthesis that is implanted into the femur to provide stability for the prosthesis. The femoral stems are designed laminar in PEEK, polysulfone, liquid crystal polymer (LCP), and polyetherimide (PEI). Due to the structural characteristics of femoral stems such as workability, flexibility, resistance to corrosion, and radiolucency, they are open to improvement [114, 141]. The use of polyetherimide (PEI) in femoral stem production is considered promising due to its excellent biocompatibility [142] The reinforcement of PEI brings features to the prosthesis such as similar stiffness to bone and similarity to the physiological structure of bone in charge transfer. It also protects the implant against breaking due to its strong structure [122, 143].

Artificial Tendons and Ligaments

Tendons and ligaments are connective tissues that are composed of collagen. While tendons are responsible for the connection of muscles to bones, ligaments bind bone to bone. Polyester and hydrogels were used in artificial tendons and ligaments. The PET-reinforced PHEMA biocomposite structure shows similar characteristics to the stress-strain curve of natural tendons under low pressure [144 - 146]. The ethylene-butene copolymer and UHMWPE biocomposite structures demonstrate prolonged and improved performance. Artificial ligaments are devices that are made from polymeric or polymer composites [22, 147]. Corrosion, bending, and torsion lead to inadequate fiber resistance and so cause damage in the long-term use of artificial ligaments [148].

Drug Delivery System

Some drugs need to proceed smoothly through the gastrointestinal system in order to reach the target tissues or organs. For this purpose, it is necessary to encapsulate these drugs within various polymer-based biocomposites. These biocomposite structures must have a sufficient resistivity property against hydrolytic enzymes. Hence, the drug molecules can proceed without problems to the desired target tissue or organs. The encapsulated tissue or organ targeted drugs are generally released by such factors as pH, temperature, ionic strength, enzyme, *etc* [149 - 152].

In recent years, polymeric biocomposite drug systems have been designed for various applications. Drugs can be released continuously and controlled over a long period of time when a polymeric biocomposite system is used as the carrier [153 - 155]. The important parameters for the design of drug delivery applications are: (i) a drug delivery matrix should have appropriate hydrophobic characteristics to prevent the degradation of the hydrophilic drug ingredient before it reaches the target zones; and (ii) with the hydrolysis of the unstable bonds in the surface layers, the matrix should be corroded from the surface [151, 156, 157].

Synthetic polymeric biocomposite drug delivery systems generally consist of PGA, PDLLA, PLLA, and poly-e-caprolactone-based biocomposite forms and their copolymers [65, 151, 153, 154]. Due to the beneficial characteristics mentioned before, the PLA/PGA copolymer biocomposite structure is widely used in controlled drug release according to the resistivity of PLA to hydrolytic attracts [158 - 160].

Polymeric biocomposites with a sufficient thermo-sensitivity property (*i.e.* copolymers of PEG/PLGA and PEO/PPO) are the most preferable biocomposite structures for use in protein/peptide drug delivery [152, 157, 160, 161]. The degradation rate of PCL is much slower than that of PLA. Therefore, PCL-based biocomposites are preferable due to the ability to maintain structural integrity during long-term usage in drug delivery systems [149, 152, 156, 158]. The other category for this application field is polyanhydride-based biocomposites. These biocomposites have the potential to allow a controllable drug delivery rate due to the adjusted surface erosion degradation mechanism. Polyanhydride-based biocomposites are used to transmit anticancer drugs to the site(s) where tumors have been removed from the brain [154, 158, 162].

Artificial Skin

Artificial skin scaffolds are not only used for wound covering and as a physical barrier to external infections, but should also induce the proliferation of dermal fibroblasts and the keratinocytes for artificial skin tissue engineering [163, 164]. Cross-linked hydrogel structures are suitable for artificial skin applications, although their lower mechanical properties limit their performance as scaffolds [22, 165].

While synthetic polymers have lower rates of cell attachment and proliferation due to the limited biological signals, hydrogel structures should be reinforced with polymers to overcome the mechanical failures [128, 163, 164]. The semi-permeable feature of PU results in this polymer being mostly used in artificial skin applications as a reinforced material. PLLA-PU is a biocomposite form with a flexible microporous structure. It is easy to handle, has good biodegradability properties, and shows perfect adherence to the wound. In addition, the PLLA-PU biocomposite material is beneficial as a barrier against bacterial penetration and provides an appropriate rate of water transport through the membrane [128, 163, 164, 166 - 168].

The attractiveness of PVA-based hydrogel structures for artificial skin applications is due to their similar mechanical characteristics to those of subcutaneous tissues like soft tissues. In order to avoid causing an undesirable tissue response, PLGA microspheres act as a carrier support for anti-inflammatory action [169 - 171]. A SPBc material that is composed of PLGA microspheres and a PVA hydrogel structure is used to coat implantable biomaterials in order to improve their biocompatibility.

This biocomposite system then provides protection against the foreign body response due to its polymeric content [169, 170]. PLGA/PVA polymeric biocomposites also promote the endothelial and platelet growth factors, which are important for the inflammatory, proliferation, and migratory phases of wound healing [152, 163, 172 - 174].

The other polymeric material that is used for artificial skin applications is pHEMA. The use of PHEMA and P[HEMA-co-(MeO-PEGMA)] biocomposites ensure a high stability in the biological environment. In order to not be biodegradable and to have a porous morphology, these synthetic polymeric biocomposite scaffolds are suitable for use in biomedical applications, especially for tissue support in tissue engineering [164, 175 - 179].

Artificial Cornea

For the replacement of central cornea, synthetic implants defined as keratoprosthesis have been designed (Fig. **7**). The utilized material should be biocompatible, colorless, transparent, and should have the ability to contain a high water content and a good mechanical strength [180 - 183]. The refractive index is another important parameter for artificial cornea applications [94, 182, 184, 185]. The central part of the artificial cornea prosthesis consists of a PMMA-based structure.

Poly(N-isopropylacrylamide-co-acrylic acid-co-acryloxy succinimide) is used as a reinforced polymer to improve the mechanical properties of the prosthesis [180, 183, 184, 186].

Due to exhibiting the necessary important characteristics (*i.e.* high mechanical strength, excellent permeability to oxygen, transparency, and biocompatibility), PDMS-based biocomposites are very popular in ophthalmic applications [48,

180]. One of the biocompatible materials most commonly used for artificial cornea applications is PVA. PVA-based biocomposites have a low cell affinity property and they are also soluble in water [94 - 96, 187].

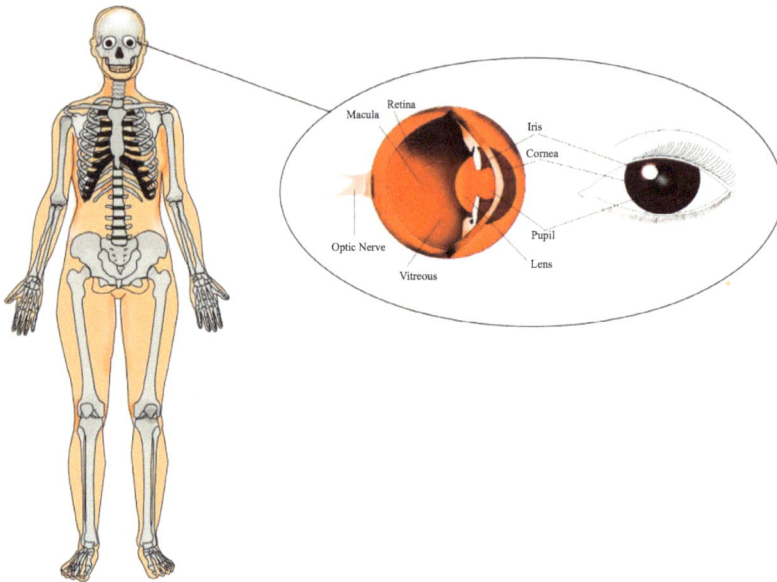

Fig. (7). Ocular applications: PMMA-based, PVA-based and PDMS-based are the polymeric biocomposites that used in ocular applications.

Surgical Sutures

Suture materials are used to bring and hold tissues together and as an artificial fiber support until the natural collagen fiber structure is synthesized.

The ideal suture material should have favorable tensile tissue handling property and should not be a catalyst for tissue reactions and bacterial growth [66, 188 - 192]. Synthetic suture materials can be categorized based on their absorbability property.

Synthetic non-absorbable biocomposite suture materials are generally based on polymers such as polyamides, polypropylene, polyesters, and expanded polytetrafluoroethylene (ePTFE) [193, 194]. Non-absorbable SPBc sutures provide permanent wound support and so are ideal options for long-term applications (*i.e.* prosthetic heart valve applications). Despite being a non-degradable material, polyamide-based SPBc suture materials can degrade *via* depolymerization in tissue after one to two years of implantation [64, 195]. After the decomposition of the polyamide coat structure, tissue fluid can penetrate through the polyamide-based suture material. Instead of using polyamide-based biocomposites for surgical suture applications, it is much more beneficial to use polypropylene and ePTFE-based biocomposites due to their resistance to absorption. In addition to being used as a non-absorbable suture material, the polypropylene polymeric structure/material is one of the least reactive materials [191, 194, 196]. This least reactiveness promotes minimal tissue reactions and histological responses after intramuscular implantation as PP/Polyamide biocomposite form [188, 193, 195].

Synthetic absorbable polymeric biocomposite suture materials include polyglactin with polyglycolic acid, poly-L-lactide, poly-ε-caprolactone, PGA, PLGA, PG (polyglyonate), polydioxanone (PDO or PDS), poly(trimethylene carbonate) (PTMC), and poly(3-hydrobutyrate) (PHB) polymers and their copolymers [64, 191, 197 - 200].

PGA-based biocomposite sutures are mostly preferred due to their good handling, high tensile strength, and knot security properties. Also, the lack of toxicity and causing minimal tissue reaction characteristics are the other reasons for selecting the PGA-based biocomposites as suture materials [64, 192, 201]. PLA has similar properties to PGA, such as non-toxicity and no tissue reaction, but the degradation time of PLA is slow because of its hydrophobic property. The copolymerization of these synthetic polymers provides controlled degradation, which is an important factor for the application of subcutaneous and intracutaneous closures, abdominal and thoracic surgeries, and also vascular grafts [64 - 66].

The natural slow absorption of PG (polyglyconate) renders this polymeric material another option for surgical sutures. Suture formations contain PG-based biocomposite structures that retain tensile strength for an adequate period for vascular healing and have a minimal tissue response. PG sutures might be suitable for the microvascular anastomosis of arteries under ordinary tension [191]. Another SPBc material that is suitable for surgical suture applications is poly(L-lactide-co-e-caprolactone). Due to the beneficial characteristics (*i.e.* good strength, adequate flexibility and improved handling, high knot-pull strength, good correlation) of PLCL-based sutures, they are more preferable in this area of application.

The surgical sutures that consist of polydioxanone-based (PDO or PDS) biocomposites have a smooth and soft surface, good handling properties, and provide adequate mechanical support for vessels to heal. In respect of these beneficial properties, PDO also provides good flexibility to the suture. PDO does not have any acute or toxic effects on implantation. Thus, no tissue or foreign body reactions were observed during degradation. PDO-based biocomposite sutures are generally useful in pediatric cardiovascular surgery and ophthalmic surgery [65, 191, 200, 202, 203].

Cardiovascular Applications

Coronary artery disease and the peripheral vascular diseases are the most common cause of severe health problems that result in death. Atherosclerosis occurs when cholesterol crystals, fatty deposits, and calcium salts accumulate on the inner walls of the vessels [2, 22, 204].

The critical issues associated with heart valve development are calcification, tissue overgrowth, and the need to use continuous anticoagulants [117, 205, 206]. Furthermore, the possibility of infection, immunological reactions to foreign materials, and thromboembolisms are the other severe problems that should be considered in artificial heart valve design [207, 208]. Using SPBc materials that are based on PGA, PLA, P3HB, and their copolymers provide a thrombo-resistant surface and the ability to remodel heart tissues (Fig. **8**). Additionally, these biocomposites increase the growth capability of host cells, have a non-inflammatory response, and prevent calcification. Thus, the mechanical properties (*i.e.* strength, flexibility, inertness, and durability) of biocomposites could be improved for the artificial heart valve leaflets [208 - 210].

Vascular grafts are used to replace diseased or blocked cardiovascular systems. The tubular structured vascular grafts are inserted into the vessel to bypass the blockages and provide blood circulation [2, 22, 211]. Porosity is the most important parameter for vascular grafts. Adequate porosity is desired in order to promote tissue growth and ensure that there is no rejection of grafts by the surrounding tissues. However, a large porosity size is an undesirable parameter because excess porosity may promote the leakage of blood. In addition to porosity, good tensile strength, resistance to degradation, a sufficient rate of tissue growth, and good handling are the most important characteristics of any material that is considered for vascular graft applications [196, 212 - 214].

In vascular applications, PET-, ePTFE-, and PU-based biocomposites are selected according to the porosity size of the material. PET-based biocomposites are blended with endothelial cells to reduce thrombogenicity, and they are generally suitable for applications involving large diameter vessels [2, 204, 205, 214, 215]. In order to have an electronegative luminar surface, ePTFE-based polymeric biocomposites improve the antithrombotic effects of the vascular grafts. Thus, this biocomposite structure is used in lower limb bypass grafts. The biocomposite that consists of PU and PELA is compliant with the natural artery and so prevents blood loss [2, 75, 76, 216].

Stents are small, hollow cylindrical devices that are inserted into the vascular lesion sites to prevent vessel restenosis in Fig. (**8**) [217, 218].

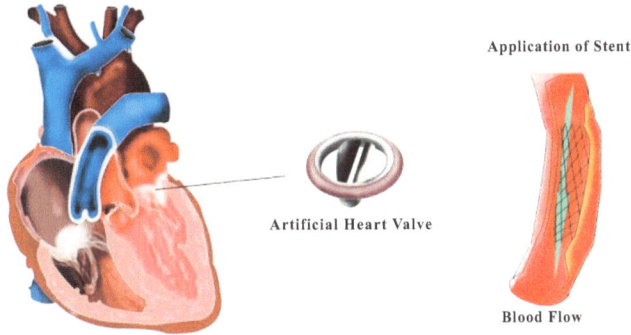

Fig. (8). Cardiovascular applications: PU/PU-PELA, PGA/PLA, PLLA/PLGA, PLLA/P4HB and PLLA/PCL are the polymeric biocomposites that used in cardiovascular applications.

It is important to have excellent flexibility and high mechanical strength in order to resist the pressure of blood on cardiovascular stents [219, 220]. Metallic stents are generally used. However, such metallic stents have disadvantageous properties, including a tendency for thrombosis formation and being damaging to the natural structure of vessel walls, and they may be a reason for the rejection of implants [76, 218]. To overcome these drawbacks, metallic stents were coated with synthetic polymer derivatives where bioactive drugs would be loaded [218, 221, 222] Drug-eluting stents prevent thrombosis formation and also provide controlled drug release over time. PLA, PGA, PCL, PLGA, and their composite forms are widely used as the reinforcing material covering stents [217, 221, 222].

Another option for stent applications is developing and using totally bioresorbable stents for cardiovascular diseases. PLLA-based polymeric stents were developed to replace metallic stents. They have a similar design and function, but PLLA-based stents can be totally degraded in two to three years after implantation [223, 224]. The critical issues that polymeric stents face are: (i) long-term degradation behavior; (ii) brittleness; (iii) low fatigue resistance; and (iv) inflammatory reactions that are provoked by the degradation of byproducts [218, 225, 226]. To prevent these problems, PLLA-based stents are reinforced with PLGA, P4HB, and PCL [217, 219, 225]. In rapid balloon expansion applications, the use of PLLA/P4HB biocomposite stents provides adequate mechanical stability and load bearing capacity to prevent stents from rupturing [219].

Biosensors

The use of polymer-based biocomposites as biosensors offers an efficient approach for immobilizing biological materials [227, 228]. The biocomposite gains particular electrochemical properties from the distribution of the conductive phase in the matrix and, consequently, on the surface of the biocomposite [229]. The SPBc materials in the different components of biosensors are mainly applied in the preparation of bio-membranes (enzyme membranes, redox membranes, *etc.*). On the other hand, they are used in receptors in the form of a polymer matrix, redox polymer, or mediator of transducers as ion-selective membranes (field effect transistors) and as optical fibers in optoelectronic sensors [228, 230].

The pH, sensitivity and thermal stability increment, minimization of measuring time, ability to reuse the enzyme, low-cost production, opportunity for continuous process, and not allowing the contamination of the analyte solution are the advantageous parameters of using polymeric biocomposite materials in biosensor applications [228].

Polyvinylpyrrolidone (PVP), polyethylene glycol (PEG), polyethylene oxide (PEO), polypropylene oxide (PPO), polyvinyl acetate (PVA), polyvinylchloride aminated (PVC-NH$_2$), polyurethane (PU), polydimethylsiloxane (PDMS), polymethyl methacrylate (PMMA), and their copolymers are the synthetic polymers used in the formation of biocomposite structures in biosensor applications, mainly in the production of protein repellent surfaces and corrosion inhibitor surfaces [61, 231 - 235]. The antifouling properties of reinforced PVP-based biocomposites are comparable to PEG reinforced surfaces. Therefore, they have a wide application area in biosensors and biochips [236]. Properties such as hydrophilicity, non-toxicity, and non-immunogenicity have also been utilized to incorporate PEG-based biocomposites in biosensors [237]. PDMS and its composite forms constitutes another useful polymeric material due to various interesting properties such as non-toxicity, biocompatibility, optical transparency, durability, chemically inert nature, and easy fabrication ability [49, 50]. Due to these properties, it is widely used in microfluidic-based biosensor devices. Biocomposite forms of PVCs (*e.g.* aminated) have been investigated for use as the electrode membrane material in order to facilitate efficient enzyme immobilization [238 - 241].

Polyethylene glycol/oxide (PEG/PEO) polymers have been described as among the most popular materials for biosensors due to their resistance to biofouling [242]. However, it is widely reported that a low adsorption of proteins occurs at the surface of these materials [242]. PEG/PEO chains are usually efficiently solvated in an aqueous system and the resulting protein molecules will experience a surface that is largely composed of water, thus mimicking the typical conditions found within biological systems. This is thought to be a major contributor to their biocompatibility.

Water-soluble copolymers of polyethylene oxide and polypropylene oxide (PEOn–PPOm) are nonionic amphiphilic, commercially available macromolecules. Due to their surface-active properties, these SPBc have been used in the dispersion stabilization of enzymes [87]. It is known that the absorbent layers of these biocomposites may act as steric barriers for nonspecific protein adsorption, which can improve the biocompatibility of a biomaterial as well as the sensitivity of a biosensor. Therefore, interest has recently been focused on studying their roles in reducing nonspecific protein adsorption and cell adhesion on biomaterial/biosensor surfaces [243 - 246].

CONCLUDING REMARKS

In this chapter, information about synthetic polymer-based biocomposites were summarized and presented along with their variety, superiority, mechanical properties, manufacturing processes, and application areas. Various polymer-based biocomposites were considered due to their significant properties (*i.e.* chemical, physical and mechanical properties, biocompatibility, tail or ability, *etc.*).

This chapter is intended to offer valuable insights for the future development of research. It is expected that due to the beneficial information content, this chapter will serve as an effective guide in the numerous application areas.

FUTURE RESEARCH

In recent years, there has been tremendous interest in the development and use of SPBc, and it can be predicted that this interest will continue to grow in future. The trend is now to design SPBc for biocompatibility, tailorability, and with unique characteristics. In the near future, SPBc will be increasingly involved in applications in the medical (*i.e.* dental, orthopedics, cardiovascular, suture, artificial skin, and cornea) and pharmaceutical arenas. The development of tailor-made polymeric biocomposites will increase the efficiency and optimized performance of materials to meet the increasing demands of biotechnology as well as biomedical applications.

With the progression of nanoscience and nanotechnology, the interest in the development of biocomposites gains new perspective. The use of polymeric nano-biocomposite materials will become increasingly popular in different areas of application as they can be synthesized with improved mechanical, physical, and chemical properties in nano-scale. Thanks to the improvements in SPBc biotechnology, science will have a new opportunity to apply biocomposites in 3D printing technology. By using SPBc, scaffolds, artificial tissue, and even artificial skin can be synthesized. In terms of future developments, the manufacture of artificial organs, articular limbs, and even diarthroses can be foreseen using SPBc and 3D printing technology.

CONFLICT OF INTEREST

The authors declare no conflict of interest, financial or otherwise.

ACKNOWLEDGEMENTS

The authors gratefully thank to Burak Ozdemir for support and Busra Gozutok for creating the pictures of this chapter.

REFERENCES

[1] Gloria A, De Santis R, Ambrosio L. Polymer-based composite scaffolds for tissue engineering. J Appl Biomater Biomech 2010; 8(2): 57-67.
[PMID: 20740467]

[2] Ramakrishna S, Mayer J, Wintermantel E, Leong KW. Biomedical applications of polymer-composite materials: a review. Compos Sci Technol 2001; 61(9): 1189-224.
[http://dx.doi.org/10.1016/S0266-3538(00)00241-4]

[3] dos Santos Rosa D, Lenz DM. Biocomposites: Influence of matrix nature and additives on the properties and biodegradation behaviour. 2013.

[4] Chand N, Fahim M. Tribology of natural fiber polymer composites. Elsevier Science 2008.
[http://dx.doi.org/10.1533/9781845695057]

[5] Kalia S, Dufresne A, Cherian BM, *et al.* Cellulose-based bio-and nanocomposites: a review 2011.
[http://dx.doi.org/10.1155/2011/837875]

[6] Karagoz A. Misel oluşturabilen, biyouyumlu, biyobozunur, pozitif yüklü polimerik malzemelerin sentezi ve karakterizasyonu [Y]. İstanbul: Yıldız Teknik üniversitesi. 2009.

[7] Peppas NA. Hydrogels in medicine and pharmacy: Polymers. CRC Press 1987.

[8] Kontrollü polimerizasyon yöntemiyle organik / anorganik polimerik kompozit malzemelerin sentezi ve karakterizasyonu. Malatya: İnönü Üniversitesi. 2011.

[9] YILDIRIM A Fonksiyonel hibrit malzemeler. Malatya: İnönü Üniversitesi 2008.

[10] Zarrabi Ahrabi A. Pet Atıkları Kullanılarak Kompozit Malzeme Üretiminin Araştırılmas. Ankara: Ankara Üniversitesi 2009.

[11] Hahn HT, Tsai SW. Introduction to composite materials. CRC Press 1980.

[12] letken poli(etilen teraftalat)/polipirol kompozit liflerinin kimyasal polimerizasyonla hazırlanması ve karakterizasyonu Ankara: Ankara Üniversitesi. 2007.

[13] Dorozhkin SV. Biocomposites and hybrid biomaterials based on calcium orthophosphates. Biomatter 2011; 1(1): 3-56.
[http://dx.doi.org/10.4161/biom.1.1.16782] [PMID: 23507726]

[14] Gravitis YA, Tééyaér R, Kallavus U, *et al.* Biocomposite structure of wood cell membranes and their destruction by explosive autohydrolysis. Mech Compos Mater 1987; 22(6): 721-5.
[http://dx.doi.org/10.1007/BF00605309]

[15] Venkatesan J, Kim S-K. Chitosan composites for bone tissue engineering--an overview. Mar Drugs 2010; 8(8): 2252-66.
[http://dx.doi.org/10.3390/md8082252] [PMID: 20948907]

[16]   Williams DF. Fundamental aspects of biocompatibility: CRC PressI Llc. 1981.

[17]   Özdemir Yön. Biyomateryaller ve Biyouyumluluk.

[18]   Ramakrishna S. An Introduction to Biocomposites. Imperial College Press 2004.
        [http://dx.doi.org/10.1142/p311]

[19]   Silver F. Biomaterials, Medical Devices and Tissue Engineering: An Integrated Approach: An
        integrated approach. Springer Netherlands 2012.

[20]   Ambrosio L. Biomedical Composites. Elsevier Science 2009.

[21]   Sarsılmaz F, Sarsılmaz C. Ortopedide kullanılan polimer esaslı kompozit malzemeler. Doğu Anadolu
        Bölgesi Araştırmaları 2003.

[22]   Salernitano E, Migliaresi C. Composite materials for biomedical applications: a review. J Appl
        Biomater Biomech 2003; 1(1): 3-18.
        [PMID: 20803468]

[23]   Cheung H-Y, Lau K-T, Lu T-P, Hui D. A critical review on polymer-based bio-engineered materials
        for scaffold development. Compos, Part B Eng 2007; 38(3): 291-300.
        [http://dx.doi.org/10.1016/j.compositesb.2006.06.014]

[24]   Ducheyne P, Healy K, Hutmacher DE, Grainger DW, Kirkpatrick CJ. Comprehensive Biomaterials.
        Elsevier Science 2015.

[25]   Fowler PA, Hughes JM, Elias RM. Biocomposites: technology, environmental credentials and market
        forces. J Sci Food Agric 2006; 86(12): 1781-9.
        [http://dx.doi.org/10.1002/jsfa.2558]

[26]   Smith WF, Hashemi J. Foundations of materials science and engineering: Mcgraw-Hill Publishing.
        2006.

[27]   Matthews F, Rawlings R. Composite materials: engineering and science. London: Chapman&Hall
        1994.

[28]   Rezwan K, Chen QZ, Blaker JJ, Boccaccini AR. Biodegradable and bioactive porous
        polymer/inorganic composite scaffolds for bone tissue engineering. Biomaterials 2006; 27(18): 3413-
        31.
        [http://dx.doi.org/10.1016/j.biomaterials.2006.01.039] [PMID: 16504284]

[29]   Langer R, Chasin M. Biodegradable polymers as drug delivery systems. New York: Marcel Dekker
        1990.

[30]   AMSC N, CMPS AA. Composite Materials Handbook. 2002.

[31]   Nicolais L, Gloria A, Ambrosio L. The mechanics of biocomposites. Biomedical Composites 2009;
        pp. 411-40.

[32]   Schwartz MM. Composite Materials Handbook. 1992.

[33]   Black J, Hastings G. Handbook of biomaterial properties. Springer Science & Business Media 2013.

[34]   Harper CA. Modern Plastics Handbook: handbook: McGraw-Hill Professional. 2000.

[35]   BRYDSON J, editor Plastics Materials; 1J. A Brydson 7th ed Library of Congress Cataloguing in
        Publication Data.

[36]   Auras RA, Lim L-T, Selke SE, Tsuji H. Poly (lactic acid): synthesis, structures, properties, processing,
        and applications. John Wiley & Sons 2011.

[37]   Ellis B, Smith R. Polymers: a property database. CRC Press 2008.

[38]   Chu CC, Moncrief G. An *in vitro* evaluation of the stability of mechanical properties of surgical suture
        materials in various pH conditions. Ann Surg 1983; 198(2): 223-8.
        [http://dx.doi.org/10.1097/00000658-198308000-00019] [PMID: 6870380]

[39]   Acton QA. Issues in Biochemistry and Biomaterials: 2011 Edition: ScholarlyEditions. 2012.

[40]   Muggli DS, Burkoth AK, Anseth KS. Crosslinked polyanhydrides for use in orthopedic applications: degradation behavior and mechanics. J Biomed Mater Res 1999; 46(2): 271-8.
[http://dx.doi.org/10.1002/(SICI)1097-4636(199908)46:2<271::AID-JBM17>3.0.CO;2-X]   [PMID: 10380006]

[41]   Lendlein A, Sisson A. Handbook of Biodegradable Polymers: Isolation, Synthesis, Characterization and Applications. Wiley 2011.
[http://dx.doi.org/10.1002/9783527635818]

[42]   Dumitriu S, Popa V. Polymeric Biomaterials: Structure and Function. CRC Press 2013.
[http://dx.doi.org/10.1201/b14913]

[43]   Engelberg I, Kohn J. Physico-mechanical properties of degradable polymers used in medical applications: a comparative study. Biomaterials 1991; 12(3): 292-304.
[http://dx.doi.org/10.1016/0142-9612(91)90037-B] [PMID: 1649646]

[44]   Hollinger JO. An Introduction to Biomaterials. Taylor & Francis 2005.

[45]   Ma D, Chen H, Shi D, Li Z, Wang J. Preparation and characterization of thermo-responsive PDMS surfaces grafted with poly(N-isopropylacrylamide) by benzophenone-initiated photopolymerization. J Colloid Interface Sci 2009; 332(1): 85-90.
[http://dx.doi.org/10.1016/j.jcis.2008.12.046] [PMID: 19168188]

[46]   Masuelli MA. Introduction of fibre-reinforced polymers −polymers and composites: Concepts, properties and processes 2013 2013-01-23.

[47]   Gil ES, Hudson SM. Stimuli-reponsive polymers and their bioconjugates. Prog Polym Sci 2004; 29(12): 1173-222.
[http://dx.doi.org/10.1016/j.progpolymsci.2004.08.003]

[48]   Liu L, Sheardown H. Glucose permeable poly (dimethyl siloxane) poly (N-isopropyl acrylamide) interpenetrating networks as ophthalmic biomaterials. Biomaterials 2005; 26(3): 233-44.
[http://dx.doi.org/10.1016/j.biomaterials.2004.02.025] [PMID: 15262466]

[49]   Bodas D, Khan-Malek C. Formation of more stable hydrophilic surfaces of PDMS by plasma and chemical treatments. Microelectron Eng 2006; 83(4): 1277-9.
[http://dx.doi.org/10.1016/j.mee.2006.01.195]

[50]   Abbasi F, Mirzadeh H, Katbab AA. Modification of polysiloxane polymers for biomedical applications: a review. Polym Int 2001; 50(12): 1279-87.
[http://dx.doi.org/10.1002/pi.783]

[51]   Roessler M, Wilke A, Griss P, Kienapfel H. Missing osteoconductive effect of a resorbable PEO/PBT copolymer in human bone defects: a clinically relevant pilot study with contrary results to previous animal studies. J Biomed Mater Res 2000; 53(2): 167-73.
[http://dx.doi.org/10.1002/(SICI)1097-4636(2000)53:2<167::AID-JBM6>3.0.CO;2-J]   [PMID: 10713563]

[52]   Radder AM, Leenders H, van Blitterswijk CA. Bone-bonding behaviour of poly(ethylene oxide)-polybutylene terephthalate copolymer coatings and bulk implants: a comparative study. Biomaterials 1995; 16(7): 507-13.
[http://dx.doi.org/10.1016/0142-9612(95)91122-F] [PMID: 7492713]

[53]   Bezemer JM, Radersma R, Grijpma DW, Dijkstra PJ, Feijen J, van Blitterswijk CA. Zero-order release of lysozyme from poly(ethylene glycol)/poly(butylene terephthalate) matrices. J Control Release 2000; 64(1-3): 179-92.
[http://dx.doi.org/10.1016/S0168-3659(99)00127-3] [PMID: 10640656]

[54]   Younes HM, Bravo-Grimaldo E, Amsden BG. Synthesis, characterization and *in vitro* degradation of a biodegradable elastomer. Biomaterials 2004; 25(22): 5261-9.

[http://dx.doi.org/10.1016/j.biomaterials.2003.12.024] [PMID: 15110477]

[55]   Shikinami Y, Okuno M. Bioresorbable devices made of forged composites of hydroxyapatite (HA) particles and poly-L-lactide (PLLA): Part I. Basic characteristics. Biomaterials 1999; 20(9): 859-77. [http://dx.doi.org/10.1016/S0142-9612(98)00241-5] [PMID: 10226712]

[56]   Patel NR, Gohil PP. A review on biomaterials: scope, applications & human anatomy significance. Int J Emerg Technol Adv Eng 2012; 2(4): 91-101.

[57]   Heise M, Schmidmaier G, Husmann I, *et al.* PEG-hirudin/iloprost coating of small diameter ePTFE grafts effectively prevents pseudointima and intimal hyperplasia development. Eur J Vasc Endovasc Surg 2006; 32(4): 418-24. [http://dx.doi.org/10.1016/j.ejvs.2006.03.002] [PMID: 16682237]

[58]   Deschamps AA, Grijpma DW, Feijen J. Poly (ethylene oxide)/poly (butylene terephthalate) segmented block copolymers: the effect of copolymer composition on physical properties and degradation behavior. Polymer (Guildf) 2001; 42(23): 9335-45. [http://dx.doi.org/10.1016/S0032-3861(01)00453-0]

[59]   Xiao YL, Riesle J, Van Blitterswijk CA. Static and dynamic fibroblast seeding and cultivation in porous PEO/PBT scaffolds. J Mater Sci Mater Med 1999; 10(12): 773-7. [http://dx.doi.org/10.1023/A:1008946832443] [PMID: 15347949]

[60]   Deschamps AA, van Apeldoorn AA, Hayen H, *et al. In vivo* and *in vitro* degradation of poly(ether ester) block copolymers based on poly(ethylene glycol) and poly(butylene terephthalate). Biomaterials 2004; 25(2): 247-58. [http://dx.doi.org/10.1016/S0142-9612(03)00495-2] [PMID: 14585712]

[61]   Li ZF, Ruckenstein E. Grafting of poly(ethylene oxide) to the surface of polyaniline films through a chlorosulfonation method and the biocompatibility of the modified films. J Colloid Interface Sci 2004; 269(1): 62-71. [http://dx.doi.org/10.1016/S0021-9797(03)00606-4] [PMID: 14651896]

[62]   Miller RA, Brady JM, Cutright DE. Degradation rates of oral resorbable implants (polylactates and polyglycolates): rate modification with changes in PLA/PGA copolymer ratios. J Biomed Mater Res 1977; 11(5): 711-9. [http://dx.doi.org/10.1002/jbm.820110507] [PMID: 893490]

[63]   Gilding D, Reed A. Biodegradable polymers for use in surgery—polyglycolic/poly (actic acid) homo- and copolymers: 1. Polymer (Guildf) 1979; 20(12): 1459-64. [http://dx.doi.org/10.1016/0032-3861(79)90009-0]

[64]   Ulery BD, Nair LS, Laurencin CT. Biomedical applications of biodegradable polymers. J Polym Sci, B, Polym Phys 2011; 49(12): 832-64. [http://dx.doi.org/10.1002/polb.22259] [PMID: 21769165]

[65]   Vainionpää S, Rokkanen P, Törmälä P. Surgical applications of biodegradable polymers in human tissues. Prog Polym Sci 1989; 14(5): 679-716. [http://dx.doi.org/10.1016/0079-6700(89)90013-0]

[66]   Barrows T. Degradable implant materials: a review of synthetic absorbable polymers and their applications. Clin Mater 1986; 1(4): 233-57. [http://dx.doi.org/10.1016/S0267-6605(86)80015-4]

[67]   Chanda M, Roy SK. Plastics technology handbook. CRC press 2006.

[68]   Ormiston JA, Webster MW, Armstrong G. First-in-human implantation of a fully bioabsorbable drug-eluting stent: the BVS poly-L-lactic acid everolimus-eluting coronary stent. Catheter Cardiovasc Interv 2007; 69(1): 128-31. [http://dx.doi.org/10.1002/ccd.20895] [PMID: 17139655]

[69]   Melvin A, Litsky A, Mayerson J, Stringer K, Melvin D, Juncosa-Melvin N. An artificial tendon to connect the quadriceps muscle to the tibia. J Orthop Res 2011; 29(11): 1775-82.

[http://dx.doi.org/10.1002/jor.21419] [PMID: 21520259]

[70]   Bernacca GM, Mackay TG, Wilkinson R, Wheatley DJ. Calcification and fatigue failure in a polyurethane heart value. Biomaterials 1995; 16(4): 279-85.
[http://dx.doi.org/10.1016/0142-9612(95)93255-C] [PMID: 7772667]

[71]   Fisher WK, Corelli J. Effect of ionizing radiation on the chemical composition, crystalline content and structure, and flow properties of polytetrafluoroethylene. Journal of Polymer Science: Polymer Chemistry Edition 1981; 19(10): 2465-93.

[72]   Hillmyer MA, Lodge TP. Synthesis and self-assembly of fluorinated block copolymers. J Polym Sci A Polym Chem 2002; 40(1): 1-8.
[http://dx.doi.org/10.1002/pola.10074]

[73]   Bosiers M, Deloose K, Verbist J, *et al.* Heparin-bonded expanded polytetrafluoroethylene vascular graft for femoropopliteal and femorocrural bypass grafting: 1-year results. J Vasc Surg 2006; 43(2): 313-8.
[http://dx.doi.org/10.1016/j.jvs.2005.10.037] [PMID: 16476607]

[74]   Kapfer X, Meichelboeck W, Groegler F-M. Comparison of carbon-impregnated and standard ePTFE prostheses in extra-anatomical anterior tibial artery bypass: a prospective randomized multicenter study. Eur J Vasc Endovasc Surg 2006; 32(2): 155-68.
[http://dx.doi.org/10.1016/j.ejvs.2005.12.015] [PMID: 16617028]

[75]   Gershon B, Cohn D, Marom G. Compliance and ultimate strength of composite arterial prostheses. Biomaterials 1992; 13(1): 38-43.
[http://dx.doi.org/10.1016/0142-9612(92)90093-4] [PMID: 1543807]

[76]   Xue L, Greisler HP. Biomaterials in the development and future of vascular grafts. J Vasc Surg 2003; 37(2): 472-80.
[http://dx.doi.org/10.1067/mva.2003.88] [PMID: 12563226]

[77]   Dickens SH, Stansbury J, Choi K, Floyd C. Photopolymerization kinetics of methacrylate dental resins. Macromolecules 2003; 36(16): 6043-53.
[http://dx.doi.org/10.1021/ma021675k]

[78]   Antonucci JM, Stansbury JW. Molecular designed dental polymer Desk reference of functional polymers: synthesis and application American Chemical Society Publication 1997:719-38.

[79]   Bowen RL. Dental filling material comprising vinyl silane treated fused silica and a binder consisting of the reaction product of bis phenol and glycidyl acrylate. Google Patents 1962.

[80]   Bowen RL. Properties of a silica-reinforced polymer for dental restorations. J Am Dent Assoc 1963; 66(1): 57-64.
[http://dx.doi.org/10.14219/jada.archive.1963.0010] [PMID: 14014600]

[81]   Leinfelder K. Five year clinical evaluation of anterior and posterior restorations of composite resin. Oper Dent 1980; 5: 57-65.

[82]   Kosonen H, Ruokolainen J, Torkkeli M, Serimaa R, Nyholm P, Ikkala O. Micro- and macrophase separation in phenolic resol resin/PEO-PPO-PEO block copolymer blends: Effect of hydrogen-bonded PEO length. Macromol Chem Phys 2002; 203(2): 388-92.
[http://dx.doi.org/10.1002/1521-3935(20020101)203:2<388::AID-MACP388>3.0.CO;2-K]

[83]   Larrañaga M, Gabilondo N, Kortaberria G, *et al.* Micro-or nanoseparated phases in thermoset blends of an epoxy resin and PEO–PPO–PEO triblock copolymer. Polymer (Guildf) 2005; 46(18): 7082-93.
[http://dx.doi.org/10.1016/j.polymer.2005.05.102]

[84]   Williams D. An introduction to medical and dental materials. Con Enc Med Den Mater 1990; pp. xvii-x.

[85]   Sun P, Dang Q, Li B, *et al.* Mobility, miscibility, and microdomain structure in nanostructured thermoset blends of epoxy resin and amphiphilic poly (ethylene oxide)-b lock-poly (propylene oxide)-

b lock-poly (ethylene oxide) triblock copolymers characterized by solid-state NMR. Macromolecules 2005; 38(13): 5654-67.
[http://dx.doi.org/10.1021/ma0505979]

[86]   Serrano E, Tercjak A, Kortaberria G, *et al.* Nanostructured thermosetting systems by modification with epoxidized styrene-butadiene star block copolymers. Effect of epoxidation degree. Macromolecules 2006; 39(6): 2254-61.
[http://dx.doi.org/10.1021/ma0515477]

[87]   Alexandridis P, Holzwarth JF, Hatton TA. Micellization of poly (ethylene oxide)-poly (propylene oxide)-poly (ethylene oxide) triblock copolymers in aqueous solutions: thermodynamics of copolymer association. Macromolecules 1994; 27(9): 2414-25.
[http://dx.doi.org/10.1021/ma00087a009]

[88]   Sionkowska A, Wisniewski M, Kaczmarek H, *et al.* The influence of UV irradiation on surface composition of collagen/PVP blended films. Appl Surf Sci 2006; 253(4): 1970-7.
[http://dx.doi.org/10.1016/j.apsusc.2006.03.048]

[89]   Lai G, Du Z, Li G. The rheological behavior of collagen dispersion/poly (vinyl alcohol) blends. Korea-Australia Rheol J 2007; 19(2): 81-8.

[90]   Bernal A, Balkova R, Kuritka I, Saha P. Preparation and characterisation of a new double-sided bio-artificial material prepared by casting of poly (vinyl alcohol) on collagen. Polym Bull 2013; 70(2): 431-53.
[http://dx.doi.org/10.1007/s00289-012-0802-2]

[91]   Onyari JM, Huang SJ. Synthesis and properties of novel polyvinyl alcohol–lactic acid gels. J Appl Polym Sci 2009; 113(4): 2053-61.
[http://dx.doi.org/10.1002/app.29909]

[92]   Tanigami T, Yano K, Yamaura K, Matsuzawa S. Anomalous swelling of poly (vinyl alcohol) film in mixed solvents of dimethylsulfoxide and water. Polymer (Guildf) 1995; 36(15): 2941-6.
[http://dx.doi.org/10.1016/0032-3861(95)94343-R]

[93]   Lakouraj MM, Tajbakhsh M, Mokhtary M. Synthesis and swelling characterization of cross-linked PVP/PVA hydrogels. Iran Polym J 2005; 14(12): 1022.

[94]   Liu K, Li Y, Xu F, *et al.* Graphite/poly (vinyl alcohol) hydrogel composite as porous ringy skirt for artificial cornea. Mater Sci Eng C 2009; 29(1): 261-6.
[http://dx.doi.org/10.1016/j.msec.2008.06.023]

[95]   Imanieh H, Aghahosseini H. Synthesis and character investigation of new collagen Hydrolysate/polyvinyl alcohol/hydroxyapatite Polymer-Nano-Porous Membranes: I. Experimental design optimization in thermal and structural properties. Syst Synth Biol 2013; 7(4): 175-84.
[http://dx.doi.org/10.1007/s11693-013-9110-x] [PMID: 24432154]

[96]   Miyashita H, Shimmura S, Kobayashi H, *et al.* Collagen-immobilized poly(vinyl alcohol) as an artificial cornea scaffold that supports a stratified corneal epithelium. J Biomed Mater Res B Appl Biomater 2006; 76(1): 56-63.
[http://dx.doi.org/10.1002/jbm.b.30332] [PMID: 16044431]

[97]   Thomas S, Joseph K, Malhotra SK, Goda K, Sreekala MS. Polymer Composites, Macro- and Microcomposites. Wiley 2012.
[http://dx.doi.org/10.1002/9783527645213]

[98]   Prasad RC, Ramakrishnan P. Composites, Science, and Technology: New Age International 2000.

[99]   Mi H-Y, Jing X, Turng L-S. Fabrication of porous synthetic polymer scaffolds for tissue engineering. J Cell Plast 2015; 51(2): 165-96.
[http://dx.doi.org/10.1177/0021955X14531002]

[100]   Kramschuster A, Turng LS. An injection molding process for manufacturing highly porous and interconnected biodegradable polymer matrices for use as tissue engineering scaffolds. J Biomed

Mater Res B Appl Biomater 2010; 92(2): 366-76.
[PMID: 19957359]

[101] Björnsson A, Johansen K, Eds. Composite manufacturing: How improvement work might lead to renewed product validation. 5th International Swedish Production Symposium (SPS 2012). 6-8 November 2012; Linköping, Sweden. 2012.

[102] Shen FC. A filament-wound structure technology overview. Mater Chem Phys 1995; 42(2): 96-100.
[http://dx.doi.org/10.1016/0254-0584(95)01554-X]

[103] Golish SR, Anderson PA. Bearing surfaces for total disc arthroplasty: metal-on-metal *versus* metal-o--polyethylene and other biomaterials. Spine J 2012; 12(8): 693-701.
[http://dx.doi.org/10.1016/j.spinee.2011.05.008] [PMID: 21700505]

[104] Kobayashi M, Chang Y-S, Oka M. A two year *in vivo* study of polyvinyl alcohol-hydrogel (PVA-H) artificial meniscus. Biomaterials 2005; 26(16): 3243-8.
[http://dx.doi.org/10.1016/j.biomaterials.2004.08.028] [PMID: 15603819]

[105] Wang H, Ren J, Hlaing A, Yan M. Fabrication and anti-fouling properties of photochemically and thermally immobilized poly(ethylene oxide) and low molecular weight poly(ethylene glycol) thin films. J Colloid Interface Sci 2011; 354(1): 160-7.
[http://dx.doi.org/10.1016/j.jcis.2010.10.018] [PMID: 21044787]

[106] Jia N, Lian Q, Wang Z, Shen H. A hydrogen peroxide biosensor based on direct electrochemistry of hemoglobin incorporated in PEO–PPO–PEO triblock copolymer film. Sens Actuators B Chem 2009; 137(1): 230-4.
[http://dx.doi.org/10.1016/j.snb.2008.10.011]

[107] Ensaff H, O'Doherty DM, Jacobsen PH. The influence of the restoration-tooth interface in light cured composite restorations: a finite element analysis. Biomaterials 2001; 22(23): 3097-103.
[http://dx.doi.org/10.1016/S0142-9612(01)00058-8] [PMID: 11603580]

[108] Moszner N, Salz U. New developments of polymeric dental composites. Prog Polym Sci 2001; 26(4): 535-76.
[http://dx.doi.org/10.1016/S0079-6700(01)00005-3]

[109] Jansen JA, de Ruijter JE, Janssen PT, Paquay YG. Histological evaluation of a biodegradable Polyactive/hydroxyapatite membrane. Biomaterials 1995; 16(11): 819-27.
[http://dx.doi.org/10.1016/0142-9612(95)94142-8] [PMID: 8527596]

[110] Ferracane JL, Condon JR. *In vitro* evaluation of the marginal degradation of dental composites under simulated occlusal loading. Dent Mater 1999; 15(4): 262-7.
[http://dx.doi.org/10.1016/S0109-5641(99)00045-7] [PMID: 10551094]

[111] Ratna D, Karger-Kocsis J. Recent advances in shape memory polymers and composites: a review. J Mater Sci 2008; 43(1): 254-69.
[http://dx.doi.org/10.1007/s10853-007-2176-7]

[112] Condon JR, Ferracane JL. Reduction of composite contraction stress through non-bonded microfiller particles. Dent Mater 1998; 14(4): 256-60.
[http://dx.doi.org/10.1016/S0109-5641(98)00036-0] [PMID: 10379253]

[113] Thomas S, Joseph K, Malhotra SK, Goda K, Sreekala MS. Polymer Composites, Biocomposites. Wiley 2013.

[114] Schedle A, Franz A, Rausch-Fan X, *et al.* Cytotoxic effects of dental composites, adhesive substances, compomers and cements. Dent Mater 1998; 14(6): 429-40.
[http://dx.doi.org/10.1016/S0300-5712(99)00018-4] [PMID: 10483406]

[115] Davy KW, Kalachandra S, Pandain MS, Braden M. Relationship between composite matrix molecular structure and properties. Biomaterials 1998; 19(22): 2007-14.
[http://dx.doi.org/10.1016/S0142-9612(98)00047-7] [PMID: 9870752]

[116] Sandner B, Baudach S, Davy KW, Braden M, Clarke RL. Synthesis of BISGMA derivatives, properties of their polymers and composites. J Mater Sci Mater Med 1997; 8(1): 39-44.
       [http://dx.doi.org/10.1023/A:1018590229166] [PMID: 15348840]

[117] Helsen JA, Missirlis Y. Biomaterials: A Tantalus Experience: Springer Berlin Heidelberg 2010.

[118] Evans SL, Gregson PJ. Composite technology in load-bearing orthopaedic implants. Biomaterials 1998; 19(15): 1329-42.
       [http://dx.doi.org/10.1016/S0142-9612(97)00217-2] [PMID: 9758033]

[119] Athanasiou KA, Agrawal CM, Barber FA, Burkhart SS. Orthopaedic applications for PLA-PGA biodegradable polymers. Arthroscopy 1998; 14(7): 726-37.
       [http://dx.doi.org/10.1016/S0749-8063(98)70099-4] [PMID: 9788368]

[120] Middleton JC, Tipton AJ. Synthetic biodegradable polymers as orthopedic devices. Biomaterials 2000; 21(23): 2335-46.
       [http://dx.doi.org/10.1016/S0142-9612(00)00101-0] [PMID: 11055281]

[121] Jayabalan M. Studies on Poly (propylene fumarate-co-caprolactone diol) Thermoset Composites towards the Development of Biodegradable Bone Fixation Devices International journal of biomaterials 2009; 2009..

[122] Chang FK, Perez JL, Davidson JA. Stiffness and strength tailoring of a hip prosthesis made of advanced composite materials. J Biomed Mater Res 1990; 24(7): 873-99.
       [http://dx.doi.org/10.1002/jbm.820240707] [PMID: 2398076]

[123] Marra KG, Szem JW, Kumta PN, DiMilla PA, Weiss LE. *In vitro* analysis of biodegradable polymer blend/hydroxyapatite composites for bone tissue engineering. J Biomed Mater Res 1999; 47(3): 324-35.
       [http://dx.doi.org/10.1002/(SICI)1097-4636(19991205)47:3<324::AID-JBM6>3.0.CO;2-Y] [PMID: 10487883]

[124] Laurencin CT, Attawia MA, Elgendy HE, Herbert KM. Tissue engineered bone-regeneration using degradable polymers: the formation of mineralized matrices. Bone 1996; 19(1) (Suppl.): 93S-9S.
       [http://dx.doi.org/10.1016/S8756-3282(96)00132-9] [PMID: 8831000]

[125] Jeon BJ, Jeong SY, Koo AN, Kim B-C, Hwang Y-S, Lee SC. Fabrication of porous PLGA microspheres with BMP-2 releasing polyphosphate-functionalized nano-hydroxyapatite for enhanced bone regeneration. Macromol Res 2012; 20(7): 715-24.
       [http://dx.doi.org/10.1007/s13233-012-0103-5]

[126] Rokkanen PU, Böstman O, Hirvensalo E, *et al.* Bioabsorbable fixation in orthopaedic surgery and traumatology. Biomaterials 2000; 21(24): 2607-13.
       [http://dx.doi.org/10.1016/S0142-9612(00)00128-9] [PMID: 11071610]

[127] Daniels AU, Chang MK, Andriano KP, Heller J. Mechanical properties of biodegradable polymers and composites proposed for internal fixation of bone. J Appl Biomater 1990; 1(1): 57-78.
       [http://dx.doi.org/10.1002/jab.770010109] [PMID: 10148987]

[128] Zhu G, Wang F, Tan H, Gao Q, Liu Y. Properties study of poly (L-lactic acid)/polyurethane-blend film. Polym Plast Technol Eng 2012; 51(15): 1562-6.
       [http://dx.doi.org/10.1080/03602559.2012.716133]

[129] Shikinami Y, Okuno M. Bioresorbable devices made of forged composites of hydroxyapatite (HA) particles and poly L-lactide (PLLA). Part II: practical properties of miniscrews and miniplates. Biomaterials 2001; 22(23): 3197-211.
       [http://dx.doi.org/10.1016/S0142-9612(01)00072-2] [PMID: 11603592]

[130] Wei G, Ma PX. Structure and properties of nano-hydroxyapatite/polymer composite scaffolds for bone tissue engineering. Biomaterials 2004; 25(19): 4749-57.
       [http://dx.doi.org/10.1016/j.biomaterials.2003.12.005] [PMID: 15120521]

[131] Tonino A, Folmer R. The clinical use of plastic plates for osteosynthesis in human fractures. Clin Mater 1987; 2(4): 275-9.
[http://dx.doi.org/10.1016/0267-6605(87)90004-7]

[132] Fujihara K, Huang Z-M, Ramakrishna S, Satknanantham K, Hamada H. Performance study of braided carbon/PEEK composite compression bone plates. Biomaterials 2003; 24(15): 2661-7.
[http://dx.doi.org/10.1016/S0142-9612(03)00065-6] [PMID: 12726720]

[133] Kotha SP, Li C, McGinn P, Schmid SR, Mason JJ. Improved mechanical properties of acrylic bone cement with short titanium fiber reinforcement. J Mater Sci Mater Med 2006; 17(12): 1403-9.
[http://dx.doi.org/10.1007/s10856-006-0616-6] [PMID: 17143773]

[134] Pourdeyhimi B, Wagner HD. Elastic and ultimate properties of acrylic bone cement reinforced with ultra-high-molecular-weight polyethylene fibers. J Biomed Mater Res 1989; 23(1): 63-80.
[http://dx.doi.org/10.1002/jbm.820230106] [PMID: 2708405]

[135] Yang JM, Huang PY, Yang MC, Lo SK. Effect of MMA-g-UHMWPE grafted fiber on mechanical properties of acrylic bone cement. J Biomed Mater Res 1997; 38(4): 361-9.
[http://dx.doi.org/10.1002/(SICI)1097-4636(199724)38:4<361::AID-JBM9>3.0.CO;2-M] [PMID: 9421758]

[136] Dalby MJ, Di Silvio L, Harper EJ, Bonfield W. Initial interaction of osteoblasts with the surface of a hydroxyapatite-poly(methylmethacrylate) cement. Biomaterials 2001; 22(13): 1739-47.
[http://dx.doi.org/10.1016/S0142-9612(00)00334-3] [PMID: 11396877]

[137] Bonfield W, Wang M, Tanner K. Interfaces in analogue biomaterials. Acta Mater 1998; 46(7): 2509-18.
[http://dx.doi.org/10.1016/S1359-6454(98)80035-9]

[138] Oosterom R, Bersee H, Beukers A. Composites for human joint replacement

[139] Katti KS. Biomaterials in total joint replacement. Colloids Surf B Biointerfaces 2004; 39(3): 133-42.
[http://dx.doi.org/10.1016/j.colsurfb.2003.12.002] [PMID: 15556342]

[140] Deng M, Shalaby SW. Properties of self-reinforced ultra-high-molecular-weight polyethylene composites. Biomaterials 1997; 18(9): 645-55.
[http://dx.doi.org/10.1016/S0142-9612(96)00194-9] [PMID: 9151996]

[141] Katoozian H, Davy DT, Arshi A, Saadati U. Material optimization of femoral component of total hip prosthesis using fiber reinforced polymeric composites. Med Eng Phys 2001; 23(7): 503-9.
[http://dx.doi.org/10.1016/S1350-4533(01)00079-0] [PMID: 11574257]

[142] Merolli A, Perrone V, Tranquilli Leali P, et al. Response to polyetherimide based composite materials implanted in muscle and in bone. J Mater Sci Mater Med 1999; 10(5): 265-8.
[http://dx.doi.org/10.1023/A:1008949311714] [PMID: 15348142]

[143] De Santis R, Ambrosio L, Nicolais L. Polymer-based composite hip prostheses. J Inorg Biochem 2000; 79(1-4): 97-102.
[http://dx.doi.org/10.1016/S0162-0134(99)00228-7] [PMID: 10830853]

[144] Okada Y, Kobayashi M, Neo M, et al. Ultrastructure of the interface between alumina bead composite and bone. J Biomed Mater Res 2000; 49(1): 106-11.
[http://dx.doi.org/10.1002/(SICI)1097-4636(200001)49:1<106::AID-JBM13>3.0.CO;2-W] [PMID: 10559752]

[145] Kolarík J, Migliaresi C, Štol M, Nicolais L. Mechanical properties of model synthetic tendons. J Biomed Mater Res 1981; 15(2): 147-57.
[http://dx.doi.org/10.1002/jbm.820150204] [PMID: 7348710]

[146] Iannace S, Sabatini G, Ambrosio L, Nicolais L. Mechanical behaviour of composite artificial tendons and ligaments. Biomaterials 1995; 16(9): 675-80.
[http://dx.doi.org/10.1016/0142-9612(95)99693-G] [PMID: 7578769]

[147] Goh JC, Ouyang H-W, Teoh S-H, Chan CK, Lee E-H. Tissue-engineering approach to the repair and regeneration of tendons and ligaments. Tissue Eng 2003; 9(4) (Suppl. 1): S31-44.
[http://dx.doi.org/10.1089/10763270360696969] [PMID: 14511469]

[148] Kazanci M, Cohn D, Marom G, Migliaresi C, Pegoretti A. Fatigue characterization of polyethylene fiber reinforced polyolefin biomedical composites. Compos, Part A Appl Sci Manuf 2002; 33(4): 453-8.
[http://dx.doi.org/10.1016/S1359-835X(02)00002-7]

[149] Dash TK, Konkimalla VB. Poly-ε-caprolactone based formulations for drug delivery and tissue engineering: A review. J Control Release 2012; 158(1): 15-33.
[http://dx.doi.org/10.1016/j.jconrel.2011.09.064] [PMID: 21963774]

[150] Braun K, Pipkorn R, Waldeck W. Development and characterization of drug delivery systems for targeting mammalian cells and tissues: a review. Curr Med Chem 2005; 12(16): 1841-58.
[http://dx.doi.org/10.2174/0929867054546672] [PMID: 16101505]

[151] Grund S, Bauer M, Fischer D. Polymers in drug delivery—state of the art and future trends. Adv Eng Mater 2011; 13(3): B61-87.
[http://dx.doi.org/10.1002/adem.201080088]

[152] Bae YH, Kim SW. Hydrogel delivery systems based on polymer blends, block co-polymers or interpenetrating networks. Adv Drug Deliv Rev 1993; 11(1): 109-35.
[http://dx.doi.org/10.1016/0169-409X(93)90029-4]

[153] Saito N, Murakami N, Takahashi J, *et al.* Synthetic biodegradable polymers as drug delivery systems for bone morphogenetic proteins. Adv Drug Deliv Rev 2005; 57(7): 1037-48.
[http://dx.doi.org/10.1016/j.addr.2004.12.016] [PMID: 15876402]

[154] Sokolsky-Papkov M, Agashi K, Olaye A, Shakesheff K, Domb AJ. Polymer carriers for drug delivery in tissue engineering. Adv Drug Deliv Rev 2007; 59(4-5): 187-206.
[http://dx.doi.org/10.1016/j.addr.2007.04.001] [PMID: 17540473]

[155] Kretlow JD, Klouda L, Mikos AG. Injectable matrices and scaffolds for drug delivery in tissue engineering. Adv Drug Deliv Rev 2007; 59(4-5): 263-73.
[http://dx.doi.org/10.1016/j.addr.2007.03.013] [PMID: 17507111]

[156] Woodruff MA, Hutmacher DW. The return of a forgotten polymer—polycaprolactone in the 21st century. Prog Polym Sci 2010; 35(10): 1217-56.
[http://dx.doi.org/10.1016/j.progpolymsci.2010.04.002]

[157] Rösler A, Vandermeulen GW, Klok H-A. Advanced drug delivery devices *via* self-assembly of amphiphilic block copolymers. Adv Drug Deliv Rev 2012; 64: 270-9.
[http://dx.doi.org/10.1016/j.addr.2012.09.026] [PMID: 11733119]

[158] Gunatillake PA, Adhikari R. Biodegradable synthetic polymers for tissue engineering. Eur Cell Mater 2003; 5(1): 1-16.
[http://dx.doi.org/10.22203/eCM.v005a01] [PMID: 14562275]

[159] Packhaeuser CB, Schnieders J, Oster CG, Kissel T. *In situ* forming parenteral drug delivery systems: an overview. Eur J Pharm Biopharm 2004; 58(2): 445-55.
[http://dx.doi.org/10.1016/j.ejpb.2004.03.003] [PMID: 15296966]

[160] Habraken WJ, Wolke JG, Jansen JA. Ceramic composites as matrices and scaffolds for drug delivery in tissue engineering. Adv Drug Deliv Rev 2007; 59(4-5): 234-48.
[http://dx.doi.org/10.1016/j.addr.2007.03.011] [PMID: 17478007]

[161] Kim S, Kim J-H, Jeon O, Kwon IC, Park K. Engineered polymers for advanced drug delivery. Eur J Pharm Biopharm 2009; 71(3): 420-30.
[http://dx.doi.org/10.1016/j.ejpb.2008.09.021] [PMID: 18977434]

[162] Pouton CW, Akhtar S. Biosynthetic polyhydroxyalkanoates and their potential in drug delivery. Adv

Drug Deliv Rev 1996; 18(2): 133-62.
[http://dx.doi.org/10.1016/0169-409X(95)00092-L]

[163] Zhong SP, Zhang YZ, Lim CT. Tissue scaffolds for skin wound healing and dermal reconstruction. Wiley Interdiscip Rev Nanomed Nanobiotechnol 2010; 2(5): 510-25.
[http://dx.doi.org/10.1002/wnan.100] [PMID: 20607703]

[164] Mogoşanu GD, Grumezescu AM. Natural and synthetic polymers for wounds and burns dressing. Int J Pharm 2014; 463(2): 127-36.
[http://dx.doi.org/10.1016/j.ijpharm.2013.12.015] [PMID: 24368109]

[165] Chen C-C, Chueh J-Y, Tseng H, Huang H-M, Lee S-Y. Preparation and characterization of biodegradable PLA polymeric blends. Biomaterials 2003; 24(7): 1167-73.
[http://dx.doi.org/10.1016/S0142-9612(02)00466-0] [PMID: 12527257]

[166] Gogolewski S, Pennings AJ. An artificial skin based on biodegradable mixtures of polylactides and polyurethanes for full□thickness skin wound covering. Makromol Chem, Rapid Commun 1983; 4(10): 675-80.
[http://dx.doi.org/10.1002/marc.1983.030041008]

[167] Luckachan GE, Pillai C. Biodegradable polymers-a review on recent trends and emerging perspectives. J Polym Environ 2011; 19(3): 637-76.
[http://dx.doi.org/10.1007/s10924-011-0317-1]

[168] Yari A, Yeganeh H, Bakhshi H. Synthesis and evaluation of novel absorptive and antibacterial polyurethane membranes as wound dressing. J Mater Sci Mater Med 2012; 23(9): 2187-202.
[http://dx.doi.org/10.1007/s10856-012-4683-6] [PMID: 22639152]

[169] Bhardwaj U, Sura R, Papadimitrakopoulos F, Burgess DJ. PLGA/PVA hydrogel composites for long-term inflammation control following s.c. implantation. Int J Pharm 2010; 384(1-2): 78-86.
[http://dx.doi.org/10.1016/j.ijpharm.2009.09.046] [PMID: 19800956]

[170] Wang Y, Papadimitrakopoulos F, Burgess DJ. Polymeric "smart" coatings to prevent foreign body response to implantable biosensors. J Control Release 2013; 169(3): 341-7.
[http://dx.doi.org/10.1016/j.jconrel.2012.12.028] [PMID: 23298616]

[171] Patil SD, Papadimitrakopoulos F, Burgess DJ. Dexamethasone-loaded poly(lactic-co-glycolic) acid microspheres/poly(vinyl alcohol) hydrogel composite coatings for inflammation control. Diabetes Technol Ther 2004; 6(6): 887-97.
[http://dx.doi.org/10.1089/dia.2004.6.887] [PMID: 15684644]

[172] Kastellorizios M. Material Biocompatibility and Applications in Metabolic Monitoring 2015.

[173] Boateng JS, Matthews KH, Stevens HN, Eccleston GM. Wound healing dressings and drug delivery systems: a review. J Pharm Sci 2008; 97(8): 2892-923.
[http://dx.doi.org/10.1002/jps.21210] [PMID: 17963217]

[174] Duan B, Wu L, Li X, *et al.* Degradation of electrospun PLGA-chitosan/PVA membranes and their cytocompatibility *in vitro.* J Biomater Sci Polym Ed 2007; 18(1): 95-115.
[http://dx.doi.org/10.1163/156856207779146105] [PMID: 17274454]

[175] Casadio YS, Brown DH, Chirila TV, Kraatz H-B, Baker MV. Biodegradation of poly(2-hydroxyethyl methacrylate) (PHEMA) and poly(2-hydroxyethyl methacrylate)-co-[poly(ethylene glycol) methyl ether methacrylate] hydrogels containing peptide-based cross-linking agents. Biomacromolecules 2010; 11(11): 2949-59.
[http://dx.doi.org/10.1021/bm100756c] [PMID: 20961104]

[176] Chirila TV, Constable IJ, Crawford GJ, *et al.* Poly(2-hydroxyethyl methacrylate) sponges as implant materials: *in vivo* and *in vitro* evaluation of cellular invasion. Biomaterials 1993; 14(1): 26-38.
[http://dx.doi.org/10.1016/0142-9612(93)90072-A] [PMID: 7678755]

[177] Young C-D, Wu J-R, Tsou T-L. High-strength, ultra-thin and fiber-reinforced pHEMA artificial skin. Biomaterials 1998; 19(19): 1745-52.

[http://dx.doi.org/10.1016/S0142-9612(98)00083-0] [PMID: 9856585]

[178] Young C-D, Wu J-R, Tsou T-L. Fabrication and characteristics of polyHEMA artificial skin with improved tensile properties. J Membr Sci 1998; 146(1): 83-93.
[http://dx.doi.org/10.1016/S0376-7388(98)00097-0]

[179] Migliaresi C, Carfagna C, Nicolais L. Laminates of poly(2-hydroxyethyl methacrylate) and polybutadiene as potential burn covering. Biomaterials 1980; 1(4): 205-8.
[http://dx.doi.org/10.1016/0142-9612(80)90018-6] [PMID: 7470575]

[180] Teichmann J, Valtink M, Nitschke M, *et al.* Tissue engineering of the corneal endothelium: a review of carrier materials. J Funct Biomater 2013; 4(4): 178-208.
[http://dx.doi.org/10.3390/jfb4040178] [PMID: 24956190]

[181] Wang J, Gao C, Zhang Y, Wan Y. Preparation and *in vitro* characterization of BC/PVA hydrogel composite for its potential use as artificial cornea biomaterial. Mater Sci Eng C 2010; 30(1): 214-8.
[http://dx.doi.org/10.1016/j.msec.2009.10.006]

[182] Chirila TV, Hicks CR, Dalton PD, *et al.* Artificial cornea. Prog Polym Sci 1998; 23(3): 447-73.
[http://dx.doi.org/10.1016/S0079-6700(97)00036-1]

[183] Xiang J, Sun J, Hong J, *et al.* T-style keratoprosthesis based on surface-modified poly (2-hydroxyethyl methacrylate) hydrogel for cornea repairs. Mater Sci Eng C 2015; 50: 274-85.
[http://dx.doi.org/10.1016/j.msec.2015.01.089] [PMID: 25746271]

[184] Zhang Q, Fang Z, Cao Y, *et al.* High refractive index inorganic–organic Interpenetrating Polymer Network (IPN) hydrogel nanocomposite toward artificial cornea implants. ACS Macro Lett 2012; 1(7): 876-81.
[http://dx.doi.org/10.1021/mz300078y]

[185] Myung D, Duhamel P-E, Cochran JR, Noolandi J, Ta CN, Frank CW. Development of hydrogel-based keratoprostheses: a materials perspective. Biotechnol Prog 2008; 24(3): 735-41.
[http://dx.doi.org/10.1021/bp070476n] [PMID: 18422366]

[186] Griffith M, Hakim M, Shimmura S, *et al.* Artificial human corneas: scaffolds for transplantation and host regeneration. Cornea 2002; 21(7) (Suppl.): S54-61.
[http://dx.doi.org/10.1097/01.ico.0000263120.68768.f8] [PMID: 12484700]

[187] Jiang H, Zuo Y, Zhang L, *et al.* Property-based design: optimization and characterization of polyvinyl alcohol (PVA) hydrogel and PVA-matrix composite for artificial cornea. J Mater Sci Mater Med 2014; 25(3): 941-52.
[http://dx.doi.org/10.1007/s10856-013-5121-0] [PMID: 24464723]

[188] Salthouse TN. Biologic response to sutures. Otolaryngol Head Neck Surg 1980; 88(6): 658-64.
[http://dx.doi.org/10.1177/019459988008800606] [PMID: 7010269]

[189] Törmälä P, Pohjonen T, Rokkanen P. Bioabsorbable polymers: materials technology and surgical applications. Proc Inst Mech Eng H 1998; 212(2): 101-11.
[http://dx.doi.org/10.1243/0954411981533872] [PMID: 9612001]

[190] Silverstein LH, Kurtzman GM. A review of dental suturing for optimal soft-tissue management. Compend Contin Educ Dent 2005; 26(3): 163-6.
[PMID: 15813570]

[191] Pillai CK, Sharma CP. Review paper: absorbable polymeric surgical sutures: chemistry, production, properties, biodegradability, and performance. J Biomater Appl 2010; 25(4): 291-366.
[http://dx.doi.org/10.1177/0885328210384890] [PMID: 20971780]

[192] Boccaccini AR, Stamboulis AG, Rashid A, Roether JA. Composite surgical sutures with bioactive glass coating. J Biomed Mater Res B Appl Biomater 2003; 67(1): 618-26.
[http://dx.doi.org/10.1002/jbm.b.10047] [PMID: 14528459]

[193] Beardsley SL, Smeak DD, Weisbrode SE. Histologic evaluation of tissue reactivity and absorption in

response to a new synthetic fluorescent pigmented polypropylene suture material in rats. Am J Vet Res 1995; 56(9): 1248-52.
[PMID: 7486407]

[194] Javed F, Al-Askar M, Almas K, Romanos GE, Al-Hezaimi K. Tissue reactions to various suture materials used in oral surgical interventions 2012.
[http://dx.doi.org/10.5402/2012/762095]

[195] Schmalz G, Arenholt-Bindslev D. Biocompatibility of dental materials. Springer 2009.

[196] Tiwari A, Cheng K-S, Salacinski H, Hamilton G, Seifalian AM. Improving the patency of vascular bypass grafts: the role of suture materials and surgical techniques on reducing anastomotic compliance mismatch. Eur J Vasc Endovasc Surg 2003; 25(4): 287-95.
[http://dx.doi.org/10.1053/ejvs.2002.1810] [PMID: 12651165]

[197] Ekholm M, Hietanen J, Lindqvist C, Rautavuori J, Santavirta S, Suuronen R. Histological study of tissue reactions to ε-caprolactone-lactide copolymer in paste form. Biomaterials 1999; 20(14): 1257-62.
[http://dx.doi.org/10.1016/S0142-9612(97)00080-X] [PMID: 10403042]

[198] Nakamura T, Shimizu Y, Matsui T, Okumura N, Hyon SH, Nishiya K. A novel bioabsorbable monofilament surgical suture made from (ε-caprolactone, L-lactide) copolymer Degradation Phenomena on Polymeric Biomaterials. Springer 1992; pp. 153-62.

[199] Mimae T, Hirayasu T, Kimura KB, Ito A, Miyata Y, Okada M. Advantage of absorbable suture material for pulmonary artery ligation. Gen Thorac Cardiovasc Surg 2010; 58(10): 511-5.
[http://dx.doi.org/10.1007/s11748-010-0608-9] [PMID: 20941564]

[200] Stewart DW, Buffington PJ, Wacksman J. Suture material in bladder surgery: a comparison of polydioxanone, polyglactin, and chromic catgut. J Urol 1990; 143(6): 1261-3.
[http://dx.doi.org/10.1016/S0022-5347(17)40250-3] [PMID: 2111412]

[201] Rokkanen PU. Absorbable materials in orthopaedic surgery. Ann Med 1991; 23(2): 109-15.
[http://dx.doi.org/10.3109/07853899109148033] [PMID: 2069786]

[202] Pulapura S, Kohn J. Trends in the development of bioresorbable polymers for medical applications. J Biomater Appl 1992; 6(3): 216-50.
[http://dx.doi.org/10.1177/088532829200600303] [PMID: 1573554]

[203] Ray JA, Doddi N, Regula D, Williams JA, Melveger A. Polydioxanone (PDS), a novel monofilament synthetic absorbable suture. Surg Gynecol Obstet 1981; 153(4): 497-507.
[PMID: 6792722]

[204] Nottelet B, Pektok E, Mandracchia D, *et al.* Factorial design optimization and *in vivo* feasibility of poly(ε-caprolactone)-micro- and nanofiber-based small diameter vascular grafts. J Biomed Mater Res A 2009; 89(4): 865-75.
[http://dx.doi.org/10.1002/jbm.a.32023] [PMID: 18465817]

[205] Castro CF, António CC, Sousa LC. On the mechanical failure of arterial prostheses.

[206] Michanetzis GP, Katsala N, Missirlis YF. Comparison of haemocompatibility improvement of four polymeric biomaterials by two heparinization techniques. Biomaterials 2003; 24(4): 677-88.
[http://dx.doi.org/10.1016/S0142-9612(02)00382-4] [PMID: 12437962]

[207] Shinoka T, Breuer CK, Tanel RE, *et al.* Tissue engineering heart valves: valve leaflet replacement study in a lamb model. Ann Thorac Surg 1995; 60(6) (Suppl.): S513-6.
[http://dx.doi.org/10.1016/0003-4975(95)00733-4] [PMID: 8604922]

[208] Schmidt D, Hoerstrup SP. Tissue engineered heart valves based on human cells. Swiss Med Wkly 2006; 136(39-40): 618-23.
[PMID: 17086507]

[209] Hoerstrup SP, Sodian R, Daebritz S, *et al.* Functional living trileaflet heart valves grown *in vitro*.

Circulation 2000; 102(19) (Suppl. 3): III44-9.
[PMID: 11082361]

[210] Dvorin EL, Wylie-Sears J, Kaushal S, Martin DP, Bischoff J. Quantitative evaluation of endothelial progenitors and cardiac valve endothelial cells: proliferation and differentiation on poly-glycolic acid/poly-4-hydroxybutyrate scaffold in response to vascular endothelial growth factor and transforming growth factor β1. Tissue Eng 2003; 9(3): 487-93.
[http://dx.doi.org/10.1089/107632703322066660] [PMID: 12857416]

[211] Desai M, Seifalian AM, Hamilton G. Role of prosthetic conduits in coronary artery bypass grafting. Eur J Cardiothorac Surg 2011; 40(2): 394-8.
[PMID: 21216613]

[212] Salacinski HJ, Goldner S, Giudiceandrea A, *et al.* The mechanical behavior of vascular grafts: a review. J Biomater Appl 2001; 15(3): 241-78.
[http://dx.doi.org/10.1106/NA5T-J57A-JTDD-FD04] [PMID: 11261602]

[213] Sarkar S, Salacinski HJ, Hamilton G, Seifalian AM. The mechanical properties of infrainguinal vascular bypass grafts: their role in influencing patency. Eur J Vasc Endovasc Surg 2006; 31(6): 627-36.
[http://dx.doi.org/10.1016/j.ejvs.2006.01.006] [PMID: 16513376]

[214] Van Damme H, Deprez M, Creemers E, Limet R. Intrinsic structural failure of polyester (Dacron) vascular grafts. A general review. Acta Chir Belg 2005; 105(3): 249-55.
[http://dx.doi.org/10.1080/00015458.2005.11679712] [PMID: 16018516]

[215] Kannan RY, Salacinski HJ, Butler PE, Hamilton G, Seifalian AM. Current status of prosthetic bypass grafts: a review. J Biomed Mater Res B Appl Biomater 2005; 74(1): 570-81.
[http://dx.doi.org/10.1002/jbm.b.30247] [PMID: 15889440]

[216] Gershon B, Cohn D, Marom G. Utilization of composite laminate theory in the design of synthetic soft tissues for biomedical prostheses. Biomaterials 1990; 11(8): 548-52.
[http://dx.doi.org/10.1016/0142-9612(90)90076-3] [PMID: 2279055]

[217] Zilberman M, Eberhart RC. Drug-eluting bioresorbable stents for various applications. Annu Rev Biomed Eng 2006; 8: 153-80.
[http://dx.doi.org/10.1146/annurev.bioeng.8.013106.151418] [PMID: 16834554]

[218] Takahashi H, Letourneur D, Grainger DW. Delivery of large biopharmaceuticals from cardiovascular stents: a review. Biomacromolecules 2007; 8(11): 3281-93.
[http://dx.doi.org/10.1021/bm700540p] [PMID: 17929968]

[219] Liu S-J, Chiang F-J, Hsiao C-Y, Kau Y-C, Liu K-S. Fabrication of balloon-expandable self-lock drug-eluting polycaprolactone stents using micro-injection molding and spray coating techniques. Ann Biomed Eng 2010; 38(10): 3185-94.
[http://dx.doi.org/10.1007/s10439-010-0075-6] [PMID: 20496003]

[220] Byrne RA, Kastrati A. Bioresorbable Drug-Eluting Stents: An Immature Technology in Need of Mature Application☐ JACC: Cardiovascular Interventions 2015;8(1_PB) 198-200.

[221] Eberhart RC, Su S-H, Nguyen KT, *et al.* Bioresorbable polymeric stents: current status and future promise. J Biomater Sci Polym Ed 2003; 14(4): 299-312.
[http://dx.doi.org/10.1163/156856203321478838] [PMID: 12747671]

[222] Peng T, Gibula P, Yao KD, Goosen MF. Role of polymers in improving the results of stenting in coronary arteries. Biomaterials 1996; 17(7): 685-94.
[http://dx.doi.org/10.1016/0142-9612(96)86738-X] [PMID: 8672630]

[223] Zilberman M, Nelson KD, Eberhart RC. Mechanical properties and *in vitro* degradation of bioresorbable fibers and expandable fiber-based stents. J Biomed Mater Res B Appl Biomater 2005; 74(2): 792-9.
[http://dx.doi.org/10.1002/jbm.b.30319] [PMID: 15991233]

[224]   Kimura T, Yokoi H, Nakagawa Y, *et al.* Three-year follow-up after implantation of metallic coronary-artery stents. N Engl J Med 1996; 334(9): 561-6.
[http://dx.doi.org/10.1056/NEJM199602293340903] [PMID: 8569823]

[225]   Zilberman M, Eberhart RC, Schwade ND. *In vitro* study of drug-loaded bioresorbable films and support structures. J Biomater Sci Polym Ed 2002; 13(11): 1221-40.
[http://dx.doi.org/10.1163/156856202320892975] [PMID: 12518801]

[226]   Nguyen K, Su S-H, Zilberman M, Bohluli P, Frenkel P, Timmons R, *et al.* Biomaterials and stent technology 2004.

[227]   Gill I, Ballesteros A. Bioencapsulation within synthetic polymers (Part 2): non-sol-gel protein-polymer biocomposites. Trends Biotechnol 2000; 18(11): 469-79.
[http://dx.doi.org/10.1016/S0167-7799(00)01493-1] [PMID: 11058788]

[228]   Geckeler KE, Müller B. Polymer materials in biosensors. Naturwissenschaften 1993; 80(1): 18-24.
[http://dx.doi.org/10.1007/BF01139752] [PMID: 8383298]

[229]   Alegret S. Rigid carbon–polymer biocomposites for electrochemical sensing. A review. Analyst (Lond) 1996; 121(12): 1751-8.
[http://dx.doi.org/10.1039/AN9962101751]

[230]   Lowe CR. As introduction to the concepts and technology of biosensors. Biosensors 1985; 1(1): 3-16.
[http://dx.doi.org/10.1016/0265-928X(85)85004-5] [PMID: 3842796]

[231]   Sun M, Deng J, Tang Z, *et al.* A correlation study of protein adsorption and cell behaviors on substrates with different densities of PEG chains. Colloids Surf B Biointerfaces 2014; 122: 134-42.
[http://dx.doi.org/10.1016/j.colsurfb.2014.06.041] [PMID: 25033433]

[232]   Freij-Larsson C, Jannasch P, Wesslén B. Polyurethane surfaces modified by amphiphilic polymers: effects on protein adsorption. Biomaterials 2000; 21(3): 307-15.
[http://dx.doi.org/10.1016/S0142-9612(99)00195-7] [PMID: 10646948]

[233]   Inoue Y, Ishihara K. Reduction of protein adsorption on well-characterized polymer brush layers with varying chemical structures. Colloids Surf B Biointerfaces 2010; 81(1): 350-7.
[http://dx.doi.org/10.1016/j.colsurfb.2010.07.030] [PMID: 20705439]

[234]   Liu P-S, Chen Q, Wu S-S, Shen J, Lin S-C. Surface modification of cellulose membranes with zwitterionic polymers for resistance to protein adsorption and platelet adhesion. J Membr Sci 2010; 350(1): 387-94.
[http://dx.doi.org/10.1016/j.memsci.2010.01.015]

[235]   Zhang F, Kang ET, Neoh KG, Wang P, Tan KL. Reactive coupling of poly(ethylene glycol) on electroactive polyaniline films for reduction in protein adsorption and platelet adhesion. Biomaterials 2002; 23(3): 787-95.
[http://dx.doi.org/10.1016/S0142-9612(01)00184-3] [PMID: 11771698]

[236]   Hasan A, Pandey L. REVIEW: Polymers, Surface Modified Polymers and Self Assembled Monolayers as Surface Modifying Agents for Biomaterials Polymer-Plastics Technology and Engineering 2015(just-accepted)

[237]   Sun C, Miao J, Yan J, *et al.* Applications of antibiofouling PEG-coating in electrochemical biosensors for determination of glucose in whole blood. Electrochim Acta 2013; 89: 549-54.
[http://dx.doi.org/10.1016/j.electacta.2012.11.005]

[238]   Wałcerz I, Koncki R, Leszczyńska E, Głąb S. Enzyme biosensors for urea determination based on an ionophore free pH membrane electrode. Anal Chim Acta 1995; 315(3): 289-96.
[http://dx.doi.org/10.1016/0003-2670(95)00313-O]

[239]   Tinkilic N, Cubuk O, Isildak I. Glucose and urea biosensors based on all solid-state PVC–NH 2 membrane electrodes. Anal Chim Acta 2002; 452(1): 29-34.
[http://dx.doi.org/10.1016/S0003-2670(01)01441-6]

[240] Altikatoglu M, Karakus E, Erci V, Pekyardımcı S, Isildak I. Novel creatine biosensors based on all solid-state contact ammonium-selective membrane electrodes. Artif Cells Nanomed Biotechnol 2013; 41(2): 131-6.
[http://dx.doi.org/10.3109/10731199.2012.696066] [PMID: 22779924]

[241] Isildak I, Cubuk O, Altikatoglu M, Yolcu M, Erci V, Tinkilic N. A novel conductometric creatinine biosensor based on solid-state contact ammonium sensitive PVC–NH 2 membrane. Biochem Eng J 2012; 62: 34-8.
[http://dx.doi.org/10.1016/j.bej.2011.10.013]

[242] Kingshott P, Griesser HJ. Surfaces that resist bioadhesion. Curr Opin Solid State Mater Sci 1999; 4(4): 403-12.
[http://dx.doi.org/10.1016/S1359-0286(99)00018-2]

[243] Amiji M, Park K. Prevention of protein adsorption and platelet adhesion on surfaces by PEO/PPO/PEO triblock copolymers. Biomaterials 1992; 13(10): 682-92.
[http://dx.doi.org/10.1016/0142-9612(92)90128-B] [PMID: 1420713]

[244] Chang Y, Chu WL, Chen WY, *et al.* A systematic SPR study of human plasma protein adsorption behavior on the controlled surface packing of self-assembled poly(ethylene oxide) triblock copolymer surfaces. J Biomed Mater Res A 2010; 93(1): 400-8.
[PMID: 19569222]

[245] Green RJ, Davies MC, Roberts CJ, Tendler SJ. A surface plasmon resonance study of albumin adsorption to PEO-PPO-PEO triblock copolymers. J Biomed Mater Res 1998; 42(2): 165-71.
[http://dx.doi.org/10.1002/(SICI)1097-4636(199811)42:2<165::AID-JBM1>3.0.CO;2-N]   [PMID: 9773812]

[246] Liou Y-B, Tsay R-Y. Adsorption of PEO–PPO–PEO triblock copolymers on a gold surface. Journal of the Taiwan Institute of Chemical Engineers 2011; 42(3): 533-40.
[http://dx.doi.org/10.1016/j.jtice.2010.09.011]

CHAPTER 3

Bioactive ACP-Based Polymeric Biocomposites

Drago Skrtic[1,*] and Joseph M. Antonucci[2]

[1] *Volpe Research Center, American Dental Association Foundation, Gaithersburg, Maryland, USA*

[2] *Biomaterials Group, Biosystems and Biomaterials Division, National Institute of Standards and Technology, Gaithersburg, Maryland, USA*

Abstract: We have led the research on polymeric dental materials based on amorphous calcium phosphate (ACP) for over two decades. The knowledge gained from systematic structure-composition-property relationship studies of ACP composites yielded a new generation of materials capable of efficiently restoring lost tooth mineral *via* sustained release of re-mineralizing calcium and phosphate ions (building blocks of both enamel and dentin). Our work has also contributed to a better understanding on how different monomer systems yield unique matrix structures and filler/matrix interactions that affect the critical properties of ACP composites and their overall performance. In this Chapter, we describe ACP filler, polymer and composite fabrication and the sequential physicochemical, mechanical and biological evaluation of ACP composites intended for different dental applications. We also discuss introducing an antimicrobial function in the formulation of ACP composites as a way of expanding their potential application beyond dentistry into area of regenerative hard tissue medicine.

Keywords: Amorphous calcium phosphate, Anti-caries agent, Dental composite, Ion release, Mechanical evaluation, Methacrylate monomers, Physicochemical evaluation, Polymerization, Remineralization potential.

INTRODUCTION

Despite significant reduction of its occurrence in some segments of population, dental caries remains one of the most prevalent diseases affecting humans [1]. Because of the concomitant concerns regarding fluorosis [2], there is a need to develop new approaches to prevent and repair dental caries and increase the efficacy of widely used fluoride without increasing its doses and/or administration frequency. Tooth demineralization/remineralization is a dynamic process that includes dissolution of calcium and phosphate ions from tooth mineral into saliva

---

* **Corresponding author Drago Skrtic:** Volpe Research Center, American Dental Association Foundation, Gaithersburg, Maryland, USA; Tel: 301.975.3541; Fax: 301.963.9143; E-mail: drago.skrtic@nist.gov

Mehdi Razavi (Ed.)

(demineralization) and their precipitation back into tooth structures (remineralization). If these processes are balanced then no net mineral loss occurs. However, local decrease in pH caused by bacterial plaque, or an overall oral acidification due to the frequent intake of acidic foods and beverages disrupts the delicate demineralization/remineralization balance and often results in generalized demineralization.

If uncontrolled, over time this demineralization leads to tooth erosion and, in advanced cases, caries. Therefore, inhibition of uncontrolled demineralization is the primary target in anti-caries therapies. For the treatment to be clinically effective it is essential that a protracted supply of remineralizing ions (calcium, phosphate, fluoride) needed to reform tooth mineral is provided and that replacement of lost mineral occurs faster than in salivary mineralization. The use of remineralizing solutions containing calcium and phosphate ions has not been successful clinically [3], particularly in the presence of fluoride ions. On the other hand, insoluble calcium phosphates (CaPs) are not easily applied and do not localize effectively at the tooth surface. One of the newer technologies introduces casein phosphopeptide-amorphous calcium phosphate (CPP-ACP) nanoclusters capable of localizing at the tooth surface and remineralizing enamel lesions [4, 5]. In addition to CPP-ACP technology, two other ACP-based technologies have been developed: one involving the unstabilized ACP and the other based on bioactive calcium sodium phosphosilicate glass. In-depth comparison of these CaP-based remineralization systems is provided in [6]. CPP-ACP technology-based commercial product has been shown to efficiently remineralize enamel lesions *in situ* and to inhibit progression of coronal caries in randomized clinical trial. These findings are consistent with the proposed anticariogenic action of CPP-ACP nanoclusters. The unstabilized ACP-based product decreased root caries increment in a clinical trial involving high risk patients. The anticariogenic action of bioglass has yet to be confirmed in animal model studies and/or clinical trials. Conclusion of the review [6] is that ACP-based remineralization technologies look promising as adjuvant therapy to topical fluoride treatment of early caries. Our group has pioneered a new generation of ACP-based dental composites. We have shown that, upon aqueous exposure, ACP filers embedded into various polymeric matrices release calcium and phosphate ions in a manner that effectively buffers free calcium and phosphate ion activities and maintain the desired state of supersaturation with respect to tooth enamel [7 - 9]. Ion release from ACP composites is accompanied by a concomitant conversion of ACP into thermodynamically stable CaP, *i.e.,* hydroxyapatite (HAP). This intra-composite ACP to HAP conversion makes ACP composites a promising anti-demineralization/remineralization tool in not only preventing the formation of new lesions, but also actively repairing existing incipient lesions. Thus, dental utility of ACP is extended beyond topical gels, toothpastes, mouth rinses and sugar-free gums [3 - 6, 10]. Foreseen dental benefits of remineralizing ACP composites and functional differences between biostable and bioactive dental restoratives are summarized in Tables **1** and **2**, respectively.

Table 1. ACP remineralizing composites: Dental benefits.

Dental Field	Foreseen Benefit
Preventive dentistry	Minimizes caries development at restoration tooth interface Particularly suitable for caries-prone patients due to radio-therapy and/or medications causing dry mouth
Orthodontics	Adhesive composite capable of reducing and/or eradicating demineralization under orthodontic brackets
Endodontics	Biocompatible material for root canal treatments

ACP: STRUCTURE, COMPOSITION, THERMODYNAMIC PROPERTIES

ACP is generally viewed as a precursor to HAP formation both *in vivo* and *in vitro* [11 - 15]. Major contributions to our understanding of the role of ACP in biological systems came from studies of its synthetic analogue, since obtaining *in vivo* information on ACP has proven difficult due to ACP's relatively high solubility and transient existence compared to crystalline CaPs. The ACP that forms initially during the rapid precipitation of CaP solids from basic solutions shows no discrete X-ray diffraction (XRD) peaks. Instead, its XRD consists of diffuse, broad bands characteristic of such commonly recognized noncrystalline substances as glasses and certain polymers. This, however, does not preclude the possibility of localized order and structure in ACP. At room temperature, ACP undergoes hydrolysis and forms a series of tricalcium orthophosphates of general formula $Ca_9(HPO_4)_x(PO_4)_{6-x}(OH)_x$ where $0<x<1$ [16]. Another model [17] proposes $Ca_9(PO_4)_6$ clusters arranged as a part of the HAP net around Ca^{2+} ions without the OH$^-$ ions at its boundary. However, in the pH range 7.4-9.3, no OH$^-$ and only small amounts of HPO_4^{2-} are present in ACP [17]. The ACP to HAP conversion can also be explained by the separate growth of octacalcium phosphate $(Ca_8H_2(PO_4)_6$; OCP) initiated by nucleation on the ACP surface and followed by *in situ* formation of OCP and HAP inter-layers [17]. An intermediate ACP phase characterized by a thermodynamic solubility product consistent with that of OCP has indeed been identified in spontaneous ACP conversion in the pH range 7.0-9.0 [18, 19]. As a result of ACP to HAP transformation, both Ca/P ratio and the crystallinity of the solids increase with time. Generally, this conversion rate is primarily dependent on the chemistry of the microenvironment and can be affected by the presence of inorganic and organic moieties. Whether the additives are inorganic anions, cations or organic molecules, the transformation is controlled initially by adsorption on the ACP surface, and followed by either incorporation into ACP's structure and/or co-precipitation [20 - 22].

Table 2. Compositional and functional differences between biostable and bioactive dental materials.

Type of Material	Activity	Components	Functions
Conventional composites	Biostable	Methacrylate monomers Glass or ceramic fillers	Form polymeric matrix Reinforce polymer phase
Glass and resin-modified ionomers	Bioactive	Polyalkenoates/resin-modified polyalkenoates Leachable glass fillers	Form polyelectrolyte/resin matrix Release F ions
ACP composites	Bioactive	Methacrylate monomers ACP fillers	Provide polymeric matrix Release Ca and PO_4 ions

EFFECT OF ADDITIVES ON PHYSICOCHEMICAL CHARACTERISTICS OF ACP

A parameter required to properly characterize any particulate system is its particle size distribution (PSD). In case of ACP spontaneously precipitated from supersaturated solutions, the PSD is highly heterogeneous and strongly affected by ACP's agglomeration. This typically uncontrolled agglomeration can hinder interfacial interactions with dental resins once ACP is incorporated into composites to provide the desired remineralization effect. One of the ensuing drawbacks is that ACP composites are generally weak and mechanically inferior to glass-reinforced dental materials [7 - 9]. In addition, state of aggregation of ACP fillers in composites may have a significant effect on the ion release kinetics of these materials. To achieve better control of ACP's PSD while maintaining a sustained release of remineralizing ions, we have modified ACP synthetic protocols by introducing *ab initio* various additives: inorganic cations, surfactants and polymers.

The rationale for introducing cations, generally known to improve adhesive bonding of composites to tooth surfaces by replacing and/or supplementing Ca ions as sites for bonding *via* either chelating or interacting with surface-active resin components [23], was the following: zinc (Zn) is as an essential trace element with stimulatory effects on bone formation [24] and a regulatory factor in dental calculus formation [25]; iron (Fe), contained in human saliva's lactoferrrin [26], may have an effect on the redox system used in free-radical polymerization of the resins; silver (Ag) may find utility as a staining agent in examining and quantifying ACP aggregation in polymers and detecting defects in the subsurface wear layer [27]; aluminum (Al) prevents topical deposition of CaF_2 in leachable glasses and develops favorable water coordination characteristics required for cementitious bonding [28]. Cation-ACP interactions are expectedly controlled by the ionic potential of additives, *i.e.*, their ionic radius, multiplicity of charges and water coordination number [28]. For the above reasons, monovalent Ag+, divalent Zn^{2+} and Fe^{2+}, and trivalent Al^{3+} and Fe^{3+} were introduced during ACP synthesis and their effects compared with the effects of tetravalent modifiers, silica (Si^{4+}) and zirconia (Zr^{4+}), used in the early stages of our research [29].

Polymers (polyelectrolytes) with multiple acid groups form the basis of modem dental cements with inherent ability to adhere to mineralized surfaces. In solution, they dissociate into polyanion chains that contain many linked charged groups and exert considerable electrostatic effect on counterions *via* ion binding. The extent of ion binding, generally depends on degree of dissociation, acid strength, conformation, distribution of ionizable groups, cooperative action between these groups and the hydration state of the molecule, is typically enhanced when the arrangements of the functional groups permit chelate formation [30]. If successfully attached to ACP during its synthesis, water soluble polymers such as polyethylene oxide [PEO; $(CH_2CH_2O)_n$] proven to stabilize cations by multiple chelation) and/or surfactants are expected to affect ACP's tendency to extensively agglomerate. Their effect is anticipated to be both structure- and size-related. These molecules may also have a profound effect on the kinetics of ACP's dissolution. Additionally, ACP formed in their presence may contain less structural water than "standard" pyrophosphate-stabilized ACP (10-15 mass % [17]). Lower water content coupled with the reduction in particle sizes size and lesser number of voids in the composites may also reduce the volumetric shrinkage upon polymerization (PS) and overall water sorption (WS) of composites.

FINE TUNING OF ACP COMPOSITES BY INTERFACE COUPLING AND POLYMER GRAFTING

To attain the desired chemical and mechanical properties of ACP composites, it is essential to achieve a fairly uniform distribution of ACP particulates in the polymer matrix, *i.e.* minimize the uneven formation of filler-rich and filler-poor areas within the composite. A major factor affecting the physicochemical and mechanical properties of polymer composites is the interfacial state between the filler and the polymer [31 - 33]. WS, important with respect to service performance in aqueous environments (reduction of mechanical properties, ion mobility, release of organic components that may be potent sensitive/irritative agents), is also affected by the critical interfacial region between the filler particles and the matrix. An important question in this regard is whether voids or non-bonding spaces in the filler/matrix interfaces can cause an increase in WS. Presumably, such spaces depend on (a) the nature of the filler particle, (b) the method of polymerization, and (c) the use of coupling agents. Furthermore, effective silane coupling agent(s) and/or surface-modification of the fillers may reduce the interfacial penetration of water between the ACP particles and polymeric matrix and, in turn, ameliorate the overall plasticization of composites.

A variety of different coupling agents have been developed to enhance filler/matrix interactions by concomitant covalent bonding of organic functionalities with the polymer matrix and hydrolyzable silane groups that can bond with the inorganic filler [34 - 37]. The silane coupling agents used in dental composites are predominantly alkyloxy silanes. Many laboratories and manufacturers use proprietary methods and there is no general consensus regarding the best method of silanation. Due to differences in the molecular structure/reactivity of organic functional groups, agents possessing vinyl, primary amine and methacryloxy functionalities are expected to have different affinities for multilayered chemisorption on ACP surfaces. These differences in affinity may affect the stability of the silane coatings and their ability to form strong, hydrophobic polysiloxane structures. It is assumed that the silane-coated ACP(s) will remain "transparent" for ionic transport in aqueous environments due to its low thickness and open flexible structure of the silane layers. If successfully applied, such coatings may provide sufficient chemical ACP/matrix bonding without weakening the properties of the interface in a composite formulation. The silane coupling agents are also expected to facilitate resin penetration into the surface cavities formed during filler particle aggregation. This penetration should enhance mechanical interlocking between the filler and the matrix of the resultant composite. In addition to mechanical improvement, it is also expected that the hydrolytic stability of the composites will be enhanced because of the hydrophobic nature of the silane coupling agents.

Filler/resin interactions may be further improved by polymer grafting without impeding the composites' remineralizing capacity. Methacrylate networks with good solvent resistance are used in a wide spectrum of dental restorative composites [38]. These are typically composed of a relatively viscous base monomer and a low viscosity diluent comonomer. The base monomer minimizes the polymerization shrinkage (PS) by virtue of its relatively large molecular volume and enhances the modulus of the cured polymer, while the diluent monomer provides good handling properties and improves copolymer conversion due to its greater flexibility and smaller molecular volume [39]. The most commonly utilized copolymers are based on the base monomer 2,2-bis[p-(2'-hydroxy-3'-methacryloxypropoxy) phenyl]-propane (Bis-GMA) and the diluent monomer triethyleneglycol dimethacrylate (TEGDMA). The hydroxyl groups of Bis-GMA and the ethylene oxide segments of TEGDMA contribute to the relatively high water sorption of Bis-GMA/TEGDMA copolymers [40]. High concentrations of the more rigid structure of Bis-GMA typically result in monomer systems with relatively low degrees of cure or vinyl conversion. PS, relatively low cure efficiency at ambient temperatures and plasticization of Bis-GMA/TEGDMA copolymers by oral fluids affect the service life of these composites. Alternative base monomers and/or diluent monomers have been explored to overcome some of the known shortcomings of the Bis-GMA/TEGDMA copolymers. Dental polymers based on ethoxylated bisphenol A dimethacrylate (EBPADMA), a relatively hydrophobic analog of Bis-GMA with a more flexible structure and lower viscosity, show higher degrees of cure and lower polymerization shrinkages than Bis-GMA/TEGDMA [41]. Another base monomer, urethane dimethacrylate (UDMA) typically reduces WS and PS while enhancing the mechanical properties of the resins [8]. The ultimate goal of the resin grafting approach is to achieve a final consistency suitable for the uniform incorporation of particulate ACP fillers, increase the degree of vinyl conversion (DVC) upon photo-curing and improve adhesion of the composite to tooth structures. Through enhanced interaction(s) with the ACP filler, multifunctional monomers improve matrix/filler coherence and provide an additional means of fine tuning the physical properties of copolymers and their composites. The physicochemical basis for the expected interactions is a Lewis acid/base reaction in which the adhesive monomer is the electron donor and the ACP is the electron acceptor [42, 43]. Polymer grafting studies are expected to provide information on the correlation(s) between the hydrophilicity, degree of cure and relative cross-link density of these polymeric matrices and the thermodynamic stability and mechanical behavior of their ACP composites.

ACP COMPOSITES: CYTOTOXICITY CONSIDERATIONS

Despite considerable research efforts, the mechanism by which the more soluble CaPs, ACP included, promote osteogenesis still remains unclear [44 - 47]. We have found that copolymers derived from highly converted resins (high DVC) also yield polymeric ACP composites with low leachability of unreacted monomeric species (which is taken as an indirect measure of high biocompatibility) and favorable calcium and phosphate ion release profiles [48, 49]. In our evaluations thus far we have routinely used the DVC as an indirect predictor of the material's biocompatibility. The majority of ACP used in our experimental composites was synthesized in the presence of Zr for the purpose of improving ACP's stability upon exposure to aqueous milieu [29]. Such ACP typically contains approx. 8.5 mass % Zr [8]. In contrast, the fast-setting CaP cements described in the literature are formulated from the solutions containing no ions other than Ca, phosphate, Na and/or K. The significance of Ca ions in bone mineralization is well established but the ability of extracellular Ca to regulate specific cell responses has been demonstrated only recently [50, 51]. The ability of osteoblasts to transport phosphate was also recognized as a prerequisite for bone mineralization [52]. Cellular receptors for both calcium and phosphate have been identified [50, 53]. There is also evidence that Si plays an important role in bone metabolism [51, 52] but a cellular receptor for Si has not been identified. At this point, no evidence on the potential role of Zr in hard tissue mineralization and its interaction(s) is available. It is, however, possible that the co-precipitation of Zr into the ACP solid could have some effect on mitochondrial dehydrogenase activity of cells cultured in the extract of Zr-ACP based composites. A series of cell viability experiments may be necessary to test this possibility.

Polymerization of composites is usually less complete than that of the corresponding unfilled resins, and almost every resin component can be detected in the extracts of polymerized materials [54, 55]. Some of the released moieties may elicit various biological effects such as genetic mutations. Among commonly used methacrylate monomers, TEGDMA has been reported as directly mutagenic in a mammalian cell gene mutation assay while no mutagenic effects were detected with UDMA and HEMA [56]. No information was available for EBPADMA. Comparative cytotoxicity toward Balb/c 3T3 mouse fibroblasts (72 h exposure) of TEGDMA, UDMA and HEMA (a concentration that suppresses the mitochondrial activity by 50%) reportedly [57] decreases in the following order: UDMA > TEGDMA > HEMA.

The chemical structure/property relations of the constituent monomers, compositional differences involving polymers and initiator systems, and the attainable DVC, especially as it relates to the leachable monomers, are important contributing factors that control the cellular response. The total residual vinyl unsaturation upon polymerization that is measured by infrared spectroscopy consists of the pendant vinyl groups in the matrix phase plus residual monomers and other leachable unsaturated species that arise from the polymerization process. Cytotoxicity is more likely to depend on leachable residual monomers and other leachable organic species in the composite. Therefore, to better understand the correlation between the cytotoxicity and DVC it is prudent to assess leachable organic moieties as well as the total vinyl unsaturation in the composite.

ACP COMPOSITES: ANTIMICROBIAL PROPERTIES

Bioactive and biocompatible ACP composites are capable of recovering tooth's anatomical form and function, and yield good aesthetics. Some concerns exist regarding their mechanical properties and abrasion resistance, as well as major drawbacks regarding the excessive PS and development of polymerization-induced stresses (PSS). Compromised bonding integrity resulting from the PS and/or PSS can lead to gaps at the restorative material/tooth interface and elevate the risk of bacterial micro-leakage and secondary caries. The release of remineralizing ions – the building blocks of enamel and dentin - can protect teeth from demineralization and even regenerate mineral lost to caries. This release, however, does not provide protection against harmful effects caused by the ingress and accumulation of microorganisms at the site of restoration. Therefore, the recurrent dental caries remains a critical issue even for this new generation of dental restoratives. Caries adjacent to restorations is usually the main cause for their replacement.

The vast majority of the commercial dental restoratives do not possess substantial antimicrobial (AM) properties [58] verifiable in clinical trials [59]. In order to make long-lasting restorations, the material should be made antimicrobial. Most of the efforts undertaken to add AM function to dental materials have been focused on controlling release of various low-molecular weight AMs such as antibiotics, zinc or silver ions, fluoride, iodine and or chlorhexidine [60 - 68]. Generally, there are numerous unresolved issues related to the AM activities of these agents: still unclear mechanism(s) of their actions, concerns about their toxicity against human cells, general risks related to their release, and questionable long-term efficiencies of their AM action. The AM effects of all low-molecular weight AM agents are typically short-lived, their release even slow-release, can lead or has led to compromised mechanical properties of the materials, and, if the dose or release kinetics are not properly controlled, toxicity to surrounding tissues becomes a serious drawback [69].

Quaternary ammonium (QA) methacrylate monomers are typically utilized to impart antibacterial activity to polymeric dental materials [58, 70]. QAs are known for their AM action against both Gram-positive and Gram-negative bacteria, but are also quite toxic [71]. Their toxicity is related primarily to the various biological effects of the QA "head" and its metabolism. It is also believed that the surfactant nature of the QAs may cause additional alterations in chemical, biological and transport phenomena. Several studies [72 - 74], aimed to understand the underlying mechanism of the QA's high toxicity for mammalian cells, have indicated that QAs destroy cell membrane integrity, and eventually lead to the complete breakdown and necrotic cell death. The AM action of most frequently researched QAs and/or quaternary phosphonium (QP) biocides [75] is associated with their cationic, surfactant characteristics and apparently depends on the type of counter-ion (bromide, chloride, fluoride, perchlorate and/or hexaflorophosphate [76 - 78]), pendant active groups [79], molecular weight, and length of the alkyl chains in QA (QP) functionality [80]. So far, these structure/performance studies [75 - 80] haven't been successfully implemented to yield dental restorative(s) with sustained AM action. Amongst QAs, a particular attention has been given to methacryloyloxydodecyl pyrimidinium bromide (MDBP) and the preparation of its acrylamide copolymer [58, 81 - 83]. The MDBP-containing primer has been commercialized and the MDBP has been suggested as potentially applicable to various restoratives. However, the composites with MDBP show poor color stability and their use is limited to the restorations of root cavities in areas where aesthetics is not an issue. Therefore, the improvements of the existing approach and/or new designs seem necessary in order to design AM material(s) ready for clinical use. Recent efforts in such direction include the use of various QAs in bonding agents and dental resin composite [84 - 86]. Dr. Antonucci has recently patented [87] his approach for synthesizing flowable, ionic dimethacrylates based on QA salts and proposed their utilization in dental applications based on the satisfactory outcome of *in vitro* screening [88]. Some of the drawbacks of currently available materials could be eliminated by incorporating into dental resins these new AM agents [87, 88]. Once established in the new experimental resins, their AM action should be extended to the remineralizing ACP composites. Successful development of these multifunctional materials will offer new tools for clinical combat against dental caries.

EXPERIMENTAL DESIGN & METHODOLOGY

ACP Filler Synthesis

ACP is precipitated instantaneously in a closed system at 23 °C upon rapidly mixing equal volumes of a 80 mmol/L $Ca(NO_3)_2$ solution and a 54 mmol/L Na_2HPO_4 solution containing 2 mol % $Na_4P_2O_7$, a known inhibitor of HAP formation. Various additives are introduced *ab initio* (cations at 10 mol % based on the Ca reactant [89], surfactants at 0.05 or 0.10 mass % and polymers at 0.25 mass % [90]) to reduce agglomeration of ACP and render fillers with narrower, more homogeneous PSD and enhanced hydrolytic stability. The reaction pH of the precipitating systems is maintained between 8.5 and 9.0. The suspensions are filtered, the solid phases washed subsequently with ice-cold ammoniated water and acetone, freeze-dried and then lyophilized. Dry solids are then used as-synthesized ACP (as-made or am-ACP) or are further treated as follows. In addition to the surface-modification by various additives, silanization of ACP with 3-aminopropyltrimethoxysilane (APTMS) or methacryloxypropyltrime-thoxysilane (MPTMS) (at 2 mass % relative to ACP [91]), grinding [92] and mechanical ball milling [94] are utilized as alternative ways to break up large ACP agglomerates that regularly form during the spontaneous formation of ACP from supersaturated solutions. To catalyze the hydrolysis of the methoxy groups, MPTMS is deposited from an aqueous/alcohol (5/95 vol %) solution adjusted to pH 5.5 by addition of acetic acid. For APTMS acidification is not necessary, since its amino group auto-catalyzed the hydrolysis/condensation reaction. Five minutes is allowed for completion of hydrolysis and silanol formation following initial mixing-in of the ACP powder and stirring for 30 min. The pH of the MPTMS/ACP slurry is then adjusted to 10 by the addition of KOH solution to facilitate the condensation and formation of siloxanols.

After filtration and drying at room temperature, the silanized ACP was heated at 100 °C for 30 min to strengthen the coating by secondary formation of polylsiloxane network structures. Unbonded silane molecules were washed-out with ethanol and the silane-coated ACPs (their amorphous character was confirmed by FTIR and XRD) were kept dry in a desiccator until used for composite preparation. Detailed descriptions of the experimental protocols employed in ACP surface modification and/or grinding and milling are provided in [89 - 93].

Formulation of Experimental Resins

The commercially available base monomers, diluent monomers, adhesive monomers and the polymerization initiator systems used to fabricate experimental resins are listed in Table **3**. Light-cure (LC) resins are formulated by first combining the selected base monomer(s) ((17-63) mass %), diluent monomers ((10-52) mass %) and adhesive monomers ((0.8-5) mass %). The chosen LC initiator(s), such as CQ and 4EDMAB (0.2 mass % and 0.8 mass %, respectively), 4265 DAROCUR (0.8 mass %), 1850 IRGACURE (1.0 mass 0%) or 369 IRGACURE (1.5 mass %)) is then blended into monomer mixture at room temperature under magnetic stirring (38 rad/s) and safe lighting until achieving a uniform consistency.

Chemical-cure (CC) resins are prepared by initially combining the monomers and homogenizing the inactivated resin *via* magnetic stirring. The resin is then split into two equal parts by mass. The individual CC components (BPO (2.0 mass %) and DHEPT (1.0 mass %) are added separately to each part and each mixture is then stirred magnetically at room temperature until fully homogenized. Dual-cure ((DC); *i.e.*, the combined LC and CC) resins required, similarly to CC resins, a preparation of a two separate batches of the same resin which are light activated (1850 IRGACURE) and contain either BPO or DHEPT. The physicochemical characterization of the unfilled resins (copolymers) typically included determination of DVC, biaxial flexure strength (BFS) and WS.

Table 3. Monomers and the polymerization-initiating systems utilized to formulate the experimental resins. Indicated acronyms are used throughout this Chapter (they are also defined in the Appendix).

Component	Chemical Nomenclature	Acronym
Base monomers	2,2-bis[p-(2'-hydroxy-3'-methacryloxypropoxy) phenyl]-propane Ethoxylated bisphenol A dimethacrylate Urethane dimethacrylate	Bis-GMA EBPADMA UDMA
Diluent monomers	Di(ethyleneglycol)methyl ether methacrylate Glyceryl methacrylate Glyceryl dimetahcrylate 2-hydroxyethyl methacrylate Hexamethylene dimethacrylate Poly(ethylene glycol) extended urethane dimethacrylate Triethyleneglycol dimethacrylate	DEGMEMA GMA GDMA HEMA HmDMA PEG-U TEGDMA
Adhesive monomers	Maleic acid Methacrylic acid Methacryloyloxyethyl phthalate Mono-4-(methacryloyloxy))ethyl trimellitate Pyromellitic glycerol dimethacrylate Vinyl phosphonic acid Zirconyl dimethacrylate	MaA MA MEP 4MET PMGDMA VPA ZrDMA
Components of chemical or photoinitiating system	Butylated hydroxytoluene (stabilizer) Benzoyl peroxide Camphorquinone Diphenyl(2,4,6-trimethylbenzoyl) phosphine oxide & 2-hydroxy-2-methyl- 1-phenyl-1-propanone N,N-dimethyl-p-toluidine Ethyl-4-N,N-dimethylaminobenzoate Bis(2,6-dimethoxybenzoyl)-2,4,4-trimethylpentyl phosphine oxide &1-hydroxycyclohexyl phenyl ketone 2-benzyl-2-(dimethylamino)-1-(4-(4-morphollinyl)phenyl)-1-butanone	BHT BPO CQ 4265 DAROCUR DMPT 4EDMAB 1850 IRGACURE 369 IRGACURE

Fabrication of ACP Composites

Composite pastes are made by combining by hand spatulation a 60 mass % resins and 40 mass % ACP. Homogenized pastes are kept under a moderate vacuum (2.7 kPa) overnight to eliminate the air entrained during the initial mixing. To make LC composite disk specimens, light-activated composite paste is first packed into Teflon molds (diameter = (15.0±0.5) mm; thickness = (1.5±0.2) mm). Each opening of the mold is then covered with Mylar film and a glass slide, and the assembly clamped in place by spring clips. The clamped specimens are photo-polymerized by irradiating sequentially each side of the mold assembly for 60 s with visible light (Triad 2000, Dentsply International). To prepare CC disk specimens, the BPO-containing paste and the DHEPT-containing paste are combined (1:1 mass ratio) and then packed into the molds where chemically-initiated polymerization occurs at room temperature. The DC specimens are prepared by combining the CC and LC procedure. All specimens are stored for 24 h in air at 23 °C before testing. The procedures identical to those used for composite disk specimen preparations are employed in fabricating unfilled copolymer specimens. Whenever the commercial materials serve as controls, their specimens are made by strictly following the manufacturer-recommended curing protocols. Besides tests routinely performed with copolymer specimens (DVC, BFS and WS: previous sub-section), the composite specimens are mapped by FTIR-m, and assessed for PS, polymerization shrinkage stress (PSS) and shear bond strength (SBS) to dentin. The DVC, PS and PSS tests are performed in the dry state. All other measurements are performed on both dry specimens and after their exposure to the aqueous environment. In addition, the release of remineralizing ions from composites into immersion medium is quantified, and, as an indicator of the potential bio-risks, leaching out of the unreacted monomers, initiators and degradation products is compared for composites and copolymer specimens.

Methods/Techniques for Validation/Characterization/Evaluation of Fillers, Copolymers and Composites

A variety of instrumental analytical techniques and procedures is utilized to evaluate (i) ACP fillers for their structure, composition, PSD, morphology and solubility, (ii) monomer systems for their curing properties and interaction(s) with coupling agents and the ACP fillers; and (iii) assess the mechanical, physicochemical and biological properties of ACP-filled composites (Table **4**). A brief description of each of the validation/characterization/evaluation techniques/methods is provided below.

Atomic Emission Spectroscopy (AES)

To determine Ca and PO_4 contents and calculate the corresponding Ca/PO_4 ratio of ACP solids they are dissolved in concentrated HCl and the solutes are analyzed by AES (Prodigy High Dispersion ICP-OES). AES is also used to follow the kinetics of ACP dissolution/transformation in aqueous media. In these experiments, powdered solids are typically dispersed in continuously stirred buffered saline (0.13 mol NaCl/L; pH=7.40) at 37 °C and aliquots for Ca and PO_4 analysis (solution only) are taken at predetermined time intervals. Solids isolated at the same time intervals are screening for conversion by XRD and FTIR. In addition, AES is used to follow the release of remineralizing ions from ACP composite specimens immersed in saline. Ion release data are corrected for variations in the total area of the disk exposed to the immersion solution using the simple relation for a given surface area, A: normalized value = measured value X (500/A). The thermodynamic stability of the solutions with the maximum Ca and PO_4 ion activities is calculated with respect to stoichiometric HAP using the Gibbs free-energy expression:

$$\Delta G° = -2.303 \ (RT/n) \ ln(IAP_{HAP}/K_{sp}) \tag{1}$$

where IAP_{HAP} is the ion activity product for HAP defined as $IAP_{HAP} = \{Ca\}^{10}\{PO_4\}^{6}\{OH\}^{2}$, K_{sp} is the corresponding thermodynamic solubility product, R is the ideal gas constant, T is the absolute temperature, and n=18 is the number of ions in the IAP. Negative $\Delta G°$ values that indicate solution supersaturated with respect to stoichiometric HAP (K_{sp}=117.2) are taken as a measure of remineralization ability [7 - 9, 29].

X-ray Diffraction (XRD)

The amorphous state of ACP is verified by powder X-ray diffraction (XRD; Rigaku X-ray diffractometer). XRD patterns are recorded from 4° to 60° 2θ with CuKα radiation (λ = 0.154 nm) at 40 kV and 40 mA. The samples are step-scanned in intervals of 0.010° 2θ at a scanning speed of 1.000 deg/min.

Table 4. Instrumental methods utilized for characterization of ACP fillers and evaluation of copolymers and ACP composites. Acronyms indicated in Table 4 are used throughout this Chapter.

Method	Measuring Parameters/Information
Atomic emission spectroscopy (AES)	Calcium, phosphate and co-cation levels in ACP solids ACP transformation and ion release from composites
Colorimetry; Confocal microscopy	Cellular response to copolymer and ACP composite extracts
Dilatometry	Polymerization shrinkage (PS) of composites
Fourier-transform infrared (FTIR) spectroscopy and microspectroscopy (m-FTIR)	Short-range structure and composition of ACP fillers and composites Degree of vinyl conversion (DVC) of copolymers and composites Surface and cross-sectional distribution of filler and polymer in composites
Gravimetry	Kinetics of water sorption (WS) of copolymers and composites
Mechanical milling	Reduction of ACP's particle size (elimination of large agglomerates) by wet (non-aqueous) milling
Mechanical strength tests	Biaxial flexure strength (BFS) of copolymers and composites; shear bond strength (SBS) of composites
Microradiography	Quantitative measure of *in vitro* remineralization efficacy of ACP composites
^{1}H-Nuclear magnetic resonance (^{1}H-NMR) spectroscopy	Identification and quantification of leachable moieties from copolymers and ACP composites

(Table 4) contd.....

Method	Measuring Parameters/Information
Particle size distribution (PSD) analysis	Number and volume distribution of ACP particles; median diameter (d_m)
Phase contract microscopy	Morphology of cells exposed to copolymers and composites
Scanning electron microscopy (SEM)	Morphological and topological characteristics of ACP fillers
Tensometry	Quantification of stresses (PSS) developed in composites due to their shrinkage upon polymerization
Thermogravimetric analysis (TGA)	Water content and thermal stability of ACP fillers
X-ray diffraction (XRD) analysis	Long-range crystalline order of ACP fillers

Fourier-Transform Infrared (FTIR) Spectroscopy

FTIR spectroscopy (Nicolet Magna-IR FTIR System 550) is used as a complementary tool for confirming amorphousness of the fillers. The FTIR spectra ($4000 \ cm^{-1}$ to $400 \ cm^{-1}$) are recorded using a KBr pellet technique (0.8 –1.0 mg solid/400 mg KBr). Near-IR is utilized to determine the DVC of the unfilled resins (copolymers) and their ACP-filled composites by monitoring the reduction in the $=CH_2$ absorption band at $6165 \ cm^{-1}$ in the overtone region. Near-IR spectra, standardized using specimen of identical thickness, are acquired before photo-cure, immediately after cure, as well as 24h and 7d post-cure. Triplicate measurements are typically performed for each experimental group.

FTIR Microspectroscopy (m-FTIR)

The FTIR micro-spectroscopy (a Nicolet Magna-IRTM 550 FTIR spectrophotometer equipped with a video camera, a liquid nitrogen cooled-mercury cadmium telluride detector, a computerized motorized mapping stage and the Omnic® Atlus™ software) is utilized to produce functional group maps in conjunction with video images of intact copolymer and composite surfaces as well as cross-sections of copolymer and composite specimens before and after exposure to aqueous environments [48].

Particle Size Distribution (PSD)

The PSD of the ACP fillers is measured using a laser light scattering particle size analyzer (CIS-100, Ankersmid). The PSD of ACP powders is measured dry and dispersed in isopropanol and utrasonicated for 10 min at room temperature prior to the analysis (triplicate runs for each experimental group). From the PSD(s), the median particle size diameter (d_m) of the sample is obtained. Changes in d_m are taken as a primary indicator of alterations in the aggregation of the ACP particulates (the higher the d_m value, the more aggregated the ACP) [93, 94]. The

PSD data are compared with the morphological screening results (SEM analysis).

Scanning Electron Microscopy (SEM)

Surface morphology/topology of ACP powders is determined by SEM using a JEOL, JSM-5400 instrument. SEM is also used to examine composite disk surfaces before, during (disks are cut perpendicular to their flat surfaces and the cut faces examined), and after immersion in the test solutions. Argon ion etching technique is utilized to observe the dentin/adhesive interphase.

^{1}H-Nuclear Magnetic Resonance (^{1}H-NMR) Spectroscopy

Following the extraction of copolymer and composite disk specimens in a series of organic solvents and measuring their total weight loss, the residual solvent-free extracts are analyzed in $CDCl_3$ by ^{1}H-NMR (GSX 270, JEOL). NMR calibration curves are calculated relative to butylated hydroxyl toluene (BHT) which is utilized as an inhibitor of monomer polymerization upon extraction. BHT's shift serves as an internal standard. Detailed descriptions of the methodology and NMR data interpretation are provided in [95].

Polymerization Shrinkage (PS)

The PS of composite samples is measured by a computer-controlled mercury dilatometer fabricated in our Center. Composite pastes are cured using a standard 60s/30s exposure and data acquisition of 60 min + 30 min. Triplicate runs are performed for each experimental group. PS of a specimen corrected for temperature fluctuations is plotted as a function of time. The overall shrinkage (volume fraction, %) is calculated based on the known mass of the sample (50 mg –100 mg) and its density. The latter is determined by means of the Archimedean displacement principle using an attachment to a microbalance.

Polymerization Stress (PSS) Development

PSS measurement device (tensometer; designed and fabricated at the VRC-ADAF) is utilized to assess stress development in experimental ACP composites [92, 96, 97]. The corresponding software program has also been developed at PRC/ADAF. The tensometer is an effective tool for investigating the PSS kinetics as well as for probing various aspects that dictate PSS developments. It is based on the cantilever beam deflection theory that a tensile force generated by the bonded shrinking sample causes a cantilever beam to deflect. The design of the sample assembly facilitates convenient sample injection, experimental reproducibility and a short preparation time between the consecutive measurements. The PSS is obtained by dividing the measured tensile force by the cross sectional area of the sample. Detailed description of a technique is given in [98].

Biaxial Flexure Strength (BFS)

BFS measurements of copolymers and composites utilize a piston-on three-ball loading cell and a computer-controlled Universal Testing Machine operated by Testworks 4 software. The BFS values are calculated according to the American Society for Testing and Materials specification F394-78 [99].

Shear Bond Strength (SBS)

SBS to dentin is tested on extracted human molars and premolars embedded with cold-cured resin in poly-carbonate cups. Exposed dentin surfaces of the tooth samples are ground flat at a 90° angle to the longitudinal axis of the polycarbonate holder. Photoactivated pyromellitic glycerol dimethacrylate /acetone solution is used to establish an adhesive layer between the dentin and composite. A brass ring (4 mm in diameter and 1.5 mm in thickness) is used as a mold for the composite. Teflon tape (0.3 mm thick) with an aperture coinciding with the hole in the ring is placed under the brass ring to prevent the ring from adhering to the dentin. Both the ring and the tape are placed in the center of the dentin surface and held down with a lead weight (450 g). The cavity in the brass ring is filled with the experimental composite, irradiated for 1 min with a commercial visible-light source, and stored (at 37 °C) immersed in distilled water, saline and/or artificial saliva solution for up to 6 months prior to debonding. The assembly is placed against the vertical surface of a nylon block and the ring-enclosed composite is sheared off at a cross-head speed of 0.5 mm/min with a flat chisel pressing against the edge of the brass ring and connected to the load cell of the testing machine. The SBS of the experimental ACP materials is typically compared to commercial control.

Water Sorption (WS) Profiles

WS of composite specimens is determined in a following manner [8, 100]. A minimum of 5 replicate disks in each experimental group is initially dried over $CaSO_4$ until a constant mass is achieved (± 0.1 mg). Specimens are then: a) exposed to an air atmosphere of 75% relative humidity (RH) at 37 °C by keeping them suspended over saturated aqueous NaCl slurry in closed systems, or b) immersed in saline solution. Gravimetric mass changes of dry-padded specimens are recorded at predetermined time intervals. The degree of WS of any individual specimen at a given time interval (t), expressed as a % mass fraction, is calculated using a simple equation:

$$WS = [(W_t - W_0)/W_0] \times 100 \tag{2}$$

where W_t represents the sample mass at the time t, and W_0 is the initial mass of dry sample.

In vitro Cytotoxicity Studies

To simulate the early interactions between the composite and osteoblastic cells, extraction experiments are performed according to the guidelines specified by the International Standard Organization [101, 102] and ANSI/ADA #41 [103]. The extracts are quantitatively assessed by measuring the viability (succinate dehydrogenase activity, MTT assay).

Cell Culture Maintenance

Osteoblast-like MC3T3-E1 cells (Riken Cell Bank, Japan) are maintained in α-modification of Eagle's minimum essential medium (Biowhittaker, USA) with a volume fraction of 10% fetal bovine serum (Gibco-BRL-Life Technologies, USA) and 60 mg/L kanamycin sulfate (Sigma, USA) in a fully humidified atmosphere with a volume fraction of 5% CO_2 at 37 °C. The medium is changed twice a week. Cultures are passaged with EDTA-containing (1 mmol/L) trypsin solution (mass fraction of 0.25%; Gibco, USA) once a week. Some cytotoxicity experiments were performed with the murine RAW 264.7 macrophage-like cell line (passages 8–12, American Type Culture Collection TIB-71). The maintenance of the RAW 264.7 cells is detailed in [88].

Extraction/Cell Viability Experiments

In experiments with MC3T3-E1 cells, disks are sterilized with 70% ethanol [104] prior to extraction experiments. After sterilization, each disk is washed with 2 mL of media for 1 h and then fresh media is placed on each disk for an overnight extraction in the cell incubator. Positive control contained only media and negative control contained media with Triton X-100 detergent (0.1mass %). In parallel, a flask of 80% confluent MC3T3-E1 cells is passaged and cells seeded with 10,000 cells per well in 2 mL of media. The "cell wells" are seeded and then placed in the incubator overnight. On the second day of the experiment, the medium from each "cell well" is removed and replaced with the 2mL of extraction medium from one of the disk specimens (or with the positive or negative control media). The cells are incubated in the extracts for 3 days, photographed (digital camera with an inverted phase contrast microscope, Nikon, USA) and then prepared for the cytotoxicity assays.

In experiments with RAW 264.7 macrophages, polymer disk specimens are also sterilized with 70% ethanol [89] before being seeded (18 000 cells/cm^2). Cells seeded on tissue culture polystyrene (TCPS) are used as negative control. After 24 h, samples are evaluated for viability by staining for 10 min with 2 μmol/L calcein acetoxymethyl ester (live cells), 2 μmol/L ethidium homodimer-1 (dead cells), and 10 μmol/L Hoechst 33342 (nuclei). Cells are visualized on an upright epifluorescent microscope (Leica Microsystems AG). Images are captured using a digital camera (Hamamatsu Photonics K.K.) and analyzed with Image-Pro Plus. Cell density is calculated as the number of cells per image. Cell viability is expressed as the number of live cells/the total number of cells per image.

Succinate Dehydrogenase Activity (Methyl-Thiazolyldipheny--Tetrazoliumbromide (MTT) Assays)

The MC3T3-E1 cells are exposed to the extracts of the samples for 24 h. Then, cell cultured in the extracts are rinsed with 1 mL phosphate buffered saline solution (PBS: 140 mmol/L NaCl, 0.34 mmol/L Na$_2$HPO$_4$, 2.9 mmol/L KCl, 10 mmol/L HEPES, 12 mmol/L NaHCO$_3$, 5 mmol/L glucose, pH = 7.4) and 0.125 mL/well of MMT solution (5 mg/mL MMT in PBS). After 2 h incubation at 37 °C, the MTT solution is removed and the insoluble formazan crystals are dissolved in 0.1 mL dimethylsulfoxide (DMSO; Sigma Aldrich). Finally, the absorbance is measured at 540 nm with a plate reader (Wallac 1420 Victor2, Perkin Elmer Life Sciences). The blank values (the well that contains only the PBS, MMT and DMSO solutions) are subtracted from each of the experimental values as background.

To determine the enzymatic activity of RAW 264.7 macrophages, the sterilized disk specimens are placed in 24-well TCPS plates, and seeded with 90 000 cells/cm^2. Wells with polymers only (no cells), cells only (no polymers) and without either cells or polymers (blanks) are used as controls. After 24 h, the growth medium is removed and polymer disks transferred to a new 24-well plate. A 300 μL MTT solution (0.5 mg/mL MTT in PBS) is added to each polymer disk and each TCPS well from which the disks were removed. The plates are incubated for 1 h at 37 °C and 5% CO$_2$. The MTT solution is then removed and replaced with 300 μL DMSO. The plates are then incubated at room temperature with gentle mixing for 20 min. After brief mixing *via* pipetting, 200 μL from each well is transferred to a 96-well plate and the optical density at 540 nm is measured. Results are normalized to the surface area exposed to cells (for disks: polymer disk area; for TCPS: well area minus the polymer disk area). Controls without cells and polymers are subtracted from all sample readings.

Bacteria Inoculation and Imaging

Streptococcus mutans (*S. mutans*; Clarke UA159 from the ATCC) are cultured in brain heart infusion (BHI) broth with 0.5 µg/mL bacitracin. Polymers are sterilized with 70% (volume fraction) ethanol for 20 min, soaked in PBS overnight, and inoculated with *S. mutans* prepared at an optical density of 0.06 in PBS containing 100 mg/L $MgCl_2·6H_2O$ and 100 mg/L $CaCl_2$. After incubating (37 °C, 5 vol. % CO_2) for 4 h, samples are washed 3X to remove non-adherent bacteria, fixed with 37 mg/mL formaldehyde, and stained for 1 h with 1 µmol/L SYTOX green. Samples are not passed through the air-liquid interface during the rinsing and fixing steps. Ultimately, samples are imaged with a Zeiss LSM 510 laser scanning confocal microscope (40× water immersion objective). Image stacks are collected at random locations on each sample, and projection images are prepared using the manufacturer's software. Custom macros in Image-Pro Plus software (Media Cybernetics, Inc.) are used to quantify each image in terms of the total surface area covered by bacteria, the area of each object, and the object density. Object density and surface coverage were plotted as a percentage of the controls.

RESULTS & DISCUSSION

Effect of Additives and Surface-Modifiers on Physicochemical Properties of ACP Fillers and Ensuing Composites

A typical XRD pattern and the corresponding FTIR spectrum of any unconverted ACP (independent of the type of additive, silanization treatment, grinding or milling) are shown in Fig. (**1a** and **1b**), respectively. These spectra confirm lack of crystalline regularity, the ACP's striking feature that distinguishes it from all other crystalline CaPs [11, 15, 17]. The XRD diffraction analysis showed only two diffuse broad bands in the $2\Theta = (4 \text{ to } 60)°$ region. Such pattern is indicative of a solid in which no translational and orientational long-range order of the atomic positions could be detected. The corresponding FTIR spectrum consisted of two wide PO_4 absorbance bands at (1200 to 900) cm^{-1} and (630 to 550) cm^{-1}, typical for phosphate stretching and phosphate bending, respectively.

Random clustering of highly agglomerated ACP particles in polymerized methacrylate matrices leads to the inferior mechanical behavior and enhanced water sorption of ACP composites upon exposure to aqueous milieus [7 - 9]. To test the hypothesis that certain additives may reduce spontaneous ACP agglomeration and, in turn, improve the hydrolytic stability of the fillers, the following additives were introduced *ab initio* during the ACP synthesis: (a) cations, (b) surfactants, and (c) polymers. The amorphous state of the solids precipitating in the presence of additives (validated by XRD and FTIR), the results of the PSD, TGA, DVC and BFS testing are compiled in Table **5** [29, 48, 89, 90].

On average, there was no change in the total water content ((13.2-19.7) mass %) or the ratio surface-bound/structurally incorporated water (2/3 of water was surface-bound and the remaining 1/3 was structurally incorporated) in cation-, surfactant- and polymer-ACPs. In cation series, mono-, di- and trivalent cations yielded ACPs with reduced median diameter (d_m =(1.4-3.8) μm) and the range of PSD (submicron to approx. 15 μm) compared to tetravalent Si- and Zr-ACP (d_m =(5.8-6.7) μm; PSD from submicron to approx. 70 μm). Observed differences in the mean values of dm between different cations would suggest slight modifications in the degree of ACP's agglomeration which seems more random than systematically related to ionic potential of cations. Fe^{2+}- and Fe^{3+}-ACPs showed early signs of conversion to crystalline HAP. In addition, significant color changes occurred in Ag^+-, Fe^{2+}- and Fe^{3+}-ACP solids. This unwanted color change was due to the co-precipitation of light-sensitive Ag- and colored Fe-phosphates with ACP. Furthermore, during the BFS testing, Ag^+-, Fe^{2+}- and Fe^{3+}-ACP based composites disintegrated upon the onset of loading. There was no significant difference between the dry BFS values of Zn-, Al, Si- and Zr-ACP based composites. After exposure to the aqueous environment, the BFS of Al- and Si-ACP specimens deteriorated (35-37) % compared to the corresponding dry BFS values. Zr-ACP composites were weakened by only 17% and Zn-ACP composite specimens did not deteriorate with soaking. The DVC of Zn-, Al, Si-ACP composites was reduced between 18% and 30% compared to the Zr-ACP counterparts. The reason(s) for this reduction in DVC of Zn-, Al, Si-ACP composite has yet to be explained.

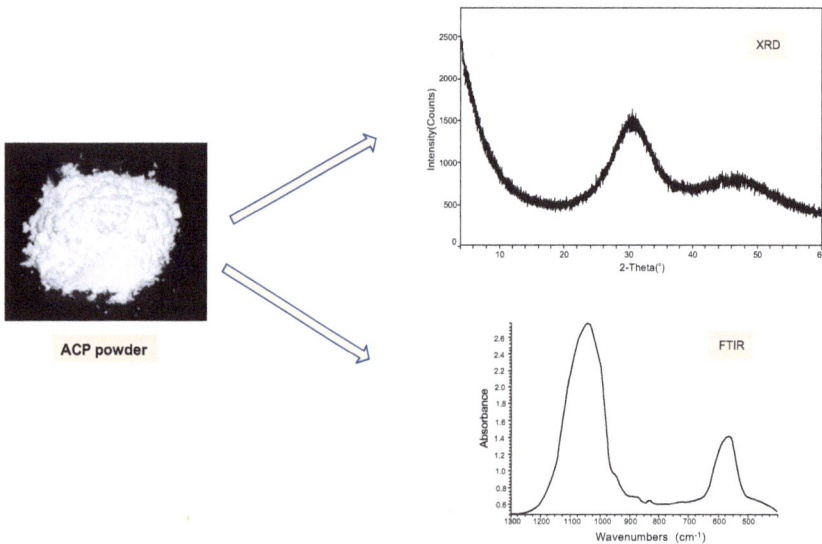

Fig. (1). Typical X-ray diffraction (XRD) pattern and Fourier-transform infrared (FTIR) spectrum of ACP.

Compared to Zr-ACP, no significant changes were detected in the PSD of Triton-, Tween- and FSN-ACP while FSN-ACP showed a 45% reduction in d_m. This reduction in d_m did not improve the mechanical performance of FSN-ACP based composites. The BFS of all surfactant-ACP based composites decreased by almost 50% or more after a month long exposure to saline solutions. Addition of polymers had an inverse effect on the PSD of ACP solids. Compared to Zr-ACP, d_m of PAA- and PEO-ACP increased 37% and 113%, respectively. The apparently higher extent of particle agglomeration in polymer-ACPs could possibly be attributed to a mechanism similar to "polymer bridging" that reportedly controls the agglomeration of HAP in the presence of high-molecular mass polymers [105]. For the reasons discussed above, Zr-ACP was chosen as a "gold standard" in all subsequent studies.

Table 5. Effect of additives on physicochemical properties of ACP fillers, and DVC and BFS of their Bis-GMA- or EBPADMA-based composites. Resin: Bis-GMA/TEGDMA/HEMA/ZrDMA (cation and polymer series) or EBPADMA/PMDGMA (surfactant series). Indicated are mean values with one standard deviation (SD) in parenthesis. Minimum number of experiments: 3/experimental group. *ACP/HAP denotes appearance of crystalline HAP in XRD and FTIR spectra due to conversion during synthesis. Nd = not determined. Um = unmeasurable (specimens disintegrated with the onset of loading).

Additive	Structure	d_m (µm)	Water Content (Mass %)	DVC (%)	BFS (MPa) Dry Wet
Cation					
Ag^+	ACP	3.5(1.9)	14.0(2.2)	63.3(1.9)	Um
Fe^{2+}	*ACP/HAP	3.8(1.9)	15.4(1.2)	65.7(1.2)	Um
Zn^{2+}	ACP	1.4(0.5)	16.6(2.5)	63.7(2.6)	44.6(13.8) 47.4(14.5)
Al^{3+}	ACP	2.2(1.3)	16.8(2.8)	56.7(2.6)	41.5(10.0) 24.6(3.2)
Fe^{3+}	*ACP/HAP	2.1(0.6)	14.1(2.3)	56.0(3.3)	Um
Si^{4+}	ACP	5.8(1.6)	13.2(1.6)	61.0(2.0)	47.7(12.4) 27.7(6.9)
Zr^{4+}	ACP	6.7(1.8)	16.1(2.0)	80.1(3.3)	43.0(10.2) 36.3(8.6)
Surfactant *Non-ionic:*					
Triton100	ACP	8.3(1.4)	16.3(1.2)	Nd	73.0(5.9) 28.2(3.0)
Tween80	ACP	8.9(2.1)	16.9(0.9)	Nd	76.1(8.2) 31.9(9.9)
FSN	ACP	6.5(1.2)	19.7(1.1)	Nd	58.2(9.9) 28.1(3.3)
Anionic:					
FSP	ACP	4.1(0.4)	17.6(2.1)	Nd	60.2(7.9) 32.3(9.7)
Polymer					
PAA	ACP	9.2(1.9)	15.8(1.0)	Nd	Nd
PEO	ACP	14.3(2.3)	13.7(0.3)	Nd	Nd

Surface modification of ACP with APTMS and MPTMS, ACP grinding and mechanical milling revealed the following. APTMS- and MPTMS-ACP were formulated into LC EBPADMA/TEGDMA/HEMA/MEP composites and their

BFS was evaluated in both dry and wet state (Fig. **2**). The BFS results for Zr-ACP/ETHM composites are shown for comparison. In dry state, MPTMS-ACP composites attained (57-58) % higher strength than APTMS-ACP and Zr-ACP control composites. Even upon soaking, the MPTMS-ACP/ETHM composites were approx. 60% stronger than the control Zr-ACP/ETHM counterparts, suggesting that the silanization of the ACP filler with MPTMS can ameliorate the overall plasticization of composites by water.

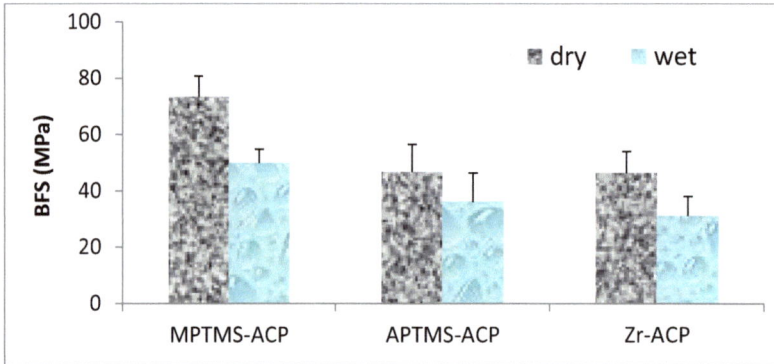

Fig. (2). Effect of filler silanization on BFS of ACP/ETHM composites. Shown are mean BFS values + SD (n≥3/group). Immersion medium: buffered saline solution (37 °C; constant magnetic stirring).

PSD of am-, g- and m-ACP are shown in Fig. (**3**). The volume fraction of fine particles decreased in following order: m-ACP > g-ACP > am-ACP. As a result, blending of g- and, particularly, m-ACP into the resin was much easier and took less time than the same process using am-ACP. Moreover, at the same filler level, pastes with g- and m-ACP were more flowable compared to the am-ACP composite paste (typically very viscous). The narrower PSD obtained through grinding and, especially, milling apparently improved dispersion of these fillers within the matrices and, in turn, the mechanical properties of g- and m-ACP composites (Table **6**). More homogeneous dispersion of g- and m-ACP fillers throughout the composites, *i.e.*, a lesser number of voids/defects existing throughout the bodies of the composite disk specimens, resulted in reduced WS in g- and m-ACP composites compared to am-ACP composites. While the levels of the mineralizing ions released into buffered saline environment from g- and m-ACP composites and the resulting supersaturations with respect to HAP were somewhat reduced compared to am-ACP composites, the conditions favorable for regenerating mineral-deficient tooth structures (ΔG^0 values $\ll 0$) were maintained in all systems.

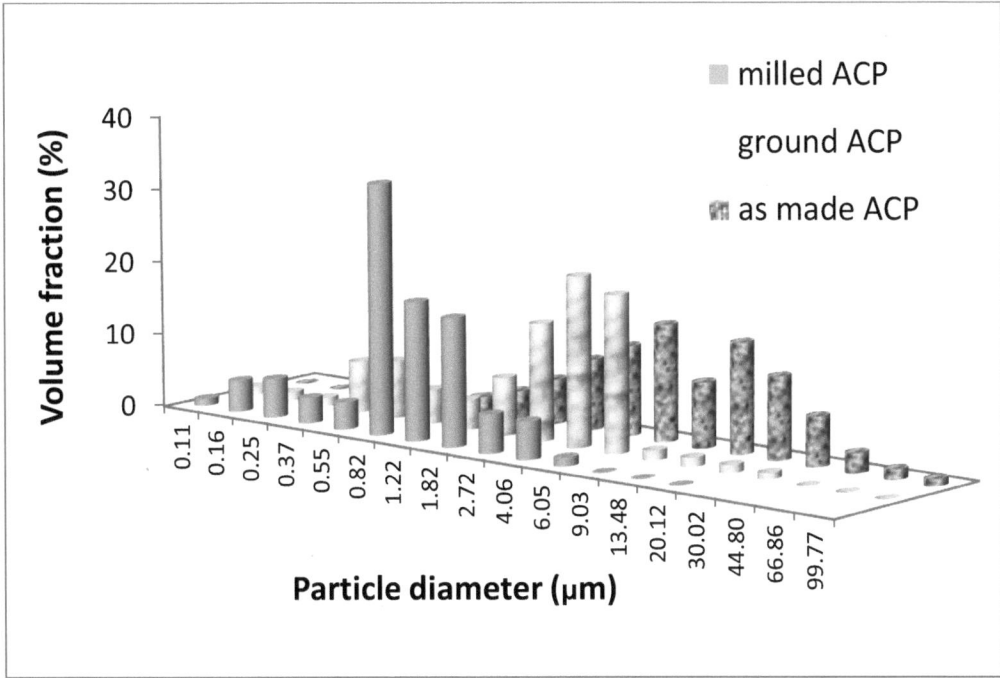

Fig. (3). Typical histograms of volume size distribution of milled, ground and as made ACP. Indicated are mean values of triplicate runs for each ACP type.

Table 6. PSD of am-, g- and m-ACP fillers, BFS (after 1 mo aqueous immersion), WS (at 75% relative humidity) and the thermodynamic stability ($\Delta G°$) of immersing solutions with respect to stoichiometric HAP of their EBPADMA/TEGDMA/HEMA/MEP resin composites. Indicated are mean values with SD in parenthesis. Number of repetitive experiments n ≥ 5.

	PSD d_m (µm) range (µm)	BFS (MPa)	WS (mass %)	$\Delta G°$ (kJ/mol)
am-ACP	6.7 (1.8) 0.4-66.9	42.2 (6.7)	3.1 (0.4)	- [5.7 (0.2)]
g-ACP	3.4 (0.8) 0.1-20.0	50.0 (8.0)	2.5 (0.5)	- [4.9 (0.6)]
m-ACP	0.9 (0.2) 0.1-9.0	56.4 (7.7)	1.7 (0.2)	- [5.1 (0.3)]

Fine-tuning of the Experimental Resins: Structure-Composition-Property Studies

In one series of structure-composition property studies, LC binary and ternary Bis-GMA-, EBPADMA- or UDMA-based experimental resins were formulated with TEGDMA, HmDMA, and/or HEMA as diluent co-monomers. These resins were intended for dental sealant and/or base/liner applications. The results of physicochemical and mechanical screening of the resins and their ACP composites are shown in Figs. (**4-6**).

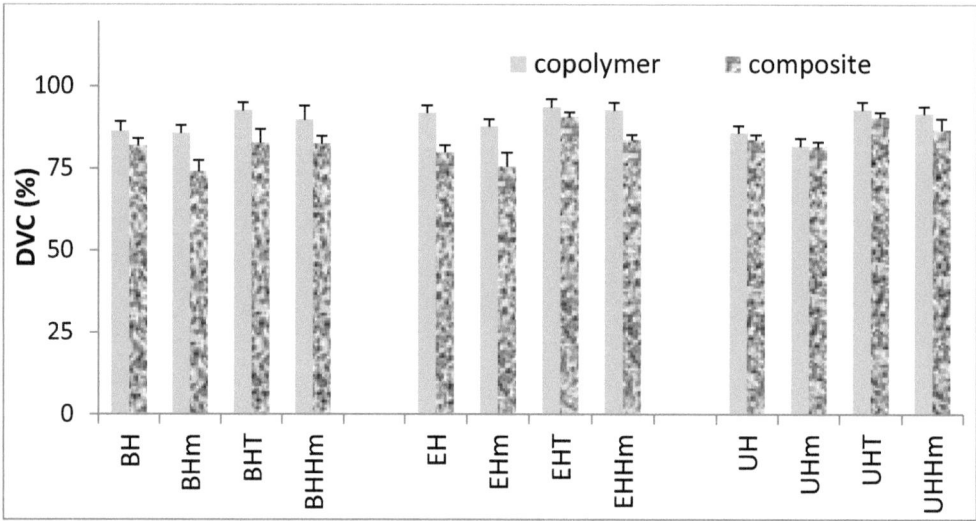

Fig. (4). DVC (24 h post curing) of binary and ternary Bis-GMA-, EBPADMA- and UDMA-based copolymers and their ACP composites. Plotted are mean values + SD (number of replicates n ≥ 7/group).

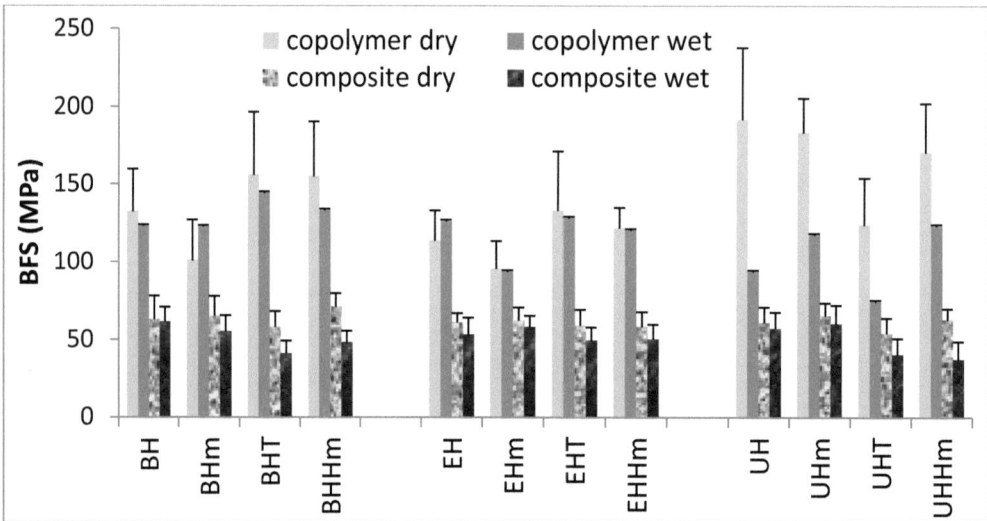

Fig. (5). BFS of dry and wet (1 mo immersion in buffered saline; pH=7.4, 37 °C) of binary and ternary Bis-GMA-, EBPADMA- and UDMA-based copolymers and their ACP composites. Indicated are mean values + SD (n ≥ 8/group).

Bis-GMA-, EBPADMA- and UDMA-based copolymers and composites generally achieved high DVC values ranging from 81.7% to 93.7% and from 74.1% to 90.7%, respectively (Fig. **4**). Regardless of the resin matrix composition, DVC values attained in UDMA-based ACP composites were marginally higher than the

DVCs of Bis-GMA- and EBPADMA-based counterparts. This trend may possibly be explained by the higher reactivity of UDMA monomer in comparison with Bis-GMA or EBPADMA [38]. Typically, higher DVC values were attained in all resins with relatively high contents of HEMA ($\geq$ 28 mass %). This effect is related to HEMA's high diffusivity and mono-functionality. Expectedly, the composites that yielded high DVCs also showed relatively high PS (on average, between 6.4 vol % and 7.4 vol % for all experimental groups; data hot shown here). The latter exceeded the PS values typically reported for highly glass-filled commercial composites (1.9 vol % to 4.1 vol %). The experimental ACP composites fell into the category of either flowable composites or adhesive resins (reported PS values (3.6 to 6.0) vol % and (6.7 to 13.5) vol %, respectively [105, 106]. These high PS values can be attributed in part to a filler level of only 40 mass % in ACP experimental materials compared to that of up to 85% of silica-based fillers in conventional composites. Based on PS results alone, the inclusion of bulkier but relatively low viscosity resins or ring-opening monomers [107, 108] into experimental resins and/or higher contents of ACP may be required to obtain composites with lower PS while maintaining satisfactory DVC.

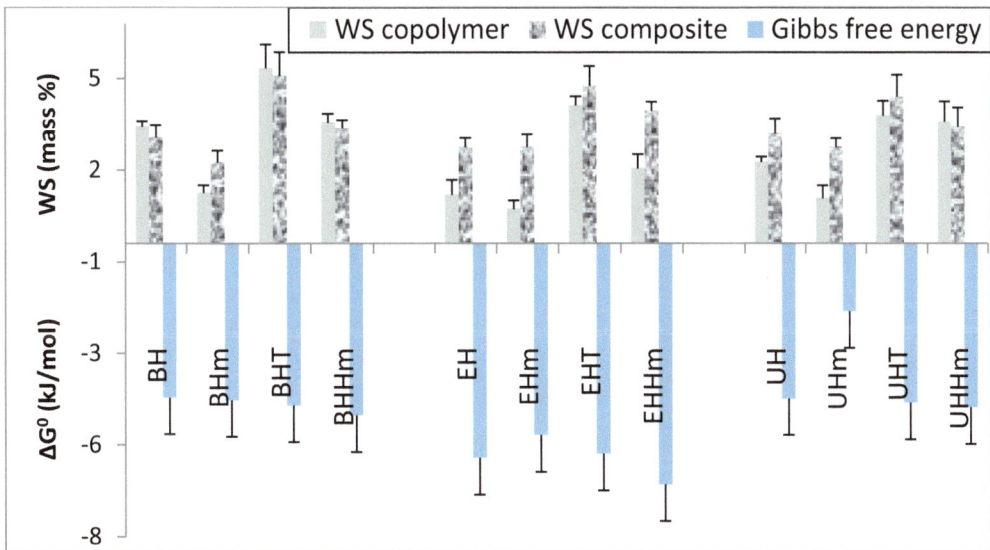

Fig. (6). WS (maximum recorded at 75% relative humidity) of binary and ternary Bis-GMA-, EBPADMA- and UDMA-based copolymers and their ACP composites and the supersaturation of the immersing solutions (ΔG°) after 1 mo immersion of composites in buffered saline). Indicated are mean values + SD (n = 4/group).

WS, if excessive, generally causes a decrease in mechanical strength, depression of the glass transition temperature of the matrix due to plasticization, solvation of the composites, reversible rupture of weak inter-chain bonds and/or irreversible disruption of the polymer matrix [109, 110]. In the case of ACP polymeric composites, the overall WS profiles are additionally affected by ACP-water interactions. WS regulates the kinetics of the intra-composite ACP to HAP conversion and, ultimately, determines the remineralizing capacity of bioactive ACP composites. WS_{max} values (Fig. **6**) for all resins and their ACP composites were reached within two weeks of saline immersion. They were generally highest for ternary formulations containing TEGDMA and HEMA, and lowest for binary resins that contained the relatively hydrophobic HmDMA. These differences are related to the relative portion of hydrophilic (HEMA and TEGDMA) or hydrophobic (HmDMA) monomer in the matrix which, ultimately, controls the overall hydrophilicity/hydrophobicity balance of the polymer matrix.

When exposed to aqueous milieu, ACP composites formulated with either of the experimental resins, released calcium and phosphate ions at such levels that the immersion solutions became highly supersaturated with respect to HAP $\Delta G^0 << 0$; (Fig. **6**). Since only marginal differences were seen in the WS of Bis-GMA-, EBPADMA- and UDMA-based copolymers, the observed trend of decreasing ΔG^0 (*i.e.*, $\Delta G^0_{EBPADMA} > \Delta G^0_{Bis-GMA} \geq \Delta G^0_{UDMA}$) is attributed to differences in the chemical structure and the composition of the monomer systems. Generally, more negative ΔG^0 values (*i.e.*, higher remineralizing potential) attained in systems containing EBPADMA as a base monomer and HEMA as a co-monomer were attributed to a more open cross-linked network structure of EBPADMA copolymer-based matrix, and the increased internal mineral saturation that allows uptake of more water and/or better accessibility of ACP filler to the water already entrained in the HEMA-rich copolymer matrix.

Bis-GMA- and EBPADMA-based copolymers did not weaken upon immersion while UDMA-based copolymers deteriorated on average 25% (Fig. **5**). Generally, dry ACP composites had substantially 49% to 63% lower BFS than the corresponding copolymers regardless of the resin composition. The strength of all but binary HmDMA-containing composites diminished further upon soaking. This 10% to 25% reduction in BFS of wet *vs* dry composites was attributed to the numerous defects/voids (resin-rich, ACP-depleted regions) and the random distribution of large am-ACP agglomerates existing in these composites [48]. These features led to an inadequate filler/resin interlocking and the mechanical inferiority of these materials.

Another structure/composition/property study focused on the effects of chemical structure and composition of the resin on BFS and DVC of LC Bis-GMA/TEGDMA/X {X=neutral comonomer (DEGMEMA, GMA, GDMA, HEMA, MEMA) or acidic comonomer (MaA, MA, 4MET, VPA)} copolymers and am-ACP composites. Results are summarized in Figs. (**7a** and **7b**). In the neutral comonomer series, DVC values decreased in the following order: BTD >

BTH, BTM > BTGm, BT control > BTGd (copolymers), and BTD > BTGm, BTH, BT control > BTGd, BTM (composites). In the acidic comonomer series, DVC values of both copolymers and composites showed no significant changes with the structural variations of the acidic comonomer. Generally, the DVCs of composites were 4.5% to 16.4% lower than DVCs of the corresponding copolymers. The only exemption is BTMa formulation, where, the reverse effect was noticed. The highest DVC values recorded in BTD formulations are most likely due to the highly flexible nature of DEGMEMA comonomer. The lower DVC in composites could primarily be attributed to the reduction in exotherm of resin polymerization by ACP phase. However, other factors, such as greater air entrapment and light scattering facilitated by the heterogeneous PSD of am-ACP may have also contributed to this reduction in DVC.

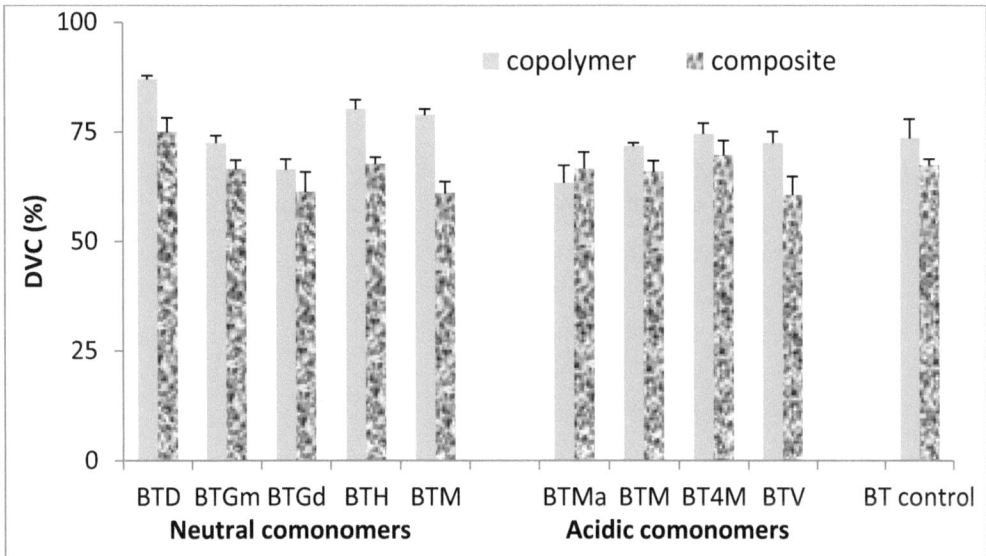

Fig. (7a). DVC values (mean + SD) attained in BTX copolymers and their composites (24 h post-LC). Number of repetitive measurements/group: n ≥ 6.

The BFS of dry and wet BTX copolymer specimens in neutral series (on average 69 MPa) was unaffected by the structure of comonomer. However, the BFS of the corresponding composites was reduced up to 23% in dry state. It deteriorated further with soaking; BFS values of wet specimens diminished additional (44-56) %. Similar trends were observed in acidic comonomer series. In this group, up to 64% drop in BFS with soaking was observed with BTMa copolymers and composites. The favorable arrangement of two carboxylic acid groups in MaA comonomer may have resulted in the enhanced cross-linking, facilitated by the increased intermolecular hydrogen bonding, in BTMa matrix and, ultimately, yielding copolymers with high dry BFS. However, presence of these two carboxylic groups in MaA also increased the overall hydrophilicity of the resin leading to easy disruption of hydrogen bond-mediated cross links by water and resulting in precipitous decline in BFS values upon immersion. Multiple factors may have caused the reduction in BFS of BTX composites: diminished ACP's integrity and/or rigidity of ACP/resin interface – possibly due to interactions between ACP and acid groups, spatial changes originating from Ca^{2+} and PO_4 ion efflux – resulting from intra-composite ACP to HAP conversion, and excessive water sorption – due to increased hydrophilicity of resins containing acidic comonomers. Significantly, the BFS of BT4M composites $\{(66.7\pm13.2)$ MPa$\}$ exceeded the BFS of all BTX formulations $\{(25.0\text{-}37.9)$ MPa$\}$ and the Bis-GMA/TEGDMA control $\{(50.1\pm6.0)$ MPa$\}$. It is, therefore, concluded that simultaneous incorporation of DEGMEMA and 4MET into polymer phase may aid in attaining high DVC while maintaining mechanical stability of composites upon aqueous exposure.

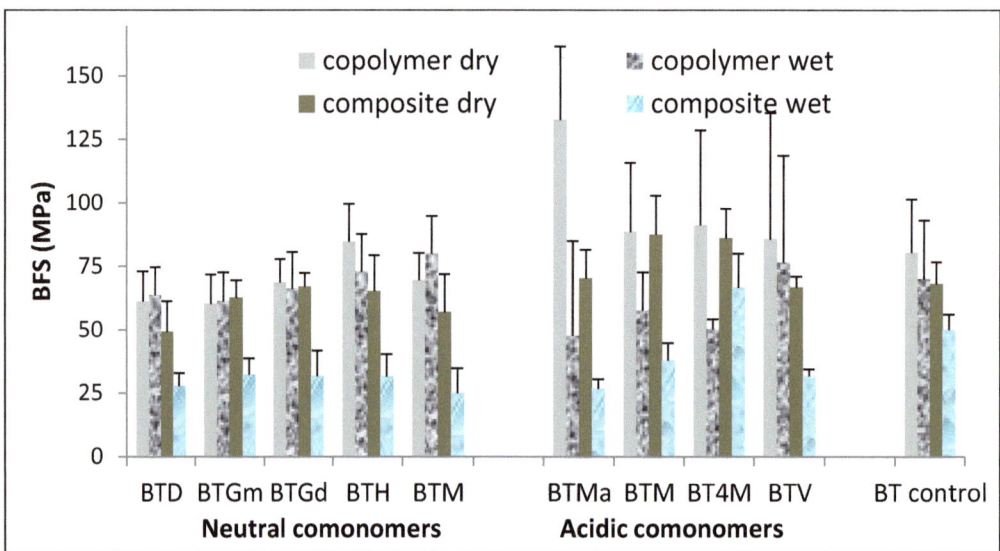

Fig. (7b). BFS (mean value + SD) of dry and wet (after 2 weeks of aqueous immersion) BTX copolymer and composite specimens (n ≥ 5).

The effect(s) of the fine-tuning of EBPADMA-based resins on the anti-demineralizing/remineralizing ability and PS of am- and m-ACP composites, and BFS, WS and DVC of both copolymers and composites were assessed in two separate studies [91, 111]. The am-ACP was blended with two types of EBPADMA/TEGDMA/HEMA/MEP (ETHM) resins: 1) EBPADMA/TEGDMA molar ratio of (0.50–0.125), a constant HEMA/MEP molar ratio of 4.28 (ETHM050, ETHM033, ETHM025 and ETHM125; photoinitiator; IRGACURE

1850), and 2) EBPADMA/TEGDMA molar ratio of (0.50–1.35) and the HEMA/MEP molar ratio of (8.26 ± 0.33) (ETHM050*, ETHM085 and ETHM135: photoinitiator: CQ and 4E). In second ETHM series, testing was expanded to include m-ACP as filler. Both ETHM formulations were intended for orthodontic application. Results of physicochemical tests are presented in Figs. (**8a - c**).

Compositional variations of the resin matrix had no significant effect on DVC, WS and BFS of am-ACP composites in ETHM013-050 series. There was, however, an effect of resin composition on PS that developed in these composites: the PS increased as the molar ratio EBPADMA/TEGDMA in the resin decreased. Apparently lower DVC (Fig. **8a**) and BFS values (Fig. **8c**) in ETHM050*-133 series compared to ETHM013-050 series were not statistically significant. Improved strength was achieved with the use of m-ACP. This improved strength together with the lower WS in m-ACP composites is due to the improved dispersion of m-ACP throughout the composite compared to am-ACP. Significantly, lower WS in m-ACP composites has only marginally affected the remineralization potential of these composites. The supersaturations with respect to HAP attained in the solutions with immersed m-ACP ETHM composites were only 8.3% to 10.3% lower than the supersaturation levels attained in am-ACP ETHM counterparts (Fig. **8b**). These values are considerably above the minimum required for HAP re-deposition ($\Delta G° < 0$), therefore, remineralization capability has been preserved in all ACP ETHM formulations.

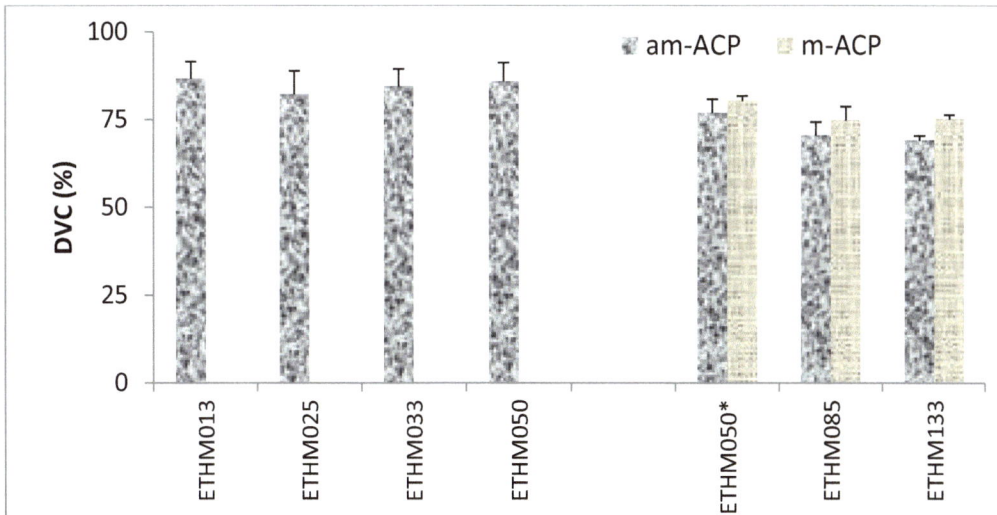

Fig. (8a). DVC (mean value + SD) attained in ETHM am- and m-ACP composites (24 h post-LC). Number of repetitive measurements/group: n ≥ 6.

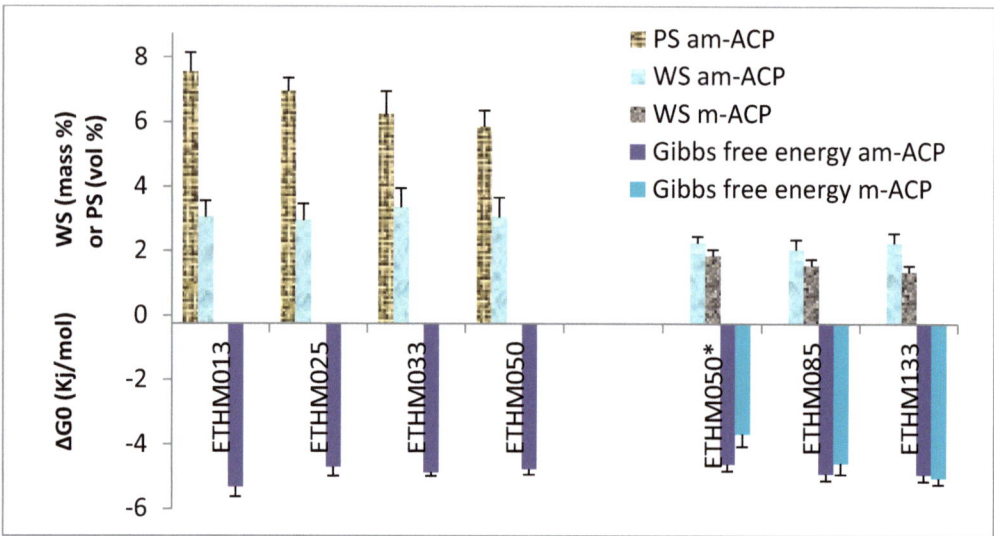

Fig. (8b). PS, WS (75% relative humidity) and the thermodynamic stability of immersing solutions at maximum calcium and phosphate concentrations released from ACP ETHM composites. Indicated are mean values + SD. Number of repetitive measurements/group: n≥3 (PS); n=5 (WS); and n=4 (ΔG°).

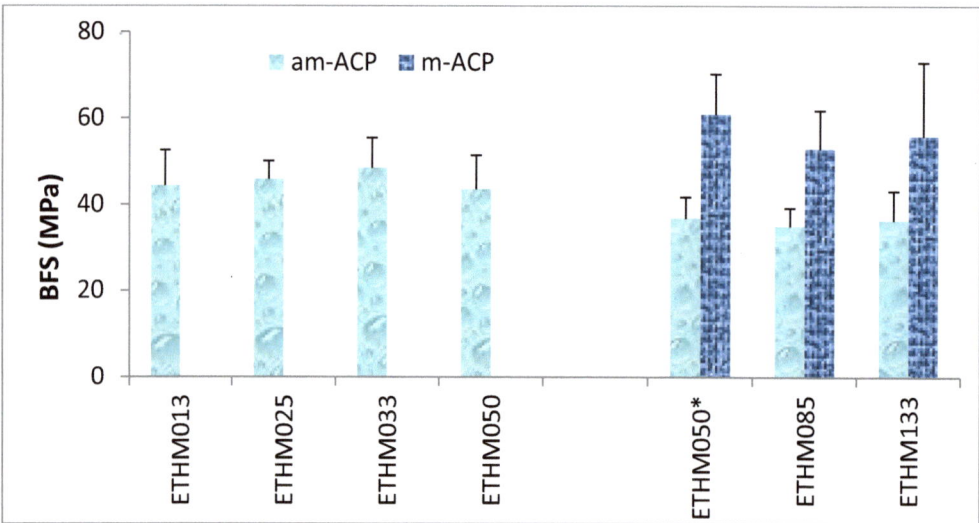

Fig. (8c). BFS (mean value +SD) of ACP ETHM composites after 1 mo immersion in buffered saline solutions. Number of repetitive measurements/group: n=5.

Results of the extensive evaluation of light-cure (LC; Irgacure 1850) and dual cure (DC; Irgacure 1850 (LC) plus BPO and DHEPT (chemical cure; CC) UDMA/PEG-U/HEMA/MEP (UPHM) resins and their am- and g-ACP composites are summarized in Figs. **(9a-9d)**.

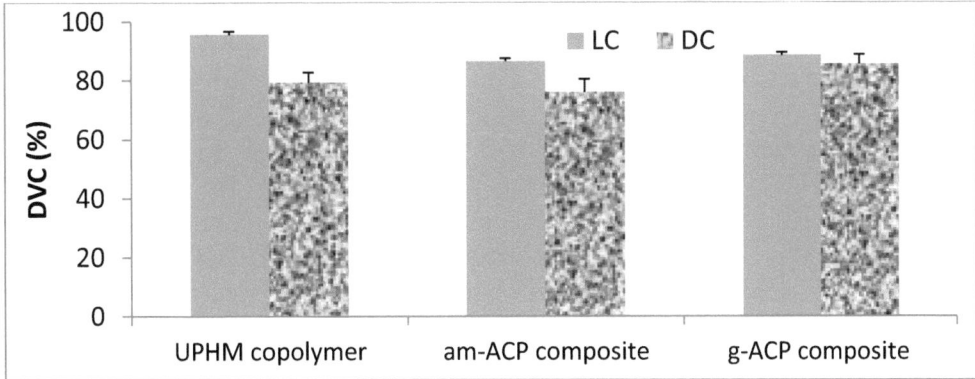

Fig. (9a). DVC (mean value + SD) attained 24 h post-cure in LC and DC UPHM copolymers and composites. Number of repetitive measurements/group: n=3.

The CC UPHM formulations were excluded from in-depth screening since, in the preliminary testing, these copolymers yielded DVC values approx. 35% lower than DVC values in LC UPHM counterparts. LC copolymers attained exceptionally high DVC values of 95.7% Fig. (**9a**). Introducing am- and g-ACP into LC UPHM resins resulted in mild reductions of DVC – 7.6% (g-ACP) and 10.0% (am-ACP). Generally, DC formulations exhibited lower DVCs than the corresponding LC specimens. The reduction in DVC ranged from 17.1% (copolymers) to 12.1% (am-ACP composites) to 3.4% (g-ACP composites). The latter was not statistically significant.

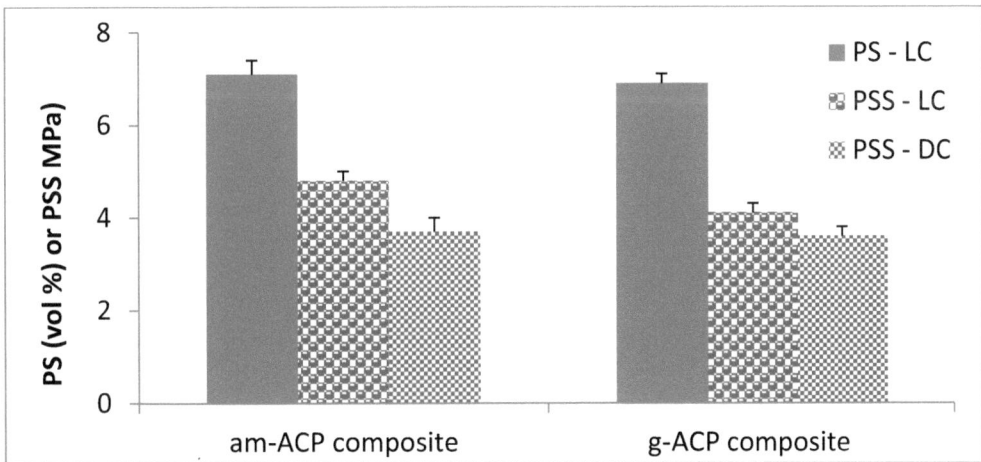

Fig. (9b). PS and PSS in LC and DC UPHM composites. Shown are mean values + SD. Number of repetitive measurements/group: n≥3.

In DC systems, a certain degree of contraction occurred immediately after combining the LC and CC paste (even before the samples were placed in tensometer) and the paste hardened within ten minutes of mixing. Consequently, DC formulations were unsuitable for tensometry measurements and PS tests were, therefore, performed on LC UPHM composites only (Fig. **9b**). The mean PS values for LC UPHM composites (7.1 vol % and 6.9 vol % for am- and g-ACP, respectively) are comparable to PS measured in LC binary and ternary EBPADMA- and UDMA-based composites (on average 7.36 MPa and 7.21 MPa, respectively (this Chapter [8, 9]). This relatively high PS is most likely caused by still relatively high content of HEMA (approx. 17 mass %) in UPHM matrices that led to the intensified hydrogen bonding and, ultimately, to densification of polymerization [96]. The PSS, generally lower in in DC compared to LC composites, decreased in going from am- to g-ACP composites. The PSS developed in LC UPHM composites {(4.1-4.8) MPa} compares well with the PSS in LC UDMA/HEMA composites (4.5 mPa on average [96];). This finding suggests that the simultaneous incorporation of HEMA and PEG-U into the UPHM resins does not increase the PSS in these matrices. In binary UDMA/HEMA *vs* UDMA/PEG-U based composites, the differences in PSS may be related to the higher relative molecular mass and more flexible character of PEG-U oligomer compared to less flexible poly(HEMA) segments. However, this same explanation cannot be applied to much more complex UPHM polymers.

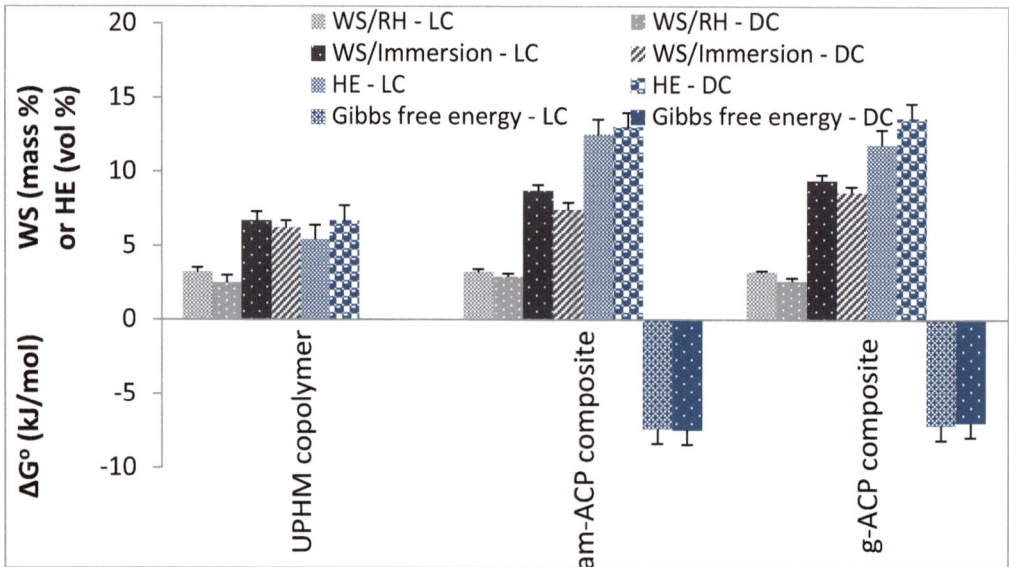

Fig. (9c). WS (at 75% relative humidity (RH) and upon aqueous immersion), hygroscopic expansion (HE) and the thermodynamic stability of immersing solutions at maximum calcium and phosphate concentrations released from LC and DC UPHM composites. Indicated are mean values + SD. Number of repetitive measurements/group: n≥3.

It appears significant that the relatively high PS in UPHM copolymers and their ACP composites is likely to be compensated by the substantial hygroscopic expansion (HE; (Fig. **9c**)) of UPHM copolymers {(5.4-6.7) vol %} and composites {(11.8-13.6) vol %}. Beneficial effects of HE on composite's performance have been demonstrated in [112, 113]. The supersaturations with respect to HAP of the immersing solutions attained with both LC and DC am-ACP and g-ACP UPHM composites {ΔG°=-(6.96-7.44) kJ/mol; (Fig. **9c**)} exceeded significantly the supersaturations resulting from similar immersion of am-ACP and m-ACP ETHM composites {ΔG°=-(4.35-5.07) kJ/mol and ΔG°=-(3.42-4.79) kJ/mol, respectively; (Fig. **8b**)} as well as binary and ternary am-ACP Bis-GMA-, EBPADMA and/or UDMA-based composites {ΔG°=-(4.21-4.70) kJ/mol, ΔG°=-(5.24-6.58) kJ/mol, and ΔG°=-(1.86-4.48) kJ/mol, respectively; (Fig. **6**)). The results of BFS testing of ACP UPHM composites (Fig. **9d**) have re-confirmed the fact that ACP-based composites are generally too weak to be considered as direct filling materials. The average BFS values across the four composite groups, {(45.5±5.3) MPa} compare well with the BFS values of am-ACP ETHM composites {(41.5±6.2) MPa; (Fig. **8c**)}. Since the UPHM formulations were primarily intended for endodontic application for which a material's mechanical performance is not the most critical property, the enhanced remineralization potential of ACP UPHM composites is likely to provide superior protection of tooth mineral under cariogenic attack thus making these experimental materials viable candidates for the intended dental use.

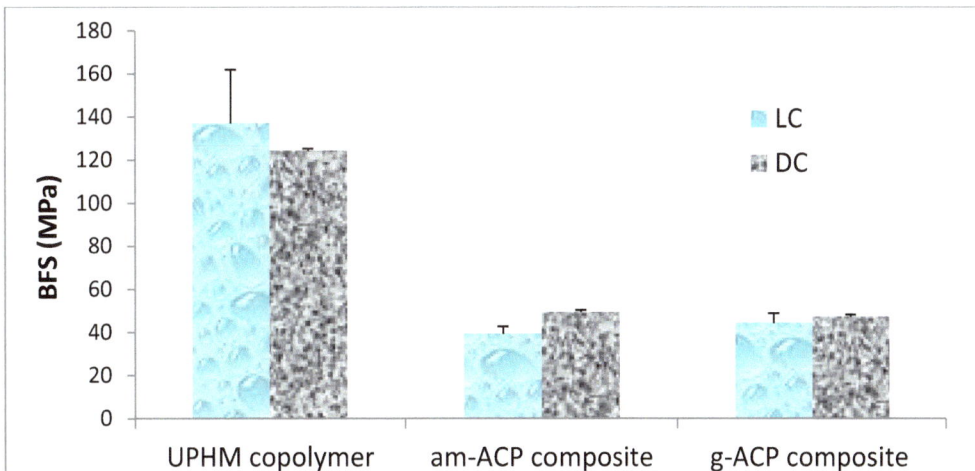

Fig. (9d). BFS (mean value +SD) of IC and DC ACP UPHM composites after 1 mo immersion in buffered saline solutions. Number of repetitive measurements/group: n≥3.

Assessing Leachable and Cytotoxicity of ACP Composites

In our structure/composition/property studies we conveniently utilized the DVC attained upon polymerization as an indirect measure of leachability of unreacted monomers and other leachable species from copolymers and composites. In order to better understand the leachability issues, it seems prudent to both qualitatively and quantitatively assess the levels of unreacted monomers and the components of polymerization initiating system. Leachability studies are typically performed by chromatographic methods, such as high-performance liquid or gas chromatography, or a combination of chromatographic and spectrometric methods, such as liquid chromatography/mass spectrometry. We have demonstrated that ^{1}H-NMR, a technique not usually utilized in leachability experiments, is equally useful for this purpose with the added benefit of simple sample preparation and data interpretation [96]. Based on the gravimetric screening study of the series of protic and aprotic solvents, acetone was chosen as a solvent for quantitative NMR evaluation. Adding acetone-d$_6$ produced spectra with clearly defined peaks that were easy to integrate. Leachability from LC UDMA/PEG-U/HEMA/MEP copolymers and the corresponding am-ACP composites are shown in Fig. (**10**). The levels of the leachable moieties from detected in acetone extracts of UPHM copolymers and composites ranged from undetectable (CQ) to minimal/low {HEMA: 0.3% (copolymer) and 0.1% (composite); PEG-U: 2.1% (copolymer) and 1.1% (composite)} to moderate {UDMA: 7.1% (copolymer) and 5.3% (composite); MEP: 14.3% (copolymer) and 10.4% (composite)} to high {4EDMAB: 33.1% (copolymer) and 24.7% (composite)}. The differences between apparently higher values seen in copolymers compared to composites became marginal once the composite leachability data are normalized with respect to the initial amount of the resins. This finding suggests that introduction of ACP filler into resins had minimal or no effect on the leachability of non-polymerized monomeric species from this experimental material. A correlation of the leachability data (Fig. **10**) with the DVC results for LC UPHM copolymers and am-ACP UPHM composites (Fig. **9a**) reveals the following. There is a 10% reduction in DVC when going from UPHM copolymers to UPHM composites. At the same time, the attained DVC values in both UPHM copolymers and composites were high enough ($\geq 85\%$) to ensure that, in terms of a cross-linked system, differences between the two groups became insignificant. In systems this highly cross-linked, the degree of polymer chain mobility is small and pathways for unreacted monomers to leach-out are, therefore, restricted. Resultantly, leachability in these systems has become practically constant.

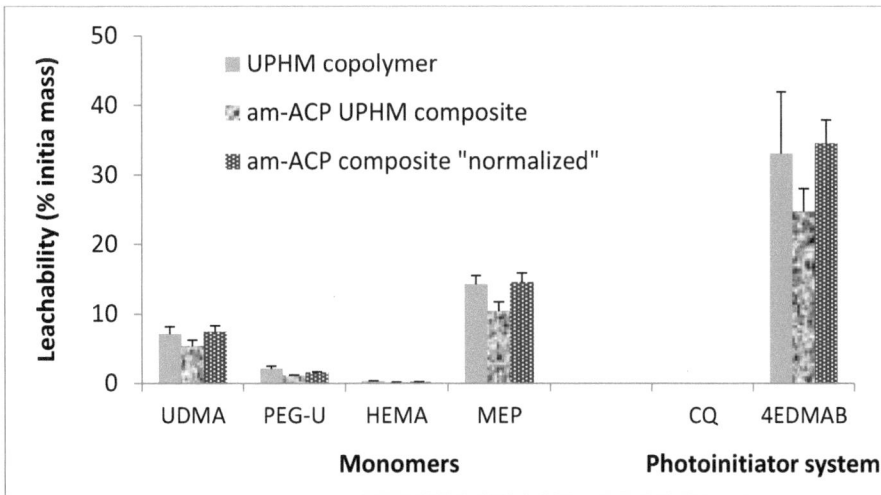

Fig. (10). A fraction (expressed as % of the initial mass; mean value + SD) of the unreacted monomers and components of the photoinitiator system leaching out from LC UPHM copolymers and their am-ACP composites. Number of repetitive measurements/group: n=3.

Whenever possible, leachability evaluation should be coupled with cytotoxicity studies. To assess cellular responses to UPHM copolymers and composites, we have cultured murine pre-osteoblast cells (MC3T3-E1) in the extracts of these specimens. Since the UPHM formulations were intended for endodontic application, a commercial endodontic sealer (CES) was utilized as a reference and media without any extracts were applied as a control. The *in situ* cell morphology examination by optical microscope revealed the spread, polygonal morphology in the control media and in the extracts of copolymers and ACP (powder only) pellets. However, contracted and spherical cell were seen in both extracts from am-ACP UPHM composites and from CES control (images not shown here). In addition to the morphological changes, cells exposed to extracts ACP UPHM composites and CES both exhibited 2.5 times slower proliferation the polygonal cells (Fig. **11**). The spherical morphology and slow proliferation of MC3T3 cells was also observed in hydrogel scaffolds for bone regeneration [114]. Alternation in cytoskeletal tension on nucleus and nucleus organization that ultimately affect the mineralization of progenitors were suggested for the observed morphological changes [115, 116]. Additional tests will be necessary to understand cellular responses to both the experimental ACP UPHM composite and the CES. However, to-date tests nevertheless indicate that the experimental ACP material is, at minimum, as good candidate for endodontic application as the chosen commercial counterpart which has a resin matrix similar to the resin phase of the ACP UPHM composite.

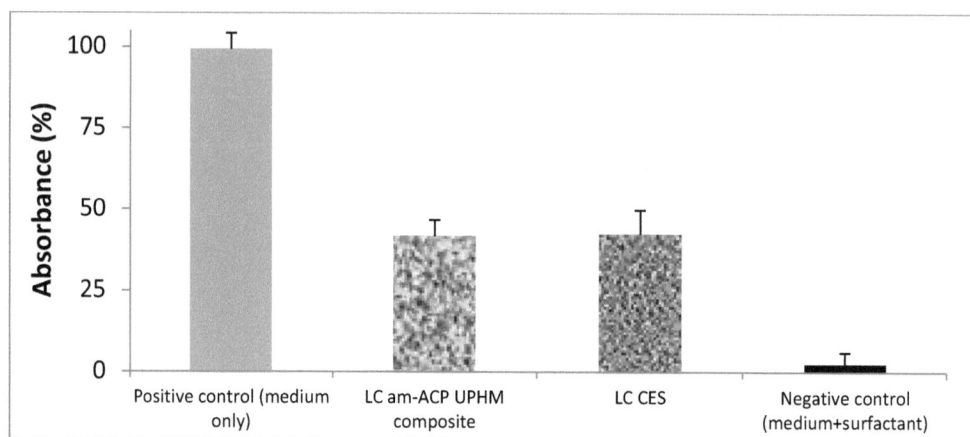

Fig. (11). Cell viability of LC am-ACP UPHM composites in comparison with commercial control (CES) positive and negative control (as indicated). Shown are mean values + SD for triplicate measurements.

Introducing AM Function: Preliminary Data

The classical Menschutkin reaction, *i.e.*, the addition reaction of tertiary amines with organo-halides [117], provides a facile approach to produce a wide variety of potentially AM monomers, oligomers, and polymers that have potential applications in a range of dental and biomedical materials. For example, step-growth polymerization based on the Menschutkin reaction yielded multiple QA functional groups in the backbone of these ionic polymers (termed ionenes) and imparted antimicrobial properties to the linear polymers [118, 119]. In our study [87], the Menschutkin reaction was adapted for the synthesis of free radical, photo-crosslinking, dimethacrylate monomers containing QA functionalities. These novel, reactive monomers can be designed to have solubility parameters similar to common dental resins and, therefore, are expected to be miscible with these resins. The resultant copolymers are expected to have lower monomer leachability and degradability due to multiple vinyl groups that lead to tighter polymer networks with increased crosslink density. Further, the class of monomers can be designed to contain one or more quaternary ammonium functionalities for reduced bacterial growth. Two cationic liquid AM monomers, bis(2-methacryloyloxy-ethyl) dimethylammonium bromide (IDMA-1) and 1,1'-bis[o-(2-methacryloyloxyethyl- 2'-methylphenylene) dimethylammonium bromide (IDMA-2) were successfully synthesized and characterized by FTIR spectroscopy (Fig. **12**). ^{1}H-NMR confirmed the assigned structures of IDMA-1 and IDMA-2.

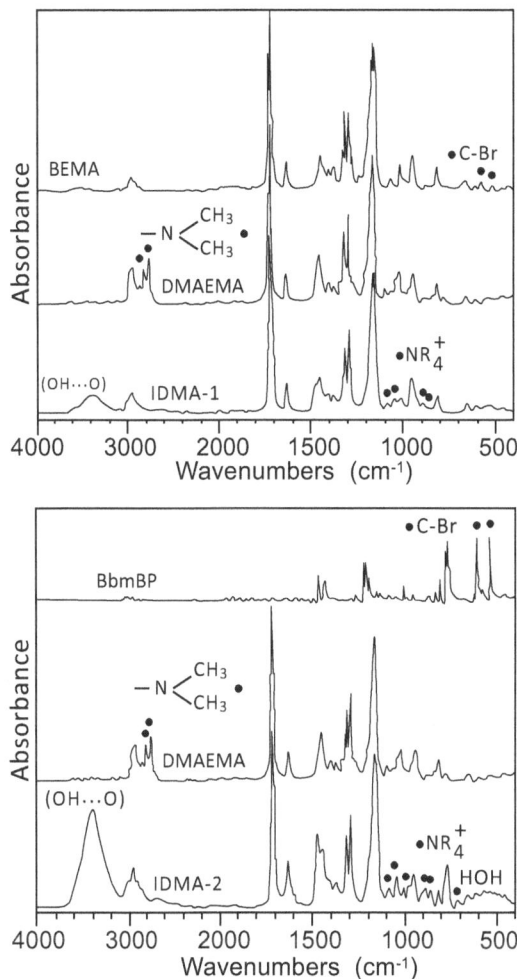

Fig. (12). FTIR spectra of reactants and low viscosity ionic dimethacrylate monomers IDMA-1 and IDMA-2 (as indicated). Both monomers displayed new bands at 1089 cm^{-1}, 1048 cm^{-1}, 886 cm^{-1}, and 858 cm^{-1}, and IDMA-2 also at 981 cm^{-1} and 712 cm^{-1}. These bands arise from vibrations of the NR^{4+} complexes [NR^{4+} groups have bands in the 1100 cm^{-1} to 450 cm^{-1} region]. Additional broad bands at 3412 cm^{-1} and 550 cm^{-1} arise from hydrogen-bonded water.

The viscosity of these monomers when incorporated into common dental monomers was characterized to assess how they affect the processability. The two dimethacrylates produced in this study were miscible with common dental resins, and the incorporation of IDMA-1 only slightly increased the viscosity of the BisGMA-TEGDMA 50:50 resin system. DVC and surface charge density both increased with the addition of IDMA-1, indicating that the charged monomer was well incorporated into the polymer network. Bis-GMA/TEGDMA resins containing various amounts of IDMA-1 were used to conduct a preliminary evaluation of the polymers' biological response in terms of both bacterial colonization and mammalian cell viability. The AM action of IDMA-1 containing Bis-GMA/ triethyleneglycol dimethacrylate (TEGDMA) resins was assessed by measuring surface charge density, bacterial attachment, macrophage viability and enzymatic activity. Fluorescein binding to the cationic QA groups revealed significant increases in the levels of QA sites on the surfaces of polymers with higher IDMA-1 content. Polymers with 30% IDMA-1 had approximately 200 times more QA sites than other formulations. IDMA-1 reduced bacteria colonization at all tested concentrations (Fig. **13**). Also, bacterial morphology on the surfaces was altered on polymers containing 30 mass % IDMA-1. Image analysis of the objects (single fluorescent entities) revealed no significant differences in object area due to IDMA-1 but confirmed that both object density and the surface coverage were significantly reduced in the presence of IDMA-1 as compared to that of 0% IDMA-1 controls. There were, however, no significant differences among the IDMA-1 levels for any quantitative bacterial adhesion parameters.

Staining was used to assess macrophage density and viability (Fig. **14**). The incorporation of 10% IDMA-1 significantly reduced cell density, and 20% and 30% IDMA-1 further reduced the density as compared to both 0% and 10% IDMA-1. Significantly, cell viability was unchanged at 10% IDMA-1 but significantly reduced by 20% and 30% IDMA-1. Therefore, although the cell density was much lower with 10% IDMA-1 as compared to 0% IDMA-1 control, the cell viability was not affected significantly. Macrophages on polymer disks (disk cells), as well as cells in the same wells as the polymer disks but adherent to the tissue culture polystyrene (TCPS) substrates, were evaluated independently (data not shown). The results for the disk cell dehydrogenase activity assay (MTT) agreed well with the viability results. At 10 mass %, IDMA-1 did not significantly affect the MTT activity while at higher IDMA-1 levels the MTT activity was significantly reduced. The results for the TCPS cells, however, showed no significant changes in MTT activity as a result of the inclusion of IDMA-1. It is clear from this screening that a desired AM effect on pathogens and the AM agent's potential cytotoxicity to mammalian cells need to be carefully balanced. These aspects will strongly impact design of a new family of AM remineralizing ACP composites.

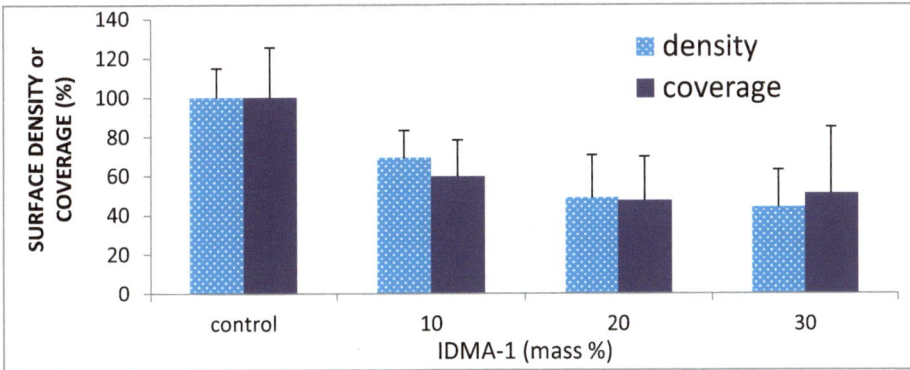

Fig. (13). Bacterial (*S. mutans*) density and surface coverage (mean value + SD; n=3) as a function of IDMA-1 concentration. Both parameters are plotted as a percentage of the control (no IDMA-1).

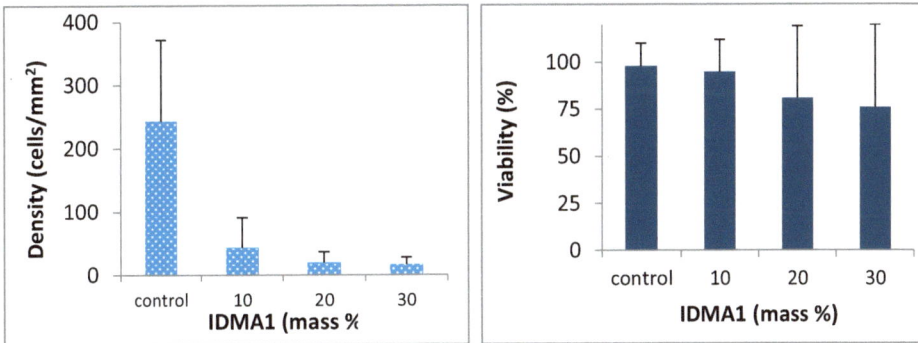

Fig. (14). Cell density (left panel) and viability (right panel) as a function of IDMA-1 concentration. Indicated are mean values + SD for six repetitive experiments in each group.

CONCLUDING REMARKS

ACP-based dental materials, generally appealing due to their biocompatibility, are especially attractive because they provide an extended supply of the remineralizing calcium and phosphate ions needed to reform damaged tooth mineral. Anti-cariogenic/remineralizing capability of ACP composites is particularly important since there is no known method for regenerating large amounts of tooth structures. Our studies of these unique materials promoted the development of hybrid and surface-modified ACPs, new polymeric chemistries and composite formulations. The comprehensive physicochemical, mechanical and biological testing improved our understanding of structure/composition/property relationships of ACP fillers and dental resins individually, as well as the interactions that control the properties of the resultant composites with their highly complex interfaces. The composite-related toxicological risks originating from materials themselves and/or from microbiological leakage are an integral part of our evaluation protocols. Lessons from our to-date studies will serve as a platform for designing a new generation of composites with dual, remineralizing and antimicrobial activity. These same lessons could also translate into development of ACP/biodegradable polymeric materials intended for generalized hard tissue regeneration.

ABBREVIATIONS

ACP	amorphous calcium phosphate
ADA	American Dental Association
ADAF	American Dental Association Foundation
AES	atomic emission spectroscopy
Ag	silver
Ag-ACP	silver-modified ACP
Al	aluminum
Al-ACP	aluminum-modified ACP
ALP	alkaline phosphatase
AM	antimicrobial
am-ACP	as-made ACP
ANOVA	analysis of variance
ANSI	American National Standards Institute
APTMS	3-aminopropyltrimethoxysilane
APTMS-ACP	APTMS-silanized ACP
ASTM	American Society for Testing and Materials
BFS	biaxial flexural strength
BH	Bis-GMA/HEMA resin
BHI	brain heart infusion
BHHm	Bis-GMA/HEMA/HmDMA resin
BHm	Bis-GMA/HmDMA resin
BHT	butylated hydroxyl toluene or Bis-GMA/HEMA/TEGDMA resin
Bis-GMA	2,2-bis[p-(2'-hydroxy-3'-methacryloxypropoxy) phenyl]propane
BPO	benzoyl peroxide
BT	Bis-GMA/TEGDMA resin
BTD	Bis-GMA/TEGDMA/DEGMEMA resin
BTGd	Bis-GMA/TEGDMA/GDMA resin
BTGm	Bis-GMA/TEGDMA/GMA resin

BTH	Bis-GMA/TEGDMA/HEMA resin
BTHZ	Bis-GMA/TEGDMA/HEMA/ZrDMA resin
BTM	Bis-GMA/TEGDMA/MA resin
BTMa	Bis-GMA/TEGDMA/MaA resin
BT4M	Bis-GMA/TEGDMA/4MET resin
BTV	Bis-GMA/TEGDMA/VPA resin
Ca	calcium
CaCl$_2$	calcium chloride
Ca(NO$_3$)$_2$	calcium nitrate
CaP	calcium phosphate
CC	chemical cure
CES	commercial endodontic sealer
COA	commercial orthodontic adhesive
CPP-ACP	casein phosphopeptide amorphous calcium phosphate
CQ	camphorquinone
4265 Darocur	commercial polymerization initiating system
DC	dual cure
DCPD	dicalcium phosphate dehydrate
DEGMEMA	di(ethylene glycol)methyl ether methacrylate
DHEPT	2,2'-dihydroxyethyl-p-toluidine
d$_m$	median particle diameter
DMSO	dimethylsulfoxide
DVC	degree of vinyl conversion
EBPADMA	ethoxylated bisphenol A dimethacrylate
4EDMAB	ethyl-4-N,N-dimethylamino benzoate
EDTA	ethylenediamine tetraacetic acid
EH	EBPADMA/HEMA resin
EHHm	EBPADMA/HEMA/HmDMA resin
EHm	EBPADMA/HmDMA resin
EHT	EBPADMA/HEMA/TEGDMA resin
ETHM	EBPADMA/TEGDMA/HEMA/MEP resin
FAP	fluoroapatite
Fe^{2+}-ACP	iron (II)-modified ACP
Fe^{3+}-ACP	iron (III)-modified ACP
FSN	non-ionic fluorosurfactant

FSP	anionic fluorosurfactant
FTIR	Fourier transform infrared spectroscopy
m-FTIR	FTIR micro-spectroscopy
ΔG°	Gibbs free energy
g-ACP	ground ACP
GMA	glyceryl methacrylate
GDMA	glyceryl dimethacrylate
HAP	hydroxyapatite
HE	hygroscopic expansion
HEMA	2-hydroxyethyl methacrylate
HEPES	4-(2-hydroxyethyl)-1-piperazineethane sulfonic acid
HmDMA	hexamethylene dimethacrylate
IAP	ion activity product
IDMA-1	bis(2-methacryloyloxyethyl) dimethylammonium bromide
IDMA-2	1,1'-bis[o-(2-methacryloyloxyethyl-2'-methylphenylene) dimethylammonium bromide
1850 Irgacure	commercial polymerization initiating system
369 Irgacure	commercial polymerization initiating system
KCl	potassium chloride
KOH	potassium hydroxide
K_{sp}	thermodynamic solubility product
LC	light cure
MA	methacrylic acid
MaA	maleic acid
m-ACP	milled ACP
MDBP	methacryloyloxydodecyl pyrimidinium bromide
MEP	methacryloyloxyethyl phthalate
4MET	mono-4-(methcryloyloxy)ethyl trimellitate
$MgCl_2 \cdot 6H_2O$	magnesium chloride hexahydrate
MPTMS	methacryloxypropyltrimethoxysilane
MPTMS-ACP	MPTMS-silanized ACP
MTT	methylthiazolyldiphenyl-tetrazolium bromide dehydrogenase activity assay
n	number of specimens (or repetitive experiments)
NaCl	sodium chloride
$NaHCO_3$	sodium hydrogen carbonate
Na_2HPO_4	sodium hydrogen phosphate

$Na_4P_2O_7$	sodium pyrophosphate
NIDCR	National Institute of Dental and Craniofacial Research
NIR	near infrared spectroscopy
NIST	National Institute of Standards and Technology
NMR	nuclear magnetic resonance
PAA	poly (acrylic acid)
PAA-ACP	PAA-modified ACP
PBS	phosphate buffered saline solution
PEG-U	poly(ethylene glycol) extended urethane dimethacrylate
PEO	polyethylene oxide
PEO-ACP	PEO-modified ACP
pH	-log (molar concentration of hydrogen ions)
PMGDMA	pyromellitic glycerol dimethacrylate
PS	polymerization shrinkage
PSD	particle size distribution
PSS	polymerization shrinkage stress
QA	quaternary ammonium
QP	quaternary phosphonium
R	ideal gas constant
RH	relative humidity
SBS	shear bond strength
SEM	scanning electron microscopy
SD	standard deviation
Si	silicon
Si-ACP	silicon-modified ACP
T	absolute temperature
TCPS	tissue culture polystyrene
TEGDMA	triethylene glycol dimethacrylate
TGA	thermogravimetric analysis
TRITON	alkyl aryl polyether alcohol (nonionic surfactant)
TWEEN	poly(oxyethylene) sorbitan monolaureate (nonionic surfactant)
UDMA	urethane dimetahcrylate
UH	UDMA/HEMA resin
UHHm	UDMA/HEMA/HmDMA resin
UHm	UDMA/HmDMA resin

UHT	UDMA/HEMA/TEGDMA resin
UPHM	UDMA/PEG-U/HEMA/MEP resin
VPA	vinyl phosphonic acid
VRC	Volpe Research Center
WS	water sorption
Wst1	mitochondrial dehydrogenase activity assay
XRD	X-ray diffraction
Zn	zinc
Zn-ACP	zinc-modified ACP
Zr	zirconia
Zr-ACP	zirconia-modified ACP
ZrDMA	zirconyl dimethacrylate

CONFLICT OF INTEREST

The authors declare no conflict of interest, financial or otherwise.

ACKNOWLEDGEMENTS

This work was supported by the American Dental Association Foundation, the National Institute of Standards and Technology and by the National Institute of Dental and Craniofacial Research (grants DE13169 and DE26122 to D. Skrtic). We gratefully acknowledge donation of the monomers from Esstech, Essington, PA, USA.

REFERENCES

[1]   Kassebaum NJ, Bernabé E, Dahiya M, Bhandari B, Murray CJ, Marcenes W. Global burden of untreated caries: a systematic review and metaregression. J Dent Res 2015; 94(5): 650-8.
        [http://dx.doi.org/10.1177/0022034515573272] [PMID: 25740856]

[2]   Pendrys DG, Stamm JW. Relationship of total fluoride intake to beneficial effects and enamel fluorosis. J Dent Res 1990; 69(Spec No): 529-38.
        [http://dx.doi.org/10.1177/00220345900690S107] [PMID: 2179311]

[3]   Reynolds EC, Black CL, Cai F, *et al.* Advances in enamel remineralization: Casein-phosphopeptid--amorphous calcium phosphate. J Clin Dent 1999; 10(2): 86-8.

[4]   Reynolds EC, Cai F, Shen P, Walker GD. Retention in plaque and remineralization of enamel lesions by various forms of calcium in a mouthrinse or sugar-free chewing gum. J Dent Res 2003; 82(3): 206-11.
        [http://dx.doi.org/10.1177/154405910308200311] [PMID: 12598550]

[5]   Reynolds EC, Cai F, Cochrane NJ, *et al.* Fluoride and casein phosphopeptide-amorphous calcium phosphate. J Dent Res 2008; 87(4): 344-8.
        [http://dx.doi.org/10.1177/154405910808700420] [PMID: 18362316]

[6]   Reynolds EC. Calcium phosphate-based remineralization systems: scientific evidence? Aust Dent J

2008; 53(3): 268-73.
[http://dx.doi.org/10.1111/j.1834-7819.2008.00061.x] [PMID: 18782374]

[7]   Antonucci JM, Skrtic D, Hailer AW, *et al.* Bioactive Polymeric Composites Based on Hybrid Amorphous Calcium Phosphate. In: Ottenbrite RM, Kim SW, Eds. Polymeric Drugs and Drug Delivery Systems. Lancaster: Technomics Publ Co 2000; pp. 301-10.

[8]   Skrtic D, Antonucci JM, Eanes ED. Amorphous calcium phosphate-based bioactive polymeric composites for mineralized tissue regeneration. J Res Natl Inst Stand Technol 2003; 108(3): 167-82.
[http://dx.doi.org/10.6028/jres.108.017] [PMID: 27413603]

[9]   Antonucci JM, Skrtic D. Physicochemical Properties of Bioactive Polymeric Composites: Effects of Resin Matrix and the Type of Amorphous Calcium Phosphate Filler. In: Shalaby SW, Salz U, Eds. Polymers for Dental and Orthopedic Applications. Boca Raton: CRC Press 2007; pp. 217-42.

[10]   Tung MS, Eichmiller FC. Dental applications of amorphous calcium phosphates. J Clin Dent 1999; 10(1 Spec No): 1-6.
[PMID: 10686850]

[11]   Eanes ED. Amorphous Calcium Phosphate. In: Chow LC, Eanes ED, Eds. Octacalcium Phosphate Monogr Oral Sci. Basel: Karger 2001; Vol. 18: pp. 130-47.
[http://dx.doi.org/10.1159/000061652]

[12]   Weiner S. Transient precursor strategy in mineral formation of bone. Bone 2006; 39(3): 431-3.
[http://dx.doi.org/10.1016/j.bone.2006.02.058] [PMID: 16581322]

[13]   Beniash E, Metzler RA, Lam RS, Gilbert PU. Transient amorphous calcium phosphate in forming enamel. J Struct Biol 2009; 166(2): 133-43.
[http://dx.doi.org/10.1016/j.jsb.2009.02.001] [PMID: 19217943]

[14]   Zhao J, Liu Y, Sun W, *et al.* First detection, characterization and application of amorphous calcium phosphate in dentistry. J Dent Sci 2012; 7: 316-23.
[http://dx.doi.org/10.1016/j.jds.2012.09.001]

[15]   Dorozhkin SV. Calcium orthophosphates in dentistry. J Mater Sci Mater Med 2013; 24(6): 1335-63.
[http://dx.doi.org/10.1007/s10856-013-4898-1] [PMID: 23468163]

[16]   Heughebaert JC, Montel G. Conversion of amorphous tricalcium phosphate into apatitic tricalcium phosphate. Calcif Tissue Int 1982; 34 (Suppl. 2): S103-8.
[PMID: 6293671]

[17]   Eanes ED. Amorphous calcium phosphate: Thermodynamic and kinetic considerations. In: Amjad Z, Ed. Calcium Phosphates in Biological and Industrial Systems. Boston: Kluwer Academic Publ. 1998; pp. 21-39.
[http://dx.doi.org/10.1007/978-1-4615-5517-9_2]

[18]   Meyer JL, Eanes ED. A thermodynamic analysis of the amorphous to crystalline calcium phosphate transformation. Calcif Tissue Res 1978; 25(1): 59-68.
[http://dx.doi.org/10.1007/BF02010752] [PMID: 25699]

[19]   Meyer JL. Phase transformations in the spontaneous precipitation of calcium phosphate. Croat Chem Acta 1983; 21(8): 753-67.

[20]   Blumenthal NC. Basic science and pathology. Mechanisms of inhibition of calcification. Clin Orhop. &. Rel Res 1989; 247: 279-89.

[21]   Abbona F, Baronnet A. A XRD abd TEM study on the transformation of amorphous calcium phosphate in the presence of magnesium. J Cryst Growth 1996; 165: 98-105.
[http://dx.doi.org/10.1016/0022-0248(96)00156-X]

[22]   LeGeros RZ. Formation and transformation of calcium phosphates: Relevance to vascular calcification. Z Kardiol 2001; 2001(Suppl 3): III/116-24.

[23]   Bowen RL. Adhesive bonding of various materials to hard tissues. VII. Metal salts and mordants for

coupling agents. In: Moskovitz HD, Ward GT, Woolridge ED, Eds. Dental Adhesive Materials. New York: Prestige Graphic Services 1974; pp. 205-21.

[24] Ito A, Kawamura H, Miyakawa S, *et al.* Fabrication of Zn containing apatite cement and its initial evaluation using human osteoblastic cells. Biometerials 2002; pp. 423-8.

[25] LeGeros RZ, Bleiwas CB, Retino M, Rohanizadeh R, LeGeros JP. Zinc effect on the *in vitro* formation of calcium phosphates: relevance to clinical inhibition of calculus formation. Am J Dent 1999; 12(2): 65-71.
[PMID: 10477985]

[26] Hidaka S, Okamoto Y, Abe K, Miyazaki K. Effects of indium and iron ions on *in vitro* calcium phosphate precipitation and crystallinity. J Biomed Mater Res 1996; 31(1): 11-8.
[http://dx.doi.org/10.1002/(SICI)1097-4636(199605)31:1<11::AID-JBM2>3.0.CO;2-T]   [PMID: 8731144]

[27] Wu W, Cobb EN. A silver staining technique for investigating wear of restorative dental composites. J Biomed Mater Res 1981; 15(3): 343-8.
[http://dx.doi.org/10.1002/jbm.820150306] [PMID: 6183267]

[28] Wilson AD, Nicholson JW. Chemistry of solid state materials 3 acid base cements their biomedical and industrial applications. Cambridge: Cambridge Univ Press 1993; pp. 56-102.
[http://dx.doi.org/10.1017/CBO9780511524813.005]

[29] Skrtic D, Antonucci JM, Eanes ED, Brunworth RT. Silica- and zirconia-hybridized amorphous calcium phosphate: effect on transformation to hydroxyapatite. J Biomed Mater Res 2002; 59(4): 597-604.
[http://dx.doi.org/10.1002/jbm.10017] [PMID: 11774320]

[30] Begala AJ, Strauss UP. Dilatomteric studies of counterion binding by polycarbonates. J Phys Chem 1972; 76: 254-60.
[http://dx.doi.org/10.1021/j100646a020]

[31] Nishiyama N, Ishizaki T, Horie K, Tomari M, Someya M. Novel polyfunctional silanes for improved hydrolytic stability at the polymer-silica interface. J Biomed Mater Res 1991; 25(2): 213-21.
[http://dx.doi.org/10.1002/jbm.820250208] [PMID: 1647393]

[32] Jones DW, Rizkalla AS. Characterization of experimental composite biomaterials. J Biomed Mater Res 1996; 33(2): 89-100. [Appl Biomater].
[http://dx.doi.org/10.1002/(SICI)1097-4636(199622)33:2<89::AID-JBM5>3.0.CO;2-H]   [PMID: 8736027]

[33] Liu Q, de Wijn JR, de Groot K, van Blitterswijk CA. Surface modification of nano-apatite by grafting organic polymer. Biomaterials 1998; 19(11-12): 1067-72.
[http://dx.doi.org/10.1016/S0142-9612(98)00033-7] [PMID: 9692805]

[34] Mohsen NM, Craig RG. Hydrolytic stability of silanated zirconia-silica-urethane dimethacrylate composites. J Oral Rehabil 1995; 22(3): 213-20.
[http://dx.doi.org/10.1111/j.1365-2842.1995.tb01566.x] [PMID: 7769516]

[35] Dupraz AM, de Wijn JR, v d Meer SA, de Groot K. Characterization of silane-treated hydroxyapatite powders for use as filler in biodegradable composites. J Biomed Mater Res 1996; 30(2): 231-8.
[http://dx.doi.org/10.1002/(SICI)1097-4636(199602)30:2<231::AID-JBM13>3.0.CO;2-P]   [PMID: 9019488]

[36] Venhoven BA, de Gee AJ, Werner A, Davidson CL. Influence of filler parameters on the mechanical coherence of dental restorative resin composites. Biomaterials 1996; 17(7): 735-40.
[http://dx.doi.org/10.1016/0142-9612(96)86744-5] [PMID: 8672636]

[37] Silane Coupling Agents. Connecting Across Boundaries Morrisville. Gelest 2003; pp. 4-5.

[38] Morgan DR, Kalachandra S, Shobha HK, Gunduz N, Stejskal EO. Analysis of a dimethacrylate copolymer (bis-GMA and TEGDMA) network by DSC and 13C solution and solid-state NMR

spectroscopy. Biomaterials 2000; 21(18): 1897-903.
[http://dx.doi.org/10.1016/S0142-9612(00)00067-3] [PMID: 10919693]

[39]   Stansbury JW, Dickens SH. Network formation and compositional drift during photoinitiated copolymerization of dimethacrylate monomers. Polymer (Guildf) 2001; 42: 6363-9.
[http://dx.doi.org/10.1016/S0032-3861(01)00106-9]

[40]   Antonucci JM, Stansbury JW. Molecularly Designed Dental Polymers. In: Arshady R, Ed. Desk Reference of Functional Polymers Syntheses and Applications. Washington, DC: ACS 1997; pp. 719-38.

[41]   Antonucci JM, Liu DW, Stansbury JW. Synthesis of hydrophobic oligomeric monomers for dental applications. J Dent Res 1993; 72: 369.

[42]   Asmussen E, Peutzfeldt A. Influence of UEDMA BisGMA and TEGDMA on selected mechanical properties of experimental resin composites. Dent Mater 1998; 14(1): 51-6.
[http://dx.doi.org/10.1016/S0109-5641(98)00009-8] [PMID: 9972151]

[43]   Morra M. Acid-base properties of adhesive dental polymers. Dent Mater 1993; 9(6): 375-8.
[http://dx.doi.org/10.1016/0109-5641(93)90060-4] [PMID: 7988771]

[44]   Kurashina K, Kurita H, Hirano M, Kotani A, Klein CP, de Groot K. *In vivo* study of calcium phosphate cements: implantation of an alpha-tricalcium phosphate/dicalcium phosphate dibasic/tetracalcium phosphate monoxide cement paste. Biomaterials 1997; 18(7): 539-43.
[http://dx.doi.org/10.1016/S0142-9612(96)00162-7] [PMID: 9105593]

[45]   Costantino PD, Friedman CD, Jones K, Chow LC, Sisson GA. Experimental hydroxyapatite cement cranioplasty. Plast Reconstr Surg 1992; 90(2): 174-85.
[http://dx.doi.org/10.1097/00006534-199290020-00003] [PMID: 1321453]

[46]   Wiltfang J, Merten HA, Schlegel KA, *et al.* Degradation characteristics of alpha and beta tri-calciu--phosphate (TCP) in minipigs. J Biomed Mater Res 2002; 63(2): 115-21.
[http://dx.doi.org/10.1002/jbm.10084] [PMID: 11870643]

[47]   Ehara A, Ogata K, Imazato S, Ebisu S, Nakano T, Umakoshi Y. Effects of alpha-TCP and TetCP on MC3T3-E1 proliferation, differentiation and mineralization. Biomaterials 2003; 24(5): 831-6.
[http://dx.doi.org/10.1016/S0142-9612(02)00411-8] [PMID: 12485801]

[48]   Skrtic D, Antonucci JM, Eanes ED, Eidelman N. Dental composites based on hybrid and surface-modified amorphous calcium phosphates. Biomaterials 2004; 25(7-8): 1141-50.
[http://dx.doi.org/10.1016/j.biomaterials.2003.08.001] [PMID: 14643587]

[49]   Antonucci JM, Skrtic D. Matrix resin effects on selected physicohemical properties of amorphous calcium phosphate composites. J Bioact Compat Polym 2005; 20: 29-49.
[http://dx.doi.org/10.1177/0883911505050082]

[50]   Yamaguchi T, Chattopadhyay N, Kifor O, Butters RR Jr, Sugimoto T, Brown EM. Mouse osteoblastic cell line (MC3T3-E1) expresses extracellular calcium ($Ca^{2+}o$)-sensing receptor and its agonists stimulate chemotaxis and proliferation of MC3T3-E1 cells. J Bone Miner Res 1998; 13(10): 1530-8.
[http://dx.doi.org/10.1359/jbmr.1998.13.10.1530] [PMID: 9783541]

[51]   Xynos ID, Edgar AJ, Buttery LD, Hench LL, Polak JM. Gene-expression profiling of human osteoblasts following treatment with the ionic products of Bioglass 45S5 dissolution. J Biomed Mater Res 2001; 55(2): 151-7.
[http://dx.doi.org/10.1002/1097-4636(200105)55:2<151::AID-JBM1001>3.0.CO;2-D]   [PMID: 11255166]

[52]   Keeting PE, Oursler MJ, Wiegand KE, Bonde SK, Spelsberg TC, Riggs BL. Zeolite A increases proliferation, differentiation, and transforming growth factor beta production in normal adult human osteoblast-like cells *in vitro*. J Bone Miner Res 1992; 7(11): 1281-9.
[http://dx.doi.org/10.1002/jbmr.5650071107] [PMID: 1334616]

[53]   Beck GR Jr, Zerler B, Moran E. Phosphate is a specific signal for induction of osteopontin gene

expression. Proc Natl Acad Sci USA 2000; 97(15): 8352-7.
[http://dx.doi.org/10.1073/pnas.140021997] [PMID: 10890885]

[54]   Pelka M, Distler W, Petschelt A. Elution parameters and HPLC-detection of single components from resin composite. Clin Oral Investig 1999; 3(4): 194-200.
[http://dx.doi.org/10.1007/s007840050101] [PMID: 10803134]

[55]   Spahl W, Budzikiewicz H, Geurtsen W. Determination of leachable components from four commercial dental composites by gas and liquid chromatography/mass spectrometry. J Dent 1998; 26(2): 137-45.
[http://dx.doi.org/10.1016/S0300-5712(96)00086-3] [PMID: 9540311]

[56]   Schweikl H, Schmalz G, Spruss T. The induction of micronuclei *in vitro* by unpolymerized resin monomers. J Dent Res 2001; 80(7): 1615-20.
[http://dx.doi.org/10.1177/00220345010800070401] [PMID: 11597020]

[57]   Ratanasathien S, Wataha JC, Hanks CT, Dennison JB. Cytotoxic interactive effects of dentin bonding components on mouse fibroblasts. J Dent Res 1995; 74(9): 1602-6.
[http://dx.doi.org/10.1177/00220345950740091601] [PMID: 7560423]

[58]   Imazato S. Bio-active restorative materials with antibacterial effects: new dimension of innovation in restorative dentistry. Dent Mater J 2009; 28(1): 11-9.
[http://dx.doi.org/10.4012/dmj.28.11] [PMID: 19280964]

[59]   Pereira-Cenci T, Cenci MS, Fedorowicz Z, Marchesan MA. Antibacterial agents in composite restorations for the prevention of dental caries. Cochrane Database Syst Rev 2009; 8(3): CD007819.
[PMID: 19588443]

[60]   Jedrychowski JR, Caputo AA, Kerper S. Antibacterial and mechanical properties of restorative materials combined with chlorhexidines. J Oral Rehabil 1983; 10(5): 373-81.
[http://dx.doi.org/10.1111/j.1365-2842.1983.tb00133.x] [PMID: 6355413]

[61]   Wiegand A, Buchalla W, Attin T. Review on fluoride-releasing restorative materials--fluoride release and uptake characteristics, antibacterial activity and influence on caries formation. Dent Mater 2007; 23(3): 343-62.
[http://dx.doi.org/10.1016/j.dental.2006.01.022] [PMID: 16616773]

[62]   Osinaga PW, Grande RH, Ballester RY, Simionato MR, Delgado Rodrigues CR, Muench A. Zinc sulfate addition to glass-ionomer-based cements: influence on physical and antibacterial properties, zinc and fluoride release. Dent Mater 2003; 19(3): 212-7.
[http://dx.doi.org/10.1016/S0109-5641(02)00032-5] [PMID: 12628433]

[63]   Takahashi Y, Imazato S, Kaneshiro AV, Ebisu S, Frencken JE, Tay FR. Antibacterial effects and physical properties of glass-ionomer cements containing chlorhexidine for the ART approach. Dent Mater 2006; 22(7): 647-52.
[http://dx.doi.org/10.1016/j.dental.2005.08.003] [PMID: 16226806]

[64]   Syafiuddin T, Hisamitsu H, Toko T, *et al.* *In vitro* inhibition of caries around a resin composite restoration containing antibacterial filler. Biomaterials 1997; 18(15): 1051-7.
[http://dx.doi.org/10.1016/S0142-9612(97)88072-6] [PMID: 9239467]

[65]   Knetsch ML, Koole LH. New strategies in the development of antimicrobial coatings: The example of increasing usage of silver and silver nanoparticles. Polymers (Basel) 2011; 3: 340-66.
[http://dx.doi.org/10.3390/polym3010340]

[66]   Dallas P, Sharma VK, Zboril R. Silver polymeric nanocomposites as advanced antimicrobial agents: classification, synthetic paths, applications, and perspectives. Adv Colloid Interface Sci 2011; 166(1-2): 119-35.
[http://dx.doi.org/10.1016/j.cis.2011.05.008] [PMID: 21683320]

[67]   Yoshida K, Tanagawa M, Atsuta M. Characterization and inhibitory effect of antibacterial dental resin composites incorporating silver-supported materials. J Biomed Mater Res 1999; 47(4): 516-22.

[http://dx.doi.org/10.1002/(SICI)1097-4636(19991215)47:4<516::AID-JBM7>3.0.CO;2-E]   [PMID: 10497286]

[68]   Kawahara K, Tsuruda K, Morishita M, Uchida M. Antibacterial effect of silver-zeolite on oral bacteria under anaerobic conditions. Dent Mater 2000; 16(6): 452-5.
[http://dx.doi.org/10.1016/S0109-5641(00)00050-6] [PMID: 10967196]

[69]   Weng Y, Guo X, Chong VJ, *et al.* Synthesis and evaluation of novel antibacterial dental resin composite with quaternary ammonium salts. J Biomed Sci Eng 2011; 4: 147-57.
[http://dx.doi.org/10.4236/jbise.2011.43021]

[70]   Li F, Chen J, Chai Z, *et al.* Effects of a dental adhesive incorporating antibacterial monomer on the growth, adherence and membrane integrity of Streptococcus mutans. J Dent 2009; 37(4): 289-96.
[http://dx.doi.org/10.1016/j.jdent.2008.12.004] [PMID: 19185408]

[71]   Bodor N, Kaminski JJ, Selk S. Soft drugs. 1. Labile quaternary ammonium salts as soft antimicrobials. J Med Chem 1980; 23(5): 469-74.
[http://dx.doi.org/10.1021/jm00179a001] [PMID: 7381846]

[72]   Inácio AS, Costa GN, Domingues NS, *et al.* Mitochondrial dysfunction is the focus of quaternary ammonium surfactant toxicity to mammalian epithelial cells. Antimicrob Agents Chemother 2013; 57(6): 2631-9.
[http://dx.doi.org/10.1128/AAC.02437-12] [PMID: 23529737]

[73]   Lichtenberg D, Opatowski E, Kozlov MM. Phase boundaries in mixtures of membrane-forming amphiphiles and micelle-forming amphiphiles. Biochim Biophys Acta 2000; 1508(1-2): 1-19.
[http://dx.doi.org/10.1016/S0304-4157(00)00004-6] [PMID: 11090815]

[74]   Prete PS, Domingues CC, Meirelles NC, *et al.* Multiple stages of detergent-erythrocyte membrane interaction: a spin label study 1808.

[75]   Kenawy ER, Worley SD, Broughton R. The chemistry and application of antimicrobial polymers: A state-of-the-art review. Biomacromolecules 2002; 8(5): 1359-84.
[http://dx.doi.org/10.1021/bm061150q]

[76]   Thorsteinsson T, Loftsson T, Masson M. Soft antibacterial agents. Curr Med Chem 2003; 10(13): 1129-36.
[http://dx.doi.org/10.2174/0929867033457520] [PMID: 12678806]

[77]   Murata H, Koepsel RR, Matyjaszewski K, Russell AJ. Permanent, non-leaching antibacterial surface--2: how high density cationic surfaces kill bacterial cells. Biomaterials 2007; 28(32): 4870-9.
[http://dx.doi.org/10.1016/j.biomaterials.2007.06.012] [PMID: 17706762]

[78]   Chen CZ, Beck-Tan NC, Dhurjati P, van Dyk TK, LaRossa RA, Cooper SL. Quaternary ammonium functionalized poly(propylene imine) dendrimers as effective antimicrobials: structure-activity studies. Biomacromolecules 2000; 1(3): 473-80.
[http://dx.doi.org/10.1021/bm0055495] [PMID: 11710139]

[79]   Ikeda T, Hirayama H, Yamaguchi H, Tazuke S, Watanabe M. Polycationic biocides with pendant active groups: molecular weight dependence of antibacterial activity. Antimicrob Agents Chemother 1986; 30(1): 132-6.
[http://dx.doi.org/10.1128/AAC.30.1.132] [PMID: 3092730]

[80]   Nonaka T, Hua L, Ogata T, *et al.* Synthesis of water-soluble thermosensitive polymers having phosphonium group from methacryloyloxyethyl trialkyl phosphonium chloride – N-isopropylacrylamide copolymers and their functions. J Appl Polym Sci 2003; 87(3): 386-93.
[http://dx.doi.org/10.1002/app.11362]

[81]   Thome T, Mayer MP, Imazato G, *et al. In vitro* analysis of the antibacterial monomer MDPB-containing restorations on the progression of secondary caries. J Dent 2009; 37: 705-11.
[http://dx.doi.org/10.1016/j.jdent.2009.05.024] [PMID: 19540033]

[82]   Imazato S, Tarumi H, Kato S, Ebisu S. Water sorption and colour stability of composites containing

the antibacterial monomer MDPB. J Dent 1999; 27(4): 279-83.
[http://dx.doi.org/10.1016/S0300-5712(98)00006-2] [PMID: 10193105]

[83]   Ebi N, Imazato S, Noiri Y, Ebisu S. Inhibitory effects of resin composite containing bactericide-immobilized filler on plaque accumulation. Dent Mater 2001; 17(6): 485-91.
[http://dx.doi.org/10.1016/S0109-5641(01)00006-9] [PMID: 11567685]

[84]   Lee SB, Koepsel RR, Morley SW, Matyjaszewski K, Sun Y, Russell AJ. Permanent, nonleaching antibacterial surfaces. 1. Synthesis by atom transfer radical polymerization. Biomacromolecules 2004; 5(3): 877-82.
[http://dx.doi.org/10.1021/bm034352k] [PMID: 15132676]

[85]   Li F, Chai ZG, Sun MN, *et al.* Anti-biofilm effect of dental adhesive with cationic monomer. J Dent Res 2009; 88(4): 372-6.
[http://dx.doi.org/10.1177/0022034509334499] [PMID: 19407160]

[86]   Beyth N, Yudovin-Farber I, Bahir R, Domb AJ, Weiss EI. Antibacterial activity of dental composites containing quaternary ammonium polyethylenimine nanoparticles against Streptococcus mutans. Biomaterials 2006; 27(21): 3995-4002.
[http://dx.doi.org/10.1016/j.biomaterials.2006.03.003] [PMID: 16564083]

[87]   Antonucci JM. Polymerizable biomedical composition. US patent No 8,217,081 B2, issued July 10 2012.

[88]   Antonucci JM, Zeiger DN, Tang K, Lin-Gibson S, Fowler BO, Lin NJ. Synthesis and characterization of dimethacrylates containing quaternary ammonium functionalities for dental applications. Dent Mater 2012; 28(2): 219-28.
[http://dx.doi.org/10.1016/j.dental.2011.10.004] [PMID: 22035983]

[89]   Antonucci JM, Skrtic D. Physicochemical and mechanical evaluation of cation-modified ACP acrylic resin composites. Polymer Prepr 2006; 47(2): 113-4.
[PMID: 24465058]

[90]   Antonucci JM, Liu DW, Skrtic D. Amorphous calcium phosphate based composites: Effect of surfactants and poly(ethylene) oxide on filler and composite properties. J Dispers Sci Technol 2007; 28(5): 819-24.
[http://dx.doi.org/10.1080/01932690701346255] [PMID: 18714365]

[91]   Antonucci JM, Skrtic D. Bioactive and biocompatible polymeric composites based on amorphous calcium phosphate. In: Ramalingam M, Tiwari A, Ramakrishna S, Kobayashi H, Eds. Integrated Biomaterials for Medical Applications. Salem: Scrivener Publishing 2012; pp. 67-119.
[http://dx.doi.org/10.1002/9781118482513.ch3]

[92]   O'Donnell JN, Skrtic D. Degree of vinyl conversion, polymerization shrinkage and stress development in experimental endodontic composite. J Biomim Biomater Tissue Eng 2009; 4: 1-12.
[http://dx.doi.org/10.4028/www.scientific.net/JBBTE.4.1] [PMID: 20411033]

[93]   Lee SY, Regnault WF, Antonucci JM, Skrtic D. Effect of particle size of an amorphous calcium phosphate filler on the mechanical strength and ion release of polymeric composites. J Biomed Mater Res B Appl Biomater 2007; 80(1): 11-7.
[http://dx.doi.org/10.1002/jbm.b.30561] [PMID: 16649181]

[94]   O'Donnell JN, Antonucci JM, Skrtic D. Illuminating the role of agglomerates on critical physicochemical properties of amorphous calcium phosphate composites. J Compos Mater 2008; 42(21): 2231-46.
[http://dx.doi.org/10.1177/0021998308094797] [PMID: 19774100]

[95]   Davis CH, O'Donnell JN, Sun J, *et al.* Fabrication and Evaluation of Bioactive Dental Composites Based on Amorphous Calcium Phosphate. In: Song DB, Ed. Resin Composites: Properties, Production and Application. Hauppauge: Nova Science Publishers 2011; pp. 55-100.

[96]   Antonucci JM, O'Donnell JN, Skrtic D. Polymerization shrinkage stress development and mechanical

strength of ACP acrylic resin composites. Polym Mater Sci Eng 2007; 96: 229-31.

[97]   Antonucci JM, Regnault WF, Skrtic D. Polymerization shrinkage and stress development in amorphous calcium phosphate/urethane dimethacrylate polymeric composites. J Compos Mater 2010; 44(3): 355-67.
        [http://dx.doi.org/10.1177/0021998309345180] [PMID: 20169007]

[98]   Lu H, Stansbury JW, Dickens SH, Eichmiller FC, Bowman CN. Probing the origins and control of shrinkage stress in dental resin-composites: I. Shrinkage stress characterization technique. J Mater Sci Mater Med 2004; 15(10): 1097-103.
        [http://dx.doi.org/10.1023/B:JMSM.0000046391.07274.e6] [PMID: 15516870]

[99]   ASTM F394-78 (re-approved 1991): Standard Test Method for Biaxial Strength (Modulus of Rupture) of Ceramic Substrates.

[100]   Skrtic D, Antonucci JM. Effect of bifunctional comonomers on mechanical strength and water sorption of amorphous calcium phosphate- and silanized glass-filled Bis-GMA-based composites. Biomaterials 2003; 24(17): 2881-8.
        [http://dx.doi.org/10.1016/S0142-9612(03)00119-4] [PMID: 12742726]

[101]   International Standard ISO 7405. Dentistry-Preclinical Evaluation of Biocompatibility of Medical Devices Used in Dentistry - Test Methods for Dental Materials 1997.

[102]   International Standard ISO 10993-5. Biological Evaluation of Medical Devices – Part 5: Tests for Cytotoxicity: *In vitro*. Methods 1992.

[103]   ANSI/ADA Specification No. 41: Recommended Standard Practices for Biological Evaluation of Dental Materials 2005.

[104]   Simon CG, Antonucci JM, Liu DW, *et al. In vitro* cytotoxicity of amorphous calcium phosphate composites. J Bioact Compat Polym 2005; 20(5): 279-95.
        [http://dx.doi.org/10.1177/0883911505051854]

[105]   Venhoven BA, de Gee AJ, Davidson CL. Polymerization contraction and conversion of light-curing BisGMA-based methacrylate resins. Biomaterials 1993; 14(11): 871-5.
        [http://dx.doi.org/10.1016/0142-9612(93)90010-Y] [PMID: 8218741]

[106]   Labella R, Lambrechts P, Van Meerbeek B, Vanherle G. Polymerization shrinkage and elasticity of flowable composites and filled adhesives. Dent Mater 1999; 15(2): 128-37.
        [http://dx.doi.org/10.1016/S0109-5641(99)00022-6] [PMID: 10551104]

[107]   Guggenberger R, Weinmann W. Exploring beyond methacrylates. Am J Dent 2000; 13(Spec No): 82D-4D.
        [PMID: 11763922]

[108]   Tilbrook DA, Clarke RL, Howle NE, Braden M. Photocurable epoxy-polyol matrices for use in dental composites I. Biomaterials 2000; 21(17): 1743-53.
        [http://dx.doi.org/10.1016/S0142-9612(00)00059-4] [PMID: 10905456]

[109]   Arima T, Hamada T, McCabe JF. The effects of cross-linking agents on some properties of HEMA-based resins. J Dent Res 1995; 74(9): 1597-601.
        [http://dx.doi.org/10.1177/00220345950740091501] [PMID: 7560422]

[110]   Garcia-Fiero JL, Aleman JV. Sorption of water by epoxide prepolymers. Macromolecules 1982; 15: 1145-9.
        [http://dx.doi.org/10.1021/ma00232a036]

[111]   Skrtic D, Antonucci JM. Dental composites based on amorphous calcium phosphate - resin composition/physicochemical properties study. J Biomater Appl 2007; 21(4): 375-93.
        [http://dx.doi.org/10.1177/0885328206064823] [PMID: 16684798]

[112]   Momoi Y, McCabe JF. Hygroscopic expansion of resin based composites during 6 months of water storage. Br Dent J 1994; 176(3): 91-6.

[http://dx.doi.org/10.1038/sj.bdj.4808379] [PMID: 7599006]

[113] Huang C, Tay FR, Cheung GS, Kei LH, Wei SH, Pashley DH. Hygroscopic expansion of a compomer and a composite on artificial gap reduction. J Dent 2002; 30(1): 11-9.
[http://dx.doi.org/10.1016/S0300-5712(01)00053-7] [PMID: 11741730]

[114] Chatterjee K, Lin-Gibson S, Wallace WE, *et al.* The effect of 3D hydrogel scaffold modulus on osteoblast differentiation and mineralization revealed by combinatorial screening. Biomaterials 2010; 31(19): 5051-62.
[http://dx.doi.org/10.1016/j.biomaterials.2010.03.024] [PMID: 20378163]

[115] Dalby MJ, Gadegaard N, Tare R, *et al.* The control of human mesenchymal cell differentiation using nanoscale symmetry and disorder. Nat Mater 2007; 6(12): 997-1003.
[http://dx.doi.org/10.1038/nmat2013] [PMID: 17891143]

[116] Dalby MJ, Biggs MJ, Gadegaard N, Kalna G, Wilkinson CD, Curtis AS. Nanotopographical stimulation of mechanotransduction and changes in interphase centromere positioning. J Cell Biochem 2007; 100(2): 326-38.
[http://dx.doi.org/10.1002/jcb.21058] [PMID: 16888806]

[117] Menschutkin N. Regarding the question on the influence of chemically indifferent solutions on reaction speed. Z Phys Chem 1890; 6: 41-57.

[118] Noguchi H, Rembaum A. Reactions of N,N,N′,N′-tetramethyl-alpha, w-diaminoalkanes with alpha, w-dihaloalkanes. I. 1-y reactions. Macromolecules 1972; 5(3): 253-60.
[http://dx.doi.org/10.1021/ma60027a006]

[119] Rembaum A. Ionene polymers for selectively inhibiting the vitro growth of malignant cells. US Patent 4013507 1977.

CHAPTER 4

Hydrogels: Types, Structure, Properties, and Applications

Amirsalar Khandan[1,*], **Hossein Jazayeri**[2], **Mina D. Fahmy**[2] and **Mehdi Razavi**[3]

[1] *Young Researchers and Elite Club, Khomeinishahr Branch, Islamic Azad University, Isfahan, Iran*

[2] *Marquette University School of Dentistry, Milwaukee, WI 53233, USA*

[3] *Department of Radiology, School of Medicine, Stanford University, Palo Alto, California 94304, USA*

Abstract: Hydrogels are one of the important biomaterials for tissue engineering applications. The hydrogel scaffolds' state-of-the-art properties for clinical applications are subject to on-going researches. Hydrogels, such as hybrid and protein-based ones, contain protein domains. Hydrogels show unique advantages compared to other polymeric materials; which made them applicable as periodontal materials and drug carriers, as well as bone matrices. The first description of its use was developed by a Scottish chemist, Thomas Graham, as a solid, jelly-like material that can have different physical and mechanical properties. Gels are defined as a substantially dilute cross-linked system, which doesn't have flow in the steady-state. Gels can be typically characterized as liquids, while they behave like solids due to a 3D cross-linked network within the liquid. The gels' IUPAC definition classifies them as a non-fluid polymer network that is expanded throughout its whole volume by a fluid. Thus, this chapter aims to describe the composition, synthesis techniques, and applications of hydrogel scaffolds for biomedical approaches.

Keywords: Biotechnology, Hydrogel, Nanomaterials, Polymers, Scaffolds, Tissue Engineering.

INTRODUCTION

These days, synthetic polymers are fabricated artificially by various synthesis methods. These techniques have some advantages by using natural polymers as these polymers are easily accessible, processable, and flexible to form into different shapes. The physiochemical characteristic of natural polymers can be easily modified by different techniques and materials. Typically, functional

---

* **Corresponding author Amirsalar Khandan:** Young Researchers and Elite Club, Khomeinishahr Branch, Islamic Azad University, Isfahan, Iran; Tel: +98 913 571 9626; E-mail: sas.khandan@iaukhsh.ac.ir

Mehdi Razavi (Ed.)
All rights reserved-© 2017 Bentham Science Publishers

groups can be incorporated. The most widely used synthetic polymers are poly(lactic acid) (PLA), poly- (glycolic acid) (PGA); polycaprolactone (PCL) and polyethylene glycol (PEG) [1 - 4]. In the field of biomaterials, hydrogels have attracted attention due to their excellent hydrophilicity, and similar structure close to the extracellular matrix (ECM). Hydrogels are popular for nanoscale tissue engineering to develop encapsulated cells *in situ* under non-cytotoxic situations. Using hydrogels for tissue engineering provides a 3D microenvironment and a suitable solute transport out of the scaffold that is biodegradable, bioactive and biocompatible. Nowadays, various techniques to fabricate hydrogel scaffolds have been reported and invented to produce pores in 3D tissues for biomaterial approaches such as freeze drying, photolithography phase separation, salt leaching, and 3D stereolithographic printing. In all the aforementioned techniques, cells grew after generation of pores in the scaffolds, limiting cell in-growth throughout the scaffolds. In every technique, non-uniform or inhomogeneous distribution of cells leads to the creation of cell coverage for biomaterials [1]. To overcome such a problem, continuous circulation of cell suspension and cell encapsulated hydrogel scaffolds were introduced. To achieve *in situ* pore formation in the presence of encapsulated cells, chemical and physical process parameters for pore generation should be selected for maintaining the cell viability and desired physical and biological functionality [1 - 3]. It is important to independently tune the physical and chemical characteristics of the hydrogel scaffold to effectively monitor 3D environments. The preparation of some fibers has been the interest of several researchers with focus on the diameter, porosity, and materials composition of the fibers for tissue engineering applications [1 - 5]. Various studies on hydrogels have described the technique, materials and applications of the material. For instance, a review of different synthetic schemes employed for hydrogel fabrication can be discovered in different chapters of a compilation edited by Peppas [5]. Recently, hydrogels produced by radiation polymerization and grafting have been reported by Khoylou [6]. Mi-Ran Park [7] which introduced the fabrication of hydrogels employed in industrial applications. Stamatialis *et al.* [8] described tailoring the hydrogels for different medical applications.

Due to the structural similarity of hydrogel-based scaffolds with natural extracellular matrices, it is a very desirable material with relevant clinical applications [9]. Physical and biological performance parameters must be optimized for an ideal scaffold in tissue regeneration. The biocompatibility of hydrogels as well as their ability to being cross-linked by different mechanisms allows them to be an effective candidate for scaffold design [10]. The ability of hydrogels to be delivered by injection into abnormally shaped defects gives them a significant advantage in tissue engineering schemes and surgical operations, especially those involving minimally invasive procedures [11]. The porosity in hydrogel-based scaffolds can be controlled to be large enough to allow diffusion of living cells and releasing the bioactive agents [12]. The hydrogels are not only water swellable and elastic similar to the native tissue, but also they are suitable for cell encapsulation due to their precursor makeup and gelation mechanism [13]. Bioactive synthetic hydrogels have variable mechanical properties and a replicable microenvironment for regenerative purposes [14]. The hydrophilic nature of hydrogels limits the entry of immunogenic molecules, so *in vivo* applications would not be restricted by a foreign body immune response [15]. For example, alginate and poly(ethylene glycol) (PEG), along with their copolymers form a more potent hydrogel complex, which reflect the characteristics of an abundant variety of polymer gels [16]. In addition to the biocompatiblity and mechanically durable nature of hydrogel-based scaffolds, its mass transport capability is essential for tissue regeneration [16]. Synthetic hydrogels are generally preferred to natural hydrogels because their mechanical properties and scaffold architecture can be more easily controlled and they are photopolymerizable [17]. Synthetic hydrogel scaffolds are also reproducible, and their structural uniformity can suspend growth factors to facilitate regeneration [18]. Given the abundance of diverse properties and advantages of the material, hydrogels are extremely suitable for scaffold design in tissue engineering applications [9].

GELS VARIETY

Organogel

One of the most important gels is called organogel. This is introduced as a non-glassy thermoplastic dense material created from an organic phase entrapped in a 3D cross-linked network. The prepared fluid can be an organic solvent, and mineral/vegetable oil. The application of organogels is varied in cosmetics, biomaterials, pharmaceuticals, and food products [19].

Xerogels

The second type of gels is xerogels, which is produced in solid form. The xerogel is produced from a gel that is dried with unhindered shrinkage. They retain with high porosity between 15 to 50% with a large surface area more than 150 m^2/g [20].

Aerogel

The third type of gel is called aerogel, which is a synthetic porous ultralight material derived from a gel. In the state of aerogel, the fluid is replaced with gas. The prepared gel is solid and has low density and thermal conductivity. Aerogels can be produced from all types of chemical compounds like air, smoke, and frozen smoke [21].

Hydrogel

A novel smart material has been recently developed and became most popular with many scientists and engineers. Hydrogels have the ability to change their structure in response to salt concentration, pH and temperature. Hydrogels are cross-linked polymers that have hydrophilic groups [3, 12, 22 - 24]. The most important polymer that aid in hydrogel preparation is sodium polyacrylate, also known by its chemical name of sodium propionate.

COMPOSITION OF HYDROGELS

The composition of hydrogels is described as a polymer network chain that is hydrophilic and is also known as a colloidal gel in which liquid (water) is the dispersion solution. Hydrogels are highly absorbent (containing more than 90% water) natural or synthetic polymeric networks. The high impact of hydrogels shows their useful application in breast implants, glue, wound healing dressings for burns. Gels that are used for wounds are useful for protecting injured cells from the moist outside environment. Hydrogels also shows high flexibility similar to natural soft tissue like skin, articular cartilage tissue due to their meaningful water component [9, 25 - 29]. The first literature about 'hydrogels' was found by Wichterle *et al.* in 1996 [30]. Hydrogels can carry human cells to repair old tissue. They can easily mimic 3D space of cells. Also, they have the ability to be used as coat. Hydrogel coats have been applied for cell culturing. Moreover, 'Intelligent Gels' are defined and used for environment sensitive [31]. These 'Intelligent hydrogels' have the ability to discover pH changes, temperature, and concentration of metabolites. Several various solutions have been utilized for hydrogels as an extender, namely water. Molecules of water are absorbed to the negative charges by H^+ bonding.

NANOCOMPOSITE HYDROGELS

Nanocomposite hydrogels (NH) have become popular in recent decades with their hybrid characteristics, and they can be introduced as highly hydrated polymeric physical networks cross-linked with each other. NHs can mimic natural tissue properties due to their interconnected porous microstructure. Several useful nanoparticles, such as carbon nano tube, polymeric and bioceramic materials can be diffused into the hydrogel structure to gain suitable properties [20 - 23].

SCAFFOLD HYDROGELS

Hydrogels carry great amounts of water without degradation. The hydrogels can keep their design and structure while they have more than 99% water in their network. This special characteristic (hydrated composition) can be used in native articular cartilages. For this reason, researchers inject hydrogels scaffolds due to their mass that is composed of water. With this useful application, hydrogels can be utilized to fill defects of an irregular shape. These advantages keep surgical intervention minimized [7, 22, 23]. Recently, hydrogels have been applied to encapsulate cells in a network of polymers, immobilizing the cells and allowing for differentiation of chondrocytes more effectively by forcing them to retain a rounded shape [22, 23]. A novel hydrogel scaffold can be designed easily to have better elasticity to recover from the compressive deformation. Also, because hydrogels can exert controlled compressive forces on encapsulated cells, they exhibit physiological and real conditions. Several polymers can be shaped and designed into hydrogels, such as collagen, alginate, agarose, chitosan, fibrin glue etc. In a contrary manner, hydrogels do not have enough stiffness to function without delay *in vivo* mechanism [23]. Hydrogels have many applications in regenerative medicine [9, 28, 29, 32], separation of cells, cellular immobilization, diagnostics, drug delivery, and barrier materials [2, 33 - 37].

HISTORY OF HYDROGELS

The first description of hydrogel properties was reported by Wichterle *et al.* in 1996 [30]. Eight years later, it was understood that the net repulsion between a polymer and a poor solvent could cause a phase transition and a change in the swelling degree. Other researchers showed a phase transition in their works induced by changes in the environment. Applications and uses of hydrogels have been changed dramatically. Several different methods have been used to synthesize hydrogels up to the present time. Lots of review articles and researchers published in this area. The scientific researchers try to present the theoretical and application of hydrogels in different areas such as molecular imprinting, micro-total analysis systems (TAS) [38]. Recently, to our knowledge, there has not been a literature article reporting porous hydrogels applications. The aim of the current chapter is to give a thorough, qualitative overview of the area, while showing recent advanced and developments of hydrogel in biomaterials engineering applications [12, 23]. Generally, hydrogel might absorb and attract more than 500 times of its water, but less salty water. Hydrogel capacity to absorb is so strong that makes the hydrogel significant for even the lining of babies' nappies. As salt diffused and mixed with hydrogel, the network chains begin to change their form and finally gel separate from the water. In addition, hydrogels are divided into different categories by their physical shapes, such as slabs, micro-nanoparticles, powder, films and biocoatings. Therefore, hydrogels are applied in a wide range for clinical surgery and medicine application [24].

HYDROGEL PRODUCT CLASSIFICATION

The hydrogel scaffold materials are divided into six groups based on:

Classification Based on Source

Natural and synthetic hydrogels are the two known sources of different hydrogels [25].

Classification Based on Composition

The method of hydrogel preparation allows for the formation of important classes of hydrogels. These can be introduced as follows:

Homopolymeric Hydrogels

Homopolymeric hydrogels are described and connected to a network of polymers which may derived from single types of monomers [26]. They might have a microstructure with cross-linked architecture based on the method of polymerization, as well as monomer composition.

Copolymeric Hydrogels

Another composition of hydrogels is comprised of two different types of monomers with at least one hydrophilic species alternating configuration during the polymer network chain [27].

Multipolymer Interpenetrating

Interpenetrating polymeric hydrogel (IPN), is created from two cross-linked synthetic/natural polymers.

Classification Based on Configuration

Both physical and chemical classification of hydrogels structure is: (a) amorphous (non-crystalline), (b) semi-crystalline: combination of amorphous and crystalline phases, (c) crystalline.

Classification Based on Cross-Linking Type

Another classification of hydrogels is based on nature of cross-link (chemical/physical nature) junctions.

Cross-linked with chemical networks have temporary junctions, although physical types have transient junctions [28].

Classification Based on Appearance

The method of polymerization shows the hydrogels appearance.

Classification Based on Charge

Presence of electrical charge for chains of crosslinks is categorised in four major groups: (a) nonionic or neutral (b) anionic/cationic (c) amphoteric (basic and acidic groups) and (d) Zwitterionic (polybetaines) including cationic and anionic groups [3].

FABRICATION TECHNIQUES FOR SCAFFOLD

In humans, the soft and hard tissues have a unique architecture that needs to be mimicked by scaffolds. To fabricate cells and tissues as functional organs, scaffolds have to be produced by different techniques to show better cell distribution and growth. There are several methods to produce scaffolds that we discuss briefly.

Solvent Casting Techniques

This method is a simple and cheap technique for scaffold fabrication. This method is used to solidify the polymer, preparing a network of polymer–porogen. There is no need for any extra or special equipment; this method deals with the evaporation of liquid (solvent) due to the shape of scaffolds by the two routes. The first step in this method is to soak the mold into a liquid polymer and allow enough time to draw off the liquid; finally the membrane polymer is prepared. The second method is to add the polymeric liquid into a mold and allow enough time to evaporate the solvent that fabricates a polymeric membrane layer. This technique is not without limitations; the toxic solvent denatures the protein which may influence other solvents. The scaffolds prepared by these methods may have toxicity incorporated in their own structures. However, the advantage of this technique is that the porous size can be tuned by making changes to the size and concentration of the particles within the prepolymer [33]. Because of some drawbacks associated with the removal and purification of solid particles from the hydrogel, solvent casting is normally restricted to the preparation of thin hydrogel sheets that are less than 500 mm. To solve toxicity problems researchers have opted to put scaffolds into a vacuum process to dry and remove all toxicity. However, these methods require extensive amounts of time, but some researchers present these methods with particulate leaching methods to produce a suitable scaffold. In the next section we will describe particulate leaching [38, 104].

Particulate-leaching Technique

Particulate-leaching is used to prepare porous scaffolds for biomaterial engineering applications [39]. Several porogen materials such as gelatine, sugars, and paraffin have been introduced with hydrogels. Salt is purified and changed into small particles and those particles that have proper size are filled into a mold and filled with the porogen. Salt, wax or sugars known as porogens are used to produce high porous channels. In the past, salt particles were used because they were cheap and largely available. It has been indicated that particles with spherical shapes lead to higher interconnected pores than other particle shapes. A polymer solution is then cast into the salt-filled mold. After the evaporation of the solvent, the salt crystals are leached away using water to form the pores of the scaffold. The process is easy to carry out. The benefit of the current technique is the starting material which needs less content of polymer to prepare the scaffold. However, important characteristics like pore shape are not possible to monitor [38, 104].

Gas Foaming

Scaffold preparation methods need both high temperature and solvent solution, while current techniques do not need the utilization of organic solvents and high temperature. High porous scaffold are designed with this technique using high pressure CO_2 (g). The utilized gas which dissolves in the polymer defines the scaffolds porosity percentages. The current method involves a high porous polymer network with CO_2 (g) at 800 psi pressure to fill the structure with CO_2 gas [40, 41]. In the present technique process, dissolving CO_2 makes the polymer network unstable and leads to different separate phase. The molecule of CO_2 becomes clustered to minimize the free energy; as a result pore nucleation is fabricated. The porous structure of the scaffolds is monitored by utilizing different porogens such as salts and sugar [41]. Several different methods like CO_2–water emulsion templating have been introduced to enhance the possibility of gas to penetrate into a polymer (hydrophilic) and create a polymer with suitable porosity. Using CO_2 as a dense gas to prepare proper porosity removes the use of unnecessary surfactant which is highly required in conventional techniques [33].

Phase Separation

This technique needs changes in temperature that separates the solution into two phases. The two phase polymeric solution for scaffold design has varying amounts of polymer concentration. Polymer material is dissolved in naphthalene, followed by dispersion of biologically active molecules in these solutions. As the temperature is lowered, the liquid-liquid phase becomes clear and separated. and then, it is quenched to form a two phase solid; the solvent is subsequently removed by extraction, evaporation and sublimation [42] to prepare scaffolds with bioactive molecules integrated into the structure [40]. The advantage of this technique is that, it can be easily combined with particulate leaching and rapid prototyping to create 3D scaffolds with suitable and enhanced morphology for biomaterials applications [43, 104].

Electrospinning

Electrospinning (ELS) is a new technology that produces soft tissues with necessity in both industrial and clinical applications due to its versatility in spinning a large variety of polymers, especially for wound healing. ELS have been utilized to prepare high porous polymeric scaffolds of polyacrylic acid [33]. The ELS method uses the electrostatic force for the production of polymeric fiber. Briefly, one electrode is settled in the polymeric fluid while another electrode remains in the collector [44, 45]. Polymeric fluid is pumped as a result of droplet formation. Subsequently, an electric field is produced, which creates a force, causing the droplets to overcome the surface tension of the liquid. The polymer jet is discharged, a jet of polymer is ejected, which fabricates the fibers, and the procedure continues after the nanofibers are deposited to the collector. Several polymers are utilized for ELS such as silk fibroin [46], collagen [47], and chitosan [48]. In the current process, a large voltage is applied to produce an electrically charged jet of polymer fluid, which shapes fibers of polymer after solidification [45, 49, 94]. The most important use of the current method is that it can prepare the porous scaffold with suitable characteristics for growth of new tissues and cells leading to tissue regeneration [50]. The desired characteristic with this method is high surface area, and possibility to monitor the geometry of the pore. The mentioned advantages and proper characteristics are suitable for improving the cellular growth [50, 104].

Porogen Leaching

This technique is used to control the scaffold porosity. It is possible in this method to use salt, wax and sugar as a porogen for dispersion either in powdered or liquid and solid form with evaporation technique [51]. Mentioned porogens act as space holder for making the porosity and interconnection in the scaffolds. This technique produces a scaffold with a high amount of porosity. Around 90% of pores, have a pore diameter higher than 500 μm [52]. The major advantages of the porogen technique are both the access to bigger pores and the increase in pore interconnectivity. Also, simplicity, geometry, ability to control the pore size and versatility are the other four benefits of this technique [53]. However, the main problem of this technique is that it is only able to fabricate thin membranes less than 3 mm thick [54, 104].

Fiber Mesh

Fiber mesh technique used for preparation of scaffolds that contain fiber interwoven into a 3D pattern of variable porosity [55]. Poly-(glycolic acid), PGA, is the primary biodegradable polymer spun into the fiber. PGA fibers are used as a synthetic suture thread. The suture thread is fabricated by the deposition of polymer liquid over a nonwoven mesh of different polymers followed by next step evaporation [41]. Aiding in both cell diffusion and growth are the vital advantages of this method [56]. However, instability of the structure is the main drawback of this technique. To solve and overcome this problem, the instable structure can be dried in a hot furnace to improve the crystallinity [44, 104].

Fiber Bonding

This method was developed in 1993 by Mikos *et al.* for fabrication of scaffolds [52]. In their study, a polymer (PLLA) was dissolved in chloroform followed by addition of a non-woven mesh of PGA fiber. The solvent was then separated by evaporation. A collagen matrix was bonded to PGA to produce the scaffolds [57]. This bonding happens along post treatments at the melting temperature of PGA. High surface area and porosity is obtained by adding PGA mesh, which ultimately provides a mass ratio for polymers [58]. The bonding created by mesh has excellent mechanical stability with suitable growth for tissues. Large surface area is one of the useful parameters in this technique that has high impact in tissue engineering applications. Therefore, the high surface area allows for better regeneration which can be obtained for cell growth in larger space [59, 104].

Self-Assembly

This technique produces synthetic/natural nanofibers with a range of less than 30 nm. Amphiphilic peptide sequence is a usual technique for the preparation of nanostructured fibrous (3D) for biomaterials engineering. In aqueous fluids, the hydrophilic domain within the peptides affects the assistance of weak non covalent bonds [60]. Polymeric dendrimers might be able to diffuse into the nanofibers with this technique [61, 104].

Rapid Prototyping (RP)

Rapid prototyping method is also called solid free-form. This advanced scaffold preparation method is connected with computer-controlled models called Computer Aided Design (CAD). The current method can easily and rapidly fabricate any product in 3D shape [62]. The researcher can design a bone defect replacement in a human's body by using a 3D model and CAD software. The 3D products are produced by using RP methods like fused deposition modelling (FDM), and selective laser sintering (SLS) layer by layer. This system is able to monitor all the necessary parameters including mechanical, biological and degradation properties of required scaffolds by integrating with the imaging [63]. One of the major disadvantages of the aforementioned technique is low resolution quality and limitation in the use of diverse polymeric materials [36, 104].

Melt Moulding

All the mentioned techniques discussed for the preparation of hydrogel scaffolds are introduced to monitor and control the geometry and interconnectivity of pores. All above methods are important for the exchange of nutrients from pore to pore. The entire scaffold prepared by this technique are like mould shape. Melt moulding technique is filling a Teflon mould with PLGA powder and gelatine microspheres in specific sizes and is continued by heating the mould above the glass transition temperature of PLGA while applying pressure to the mixture [33, 64]. This process leads the PLGA particles to join together. When the mould is removed, the gelatine microspheres are dissolved by soaking the mixture in water and the scaffolds are then dried [104].

Membrane Lamination

Lamination membrane is one of the new techniques for preparation of 3D foam polymer scaffolds with suitable anatomical forms. This technique is performed by both particle leaching and solvent casting. Porous polymer with suitable anatomical form are generated during this method as it is possible to use computer software to model the conjured design for required bone implant or soft tissues [63]. The created membranes are immerged into the solvent, and then stacked up in 3D assemblies with morphology [65]. The drawback for this technique is that porous sheets, cause in lesser interconnectivity and is very time consuming [63, 104].

Freeze Drying

The easy method for fabrication of porous scaffolds is freeze drying [66]. The freeze drying method is used according to the sublimations principle. The procedure is described simply with dissolved polymer in a solvent to prepare a liquid/solution with required concentrations. The fabricated solution is then frozen with lyophilisation solvent removed under the high vacuum condition [67]. Several researchers applied this method for various polymers including silk proteins, PLGA, PLLA, PGA, and PLGA/PPF blends [68]. In this technique, the porosity is controlled by the rate of freezing and pH. The freezing rate and pH produce smaller pores [33]. The major advantage of the freeze-drying method is that a low temperature is required and there is a mixed leaching step. On the other hand, this technique produces small pore size and is very time consuming. (Table 1) shows hydrogels fabrication methods with their significant advantages and disadvantages for tissue engineering applications. However, the most notable limitations of hydrogels are their weak mechanical strength and high degradability [12, 104].

Table 1. The general information about hydrogels fabrications methods.

Methods	Advantageous	Disadvantageous
Particulate leaching	Control over porosity, pore size and crystallinity	Limited mechanical property, residual solvents and porogen materials
Porogen leaching	Controlled over porosity and pore geometry	Inadequate pore size and pore interconnectivity
Gas foaming	Free of harsh organic solvents, control over porosity and pore size	Limited mechanical property, inadequate pore interconnectivity
Self-assembly	Control over porosity, pore size and fiber diameter	Expensive material, complex design parameters
Electrospinning	Control over porosity, pore size and fiber diameter	Limited mechanical property, pore size decrease with fiber thickness
Phase separation	No decrease in the activity of the molecule	Difficult to control precisely scaffold morphology
Rapid prototyping	Excellent control over geometry, porosity, no supporting material required	Limited polymer type, highly expensive equipment
Fiber mesh	Large surface area for cell attachment, rapid nutrient diffusion	Lack the structural stability
Fiber bonding	High surface to volume ratio, high porosity	Poor mechanical property, limited applications to other polymers
Melt molding	Independent control pore porosity and pore size	Required high temperature for nonamorphous polymer
Membrane lamination	Provide 3D matrix	Lack required mechanical strength inadequate pore interconnectivity
Freeze drying	High temperature and separate leaching step not required	Small pore size and long processing time

HYDROGELS APPLICATIONS

In this section, we attempt to describe hydrogels' applications from different reviews. Hydrogels have various clinical applications such as angiogenesis, wound repair, liver regeneration, sensing, nerve regeneration, drug delivery, and control of fluid and artificial muscles [37]. Researchers around the world are actively working on tissue replacement materials which are derived from hydrogels, to use as degradable or non-degradable (temporary/permanent) implants. Other applications of hydrogels exist naturally in the human body and include: mucus, blood clots, vitreous humor, cartilage, and tendons. The first and most attractive application of hydrogels is their sensing capability (*i.e.* pH sensors) [9]. Some of hydrogels application represent in Fig. (**1**).

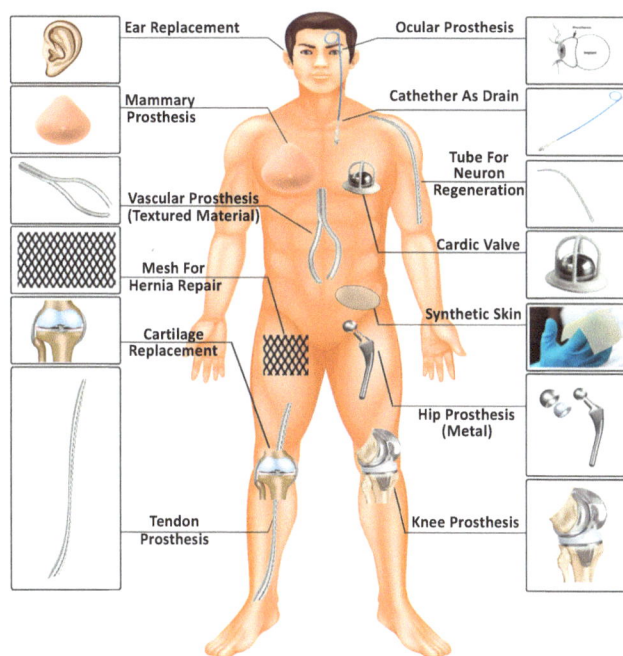

Fig. (1). All hydrogel application in different human's body place.

Scaffolds for Growth Factor Release

The high impact of polymer scaffolds is due to their good function in tissue regeneration and also remodelling by incorporating growth factors (GF). It is possible to incorporate GF into the scaffold tissue matrix with specific bulk encapsulation and addition of microspheres [3].

Angiogenesis

Therapeutic angiogenesis is an important treatment of ischemic wound repair and heart diseases. The formation of blood vessels is vital for the growing organ. Different angiogenic GFs, like vascular endothelial GF, and acidic fibroblast GF have been diffused and incorporated into 3D matrices. Incorporation of angiogenic GF was discovered by preparing the tissue or scaffold using a water-in-oil emulsion [3].

Bone Formation

Hydrogels aid bone formation which needs stimulation by growth factors. The formation of bone and expression of a large number of bone morphogenic proteins are vital in osteogenesis. The osteogenic factor released from the matrix improved osteoprogenitor proliferation when introduced *ex vivo* in a chorioallantoic layer, and *in vivo* diffusion chambers [3].

Wound Healing Repair

GF helps the wound to heal better for those who suffer from diabetic foot ulcers or burns. Hydrogels and other soft tissues are developed by scientists to attain suitable wound dressings for patients. Wound tissues are normally comprised of an inner hydrogel [3].

Regeneration of Liver

Growth factors that are important for enhancing rapid growth of hepatocytes include epidermal growth factor (EGF) and hepatocyte growth factor (HGF). Epidermal growth factor released from Poly-(glycolic acid) mesh force the aggregation and densification of hepatocytes linked to the matrix. Because blood supply shows a key role in function and regeneration of liver, hepatocyte culture has been frequently connected with angiogenesis [3].

Neural Tissue Engineering

Engineering of tissue includes the implant of a polymeric help conduit at the place of neural wound to promote the regeneration action. Neurotrophic factors like brain-derived neurotrophic factor (BDNF), nerve growth factor (NGF), and glial growth factor (GGF) have been utilized to enhance migration, ingrowth and proliferation of neural cells. Recently, ECM materials are attracting the attention of researchers for delivery of neurotrophic factors. Several synthetic materials like hydrogels have been discovered for nerve repair applications [3].

Drug Delivery Application

One of the most important drug delivery applications is for small molecular weight that shows differentiation and ingrowths of cells to penetrate into biodegradable polymeric scaffolds to help the tissue remodelling [3].

HYDROGEL PROPERTIES

Biocompatibility Hydrogel Scaffold

The biocompatibility of hydrogel products in the human body show important effects in biomaterials engineering applications, which define the prepared and implanted materials, as useful and proper for use in the endogenous fluids. An implant to help and repair the defected tissue is designed and the proliferation and regeneration of implanted tissue for wound and bone formation sites needs to be biocompatible, *i.e.*, the implanted part should not cause any inflammatory, cytotoxicity and immunogenicity reaction to the host cells or organs [22, 23]. Biocompatibility is described to prevent unnecessary host tissue feedback to the bone implant [39]. Scaffolds with high interconnected pores are suitable to help and support infiltration of cells [63].

Hydrogels are indeed biocompatible materials that have characteristics of porosity while also displaying a soft, consistency that allows for reduction of friction and irritation upon implantation [69]. Furthermore, hydrogels have good tissue compatibility and are minimally thrombogenic with blood contact. Studies have indicated that hydrogels obtained from synthetic polymers have the required biocompatibility and can be used for such things as drug delivery [70, 71]. In one study biocompatibility was tested and results showed that when acrylamide-based hydrogels were tested against biochemical human parameters such as post-prandial blood glucose, cholesterol, blood urea nitrogen, creatine, albumin, alkaline phosphate, alanine transaminase, bilirubin, chlorine, sodium and potassium, there was no significant difference in values before and after contacting these area with the hydrogels. It was concluded from this study that acrylamide/crotonic acid and acrylamide/itaconic acid hydrogels show biocompatibility with the tested biochemical parameters [69 - 72].

Although there are numerous combinations of materials that can be explored and investigated for use in drug delivery systems (DDS), research is limited by the material's biocompatibility, potentially toxic byproducts and cost of manufacturing process. Chitosan, an amino-polysaccharide obtained from chitin has the sought after characteristics of biocompatibility, low toxicity and degradability by human enzymes [72, 73]. Chitosan has been studied extensively and the level of biocompatibility seems to vary widely depending on the degree of deacetylation (DDA) among other factors. Chitosan-based hydrogels have been used in *in-vivo* experiments of injectable biomaterials. From several studies, it is known that chitosan salts that are of lower degree of acetylation are more easily degraded because of the existence of acetyl groups [74 - 76]. This increased degradation may be responsible for acute inflammatory responses. In a study by

Hidaka and colleagues, membranes that were made of different percentages (65%, 70%, 80%, 94% and 100%) of deacetylated chitin were implanted subperiosteally above rat calvaria. It was found that those membranes prepared with 65%, 70% and 80% deacetylated chitin stimulated inflammatory reactions while membranes made of 94% deacetylated chitin showed mild inflammation [77]. Bhattarai et al, note that researchers have looked at developing different hydrogels using chitosan co-polymers with poly(N—isopropyl acrylamide) (PNi-PAM) [78]. PNi-PAM modified with chitosan, and other natural polymers such as collagen allows for the adjusting of gelation temperatures closer to normal physiological temperatures, thereby increasing strength, and improving biocompatibility of the hydrogel [79].

Small molecule cross-linkers have been used to cross-link chitosan polymers, generally these hydrogels have improved mechanical properties when reinforced with such chemical cross-linkers [80]. However, the biocompatibility of many cross-linkers is unknown while some have been found to be toxic. Thus, constructed hydrogels must undergo purification cycles before administration. These cross-linkers may also deactivate or limit the therapeutic action of hydrogels. Limitations caused by these covalent cross-linkers represent the main drawback of hydrogels. Of major importance is the fact that, although the chitosan polymer may be biocompatible, a chitosan polymer with a reactive group may have cytotoxic properties. Despite this, genipin has been investigated and reported to be a biocompatible cross-linking agent [81].

For wound healing, there needs to be a dressing that protects the wound from bacteria, while providing a moist, biocompatible environment [82]. Chitosan has been shown to induce more rapid wound healing, as well as allow for smoother scarring, perhaps due to augmented vascularisation [83, 84]. Due to its flexibility in its use in several "intelligent" delivery systems, chitosan-based hydrogel formulations have been a major area of research. In work by Draye et al, the biosafety of a wound dressing material made of dextran dialdehyde cross-linked gelatin hydrogel films was examined [85]. They evaluated cross-linked gelatin hydrogel cytotoxicity on keratinocyte, fibroblast and endothelial cell cultures. It was found that semi-occlusive polyurethane dressings showed low cytotoxicity while hydrocolloid dressings induced high cytotoxicity in keratinocyte cultures [86, 87]. In both fibroblast and endothelial cell cultures, hydrogel and hydrocolloid dressings were much less toxic than in keratinocyte cultures. In addition, *in vitro* experimentation showed that fibroblasts were indeed capable of growing on cross-linked gelatin hydrogels [85].

Biodegradability Hydrogel Scaffold

Another important parameter in implantation of hydrogels in the biomaterials field is biodegradability of polymers like hydrogels to have a fast growing and avoiding dissolution. A biodegradable polymer can be naturally decomposed but their dissolute parts will remain within the human body. For such a bioresorbable polymer, degradation occurs after implantation at certain period of time, and non-toxic parts will be fabricated when the metabolism eliminate [23, 24]. Controlling the biodegradability is important to support the creation of new tissue [88].

Surface Morphology Hydrogel Scaffold

The modification of surface morphology for biodegradable polymer is based on the ability to be retained at the implantation site while maintaining its mechanical, physical and chemical properties. The porous scaffold degradability should be correlated with the neo-tissue fabrication rate to produce a smooth transition of the load transfer from the scaffold to the tissue. Hydrogels surface morphology is important for cartilage joints. Basically, there are four types of polymer-based materials used for cartilage joints, they are polymers types (a) natural, (b) hydrogels, (c) nanocomposites and (d) synthetic [23].

Physical Properties Hydrogel Scaffold

The physical properties of hydrogels are inherent to the prosperity of the scaffold. Crosslinking properties like amount, type, and size of crosslinking molecules are prescribed by the intrinsic properties of the main polymer chains and environmental conditions. Usual preparation of hydrogel processes which effect hydrogel properties such as temperature increases, pH changes, and various solvents can denature proteins and cause cell damage or death [9].

Mechanical Properties Hydrogel Scaffold

Hydrogel mechanical properties have been developed recently, with a vast area of applicability in biomaterials. The main achievements and fundamentals of sliding crosslinking agents and nanocomposite hydrogels are enhanced with nanoclays [5, 45, 89] Okumura *et al.* described a new type of chain crosslinking agents. Such nanocomposite hydrogels are a type of organic-inorganic hybrids. They can have high surface hydrophobicities, as shown by contact angle assessment [28, 95]. Mechanical properties need to be protected immediately after the implantation and during the remodeling process [89]. It must obtain the proper mechanical properties to provide an enhanced environment for cells to repair within the defected site and be active as a function of newly formed tissue [63].

Biological Properties Hydrogel Scaffold

Hydrogels fabricated to apply in human's body must satisfy all desirable biological functions like proliferation and differentiation for a tissue engineering application. Polymer hydrogel is created to be nontoxic to the surrounding the tissue. Collagen and hydroxyapatite (HA) are the most important components of human hard tissues [90 - 96, 105, 106]. HA and collagen must interact favourably within the humans body [44]. One of the famous polymers, chitosan, has been shown to be nontoxic despite its chemotaxic influence on neutrophils. Several types of hydrogels are nontoxic and cannot activate a chronic immune response and cannot promote cellular adhesion. As collagen is a natural ECM protein, most cells do not have receptors to hydrogel forming polymers and thus cannot adhere. Thus, as hydrogels have hydrophilic nature, numerous ECM proteins including fibronectin, laminin, vitronectin, and collagen do not adhere to the surface of gel [97 - 100]. The mentioned application has been exploited in post-operative adhesion barriers. A novel technique to fabricate and design a surface with high specific adhesive is to covalently couple an entire ECM protein to the polymer [9].

In vivo Evaluation Hydrogel Scaffold

An in vivo test is required for osteochondral scaffolds [100 - 102]. In the *in vivo* examination the cartilage and bone implant are joined and connected using different techniques like fibrin adhesive bonding and suturing, however the problem of scaffold dislocation suggests that the joining strength between cartilage and bone implant tissues of these methods is not adequate. The connection must be strong enough to keep the scaffold stable and prevent delamination or dislocation in the natural *in vivo* space. Also, investigation of bone tissue regeneration rate or bone-like apatite formation is required [35]. The bone implants work as an anchor to prepare suitable mechanical stability to cartilage in an osteochondral scaffold [90 - 95]. Another factor is that tissues made of bone should be regenerated quickly. Although, most bone tissues have been prepared from synthesis or natural polymers and have less ability for tissue restoration and regeneration than bone scaffolds created from bio-ceramic materials [44, 90, 91]. Although ceramic biomaterials have been developed to prepare scaffolds for bone regeneration, bone ingrowths are gradual in such scaffolds due to their pore-interconnectivity [32]. Applying alginate to hydrogels, researchers find hybrid scaffolds for cartilage tissue repair [32]. These alginate-hydrogel scaffolds contain both hydrogels and ceramics. The *in vivo* study of hydrogels consisted of three layer application: a bioceramic layer for the bone area, a nanocomposite biolayer of ceramic and alginate for calcified zone, and an alginate hydrogel layer for the articular cartilage zone [44, 92 - 94]. Hybrid scaffolds of 4 mm diameter and 6 mm height were successfully fabricated according to the literature [29]. The prepared scaffold tissue must be able to tolerate fibroblasts, osteoblasts and chondrocytes, harvested from the donor site

[102 - 106]. The consequence of created scaffold with a culture of cells will contain of a bone-integrative side. Scaffolds must be inserted into the defected zone from the bone-integrative side, while the soft tissue-integrative piece of it stays within the joint cavity the soft tissue. The chemical and cell stability of this part can be increased with biodegradable screws for mechanical fixation of the graft to the body tissues [35]. Silicate ceramic containing Si, Ca, and Mg, akermanite, baghdadite, diopside have shown bioactive feature in both *in vivo* and *in vitro* conditions [107, 108].

Cell Culture of Hydrogel Scaffold

3D cell culture experiments are used for hydrogels scaffolds as they have structures with high swollen stability [100]. Scaffolds made of hydrogels are tested by 3D cell culture to recognize these characteristics. Several studies showed that hydrogel scaffold is derived from ECM components such as decellulized tissue and matrigel, like collagen and gelatin. Investigating the 3D cell cultures of these materials is important due to their high impact and application in biomaterials. Some techniques have been used to prepare scaffolds with controlled environments from nanofiber tissue scaffolds such as natural and synthetic polymers to create hydrogels. Normally, scaffold made of hydrogel in 3D form systems must use mild fabrication conditions and permit for tunable biochemical parameters of the cellular microenvironment. Cell delivery is one of the hydrogel scaffolds characterization in tissue engineering because tissues require investigation of their 3D networks of polymers that produce a site for cells to differentiate and adhere [98 - 100]. Recently, hydrogel scaffolds are being applied in a wide range of engineering applications, including cartilage tissue, dental bone implant, neurons, liver, and wound healing. It is clear that hydrogels have similar structure and macromolecular to cartilage tissues. Today, several types of hydrogel scaffolds are replaced with chondrocytes that have been fabricated and examined by both *in vitro* and *in vivo* evaluation [101 - 103]. Thus, to develop new technique to enhance the function and structure of scaffolds we discuss these techniques in the current chapter. This chapter introduces the various fabrication techniques to prepare scaffolds using several synthetic and natural polymers, including all the above techniques.

CONCLUDING REMARKS

In this chapter we briefly represented the basic principles of fabrication and preparation of hydrogel materials for tissue engineering applications. Hydrogels have the ability to have different characteristics due to their essential applications. The soft nature of hydrogels helps them to be suitable candidates in biomedical applications. Also, their excellent biodegradability and biocompatibility bring them to the attention of scientific investigators. For example we introduced in the current chapter their applications which include nerve regeneration, wound healing and drug delivery applications. However, one of their disadvantages is the gradual response due to the time. This problem separates them from useful materials and makes them unsuitable for large-scale situations like using in sensors or artificial muscles that requires high reaction. However, no one can ignore their suitable application in biomedical devices and materials.

FUTURE RESEARCH

Many techniques have been used to design porous scaffold architecture. All of the mentioned fabrication techniques are used to prepare scaffolds of hydrogels, ceramics, and polymers for biomaterials applications. These created porous scaffolds show more suitable mechanical properties than scaffolds processed using other methods. Designers of these scaffolds have achieved better bone regeneration compared with other scaffolds, because of their excellent interconnected porosity. Cell attachment is important for bone repair and critical for neural regeneration. According to preparation and characterization of scaffolds design and amount of optimal material for regeneration of tissues, several important questions arise. How should different materials be able to generate on the surface tissues. Development of new hydrogel is due to joining them with nanofiber gradient networks that show enhanced flexibility, better mechanical and functional properties. Hydrogels and other biomaterials are able to be used with complex gradients to mimic the signals that are graded in the environment.

CONFLICT OF INTEREST

The authors declare no conflict of interest, financial or otherwise.

ACKNOWLEDGEMENTS

Declared none.

REFERENCES

[1]   Hwang CM, Sant S, Masaeli M, *et al.* Fabrication of three-dimensional porous cell-laden hydrogel for tissue engineering. Biofabrication 2010; 2(3): 035003.
      [http://dx.doi.org/10.1088/1758-5082/2/3/035003] [PMID: 20823504]

[2]   Wheeldon I, Farhadi A, Bick AG, Jabbari E, Khademhosseini A. Nanoscale tissue engineering: spatial control over cell-materials interactions. Nanotechnology 2011; 22(21): 212001.
      [http://dx.doi.org/10.1088/0957-4484/22/21/212001] [PMID: 21451238]

[3]   Ahmed EM. Hydrogel: preparation, characterization, and applications. J Adv Res 2013.
      [PMID: 25750745]

[4]   Makadia HK, Siegel SJ. Poly lactic-co-glycolic acid (PLGA) as biodegradable controlled drug delivery carrier. Polymers (Basel) 2011; 3(3): 1377-97.

[http://dx.doi.org/10.3390/polym3031377] [PMID: 22577513]

[5]   Peppas NA, Mikos AG. Preparation methods and structure of hydrogels. Hydrogels in medicine and pharmacy 1986; 1: 1-27.

[6]   Khoylou F, Naimian F. Radiation synthesis of superabsorbent polyethylene oxide/tragacanth hydrogel. Radiat Phys Chem 2009; 78(3): 195-8.
        [http://dx.doi.org/10.1016/j.radphyschem.2008.11.008]

[7]   Park MR, Chun C, Ahn SW, Ki MH, Cho CS, Song SC. Sustained delivery of human growth hormone using a polyelectrolyte complex-loaded thermosensitive polyphosphazene hydrogel. J Control Release 2010; 147(3): 359-67.
        [http://dx.doi.org/10.1016/j.jconrel.2010.07.126] [PMID: 20713099]

[8]   Stamatialis DF, Papenburg BJ, Gironés M, *et al.* Medical applications of membranes: drug delivery, artificial organs and tissue engineering. J Membr Sci 2008; 308(1): 1-34.
        [http://dx.doi.org/10.1016/j.memsci.2007.09.059]

[9]   Drury JL, Mooney DJ. Hydrogels for tissue engineering: scaffold design variables and applications. Biomaterials 2003; 24(24): 4337-51.
        [http://dx.doi.org/10.1016/S0142-9612(03)00340-5] [PMID: 12922147]

[10]   Lee KY, Mooney DJ. Hydrogels for tissue engineering. Chem Rev 2001; 101(7): 1869-79.
        [http://dx.doi.org/10.1021/cr000108x] [PMID: 11710233]

[11]   Ma PX. Scaffolds for tissue fabrication. Mater Today 2004; 7(5): 30-40.
        [http://dx.doi.org/10.1016/S1369-7021(04)00233-0]

[12]   Hoffman AS. Hydrogels for biomedical applications. Adv Drug Deliv Rev 2012; 64: 18-23.
        [http://dx.doi.org/10.1016/j.addr.2012.09.010] [PMID: 11755703]

[13]   Nicodemus GD, Bryant SJ. Cell encapsulation in biodegradable hydrogels for tissue engineering applications. Tissue Eng Part B Rev 2008; 14(2): 149-65.
        [http://dx.doi.org/10.1089/ten.teb.2007.0332] [PMID: 18498217]

[14]   Zhu J, Marchant RE. Design properties of hydrogel tissue-engineering scaffolds. Expert Rev Med Devices 2011; 8(5): 607-26.
        [http://dx.doi.org/10.1586/erd.11.27] [PMID: 22026626]

[15]   Sharma B, Elisseeff JH. Engineering structurally organized cartilage and bone tissues. Ann Biomed Eng 2004; 32(1): 148-59.
        [http://dx.doi.org/10.1023/B:ABME.0000007799.60142.78] [PMID: 14964730]

[16]   Brandl F, Sommer F, Goepferich A. Rational design of hydrogels for tissue engineering: impact of physical factors on cell behavior. Biomaterials 2007; 28(2): 134-46.
        [http://dx.doi.org/10.1016/j.biomaterials.2006.09.017] [PMID: 17011028]

[17]   Zhu J. Bioactive modification of poly(ethylene glycol) hydrogels for tissue engineering. Biomaterials 2010; 31(17): 4639-56.
        [http://dx.doi.org/10.1016/j.biomaterials.2010.02.044] [PMID: 20303169]

[18]   Fedorovich NE, Alblas J, de Wijn JR, Hennink WE, Verbout AJ, Dhert WJ. Hydrogels as extracellular matrices for skeletal tissue engineering: state-of-the-art and novel application in organ printing. Tissue Eng 2007; 13(8): 1905-25.
        [http://dx.doi.org/10.1089/ten.2006.0175] [PMID: 17518748]

[19]   Jung JH, Ono Y, Hanabusa K, Shinkai S. Creation of both right-handed and left-handed silica structures by sol-gel transcription of organogel fibers comprised of chiral diaminocyclohexane derivatives. J Am Chem Soc 2000; 122(20): 5008-9.
        [http://dx.doi.org/10.1021/ja000449s]

[20]   Hoffman DW. Roy R, Komarneni S. Diphasic Xerogels, A New Class of Materials: Phases in the System Al2o3-Sio2. J Am Ceram Soc 1984; 67(7): 468-71.

[http://dx.doi.org/10.1111/j.1151-2916.1984.tb19636.x]

[21]   Schaefer DW, Keefer KD. Structure of random porous materials: Silica aerogel. Phys Rev Lett 1986; 56(20): 2199-202.
[http://dx.doi.org/10.1103/PhysRevLett.56.2199] [PMID: 10032916]

[22]   Sridhar V, Takahata K. A hydrogel-based passive wireless sensor using a flex-circuit inductive transducer. Sens Actuators A Phys 2009; 155(1): 58-65.
[http://dx.doi.org/10.1016/j.sna.2009.08.010]

[23]   Cheung HY, Lau KT, Lu TP, Hui D. A critical review on polymer-based bio-engineered materials for scaffold development. Compos, Part B Eng 2007; 38(3): 291-300.
[http://dx.doi.org/10.1016/j.compositesb.2006.06.014]

[24]   Hoare TR, Kohane DS. Hydrogels in drug delivery: progress and challenges. Polymer (Guildf) 2008; 49(8): 1993-2007.
[http://dx.doi.org/10.1016/j.polymer.2008.01.027]

[25]   Zhao W, Jin X, Cong Y, Liu Y, Fu J. Degradable natural polymer hydrogels for articular cartilage tissue engineering. J Chem Technol Biotechnol 2013; 88(3): 327-39.
[http://dx.doi.org/10.1002/jctb.3970]

[26]   Iizawa T, Taketa H, Maruta M, Ishido T, Gotoh T, Sakohara S. Synthesis of porous poly (N☐isopropylacrylamide) gel beads by sedimentation polymerization and their morphology. J Appl Polym Sci 2007; 104(2): 842-50.
[http://dx.doi.org/10.1002/app.25605]

[27]   Yang L, Chu JS, Fix JA. Colon-specific drug delivery: new approaches and *in vitro/in vivo* evaluation. Int J Pharm 2002; 235(1-2): 1-15.
[http://dx.doi.org/10.1016/S0378-5173(02)00004-2] [PMID: 11879735]

[28]   Slaughter BV, Khurshid SS, Fisher OZ, Khademhosseini A, Peppas NA. Hydrogels in regenerative medicine. Adv Mater 2009; 21(32-33): 3307-29.
[http://dx.doi.org/10.1002/adma.200802106] [PMID: 20882499]

[29]   Kopeček J. Hydrogel biomaterials: a smart future? Biomaterials 2007; 28(34): 5185-92.
[http://dx.doi.org/10.1016/j.biomaterials.2007.07.044] [PMID: 17697712]

[30]   Wichterle O. Inventor; Ceskoslovenska Akademie Ved, assignee. Method of centrifugally casting thin edged corneal contact lenses. United States patent US 3,660,545 1972. May, 2.

[31]   Qiu Y, Park K. Environment-sensitive hydrogels for drug delivery. Adv Drug Deliv Rev 2012; 64: 49-60.
[http://dx.doi.org/10.1016/j.addr.2012.09.024] [PMID: 11744175]

[32]   Seol YJ, Park JY, Jeong W, Kim TH, Kim SY, Cho DW. Development of hybrid scaffolds using ceramic and hydrogel for articular cartilage tissue regeneration. J Biomed Mater Res A 2015; 103(4): 1404-13.
[http://dx.doi.org/10.1002/jbm.a.35276] [PMID: 25044835]

[33]   Annabi N, Nichol JW, Zhong X, *et al.* Controlling the porosity and microarchitecture of hydrogels for tissue engineering. Tissue Eng Part B Rev 2010; 16(4): 371-83.
[http://dx.doi.org/10.1089/ten.teb.2009.0639] [PMID: 20121414]

[34]   Hollister SJ. Porous scaffold design for tissue engineering. Nat Mater 2005; 4(7): 518-24.
[http://dx.doi.org/10.1038/nmat1421] [PMID: 16003400]

[35]   Seidi A, Ramalingam M, Elloumi-Hannachi I, Ostrovidov S, Khademhosseini A. Gradient biomaterials for soft-to-hard interface tissue engineering. Acta Biomater 2011; 7(4): 1441-51.
[http://dx.doi.org/10.1016/j.actbio.2011.01.011] [PMID: 21232635]

[36]   Morais MG, Vaz BD, Morais EG, Costa JA. Biological effects of Spirulina (Arthrospira) biopolymers and biomass in the development of nanostructured scaffolds BioMed research international, 2014 Jul

23 2014.

[37]   Chung HJ, Park TG. Surface engineered and drug releasing pre-fabricated scaffolds for tissue engineering. Adv Drug Deliv Rev 2007; 59(4-5): 249-62.
       [http://dx.doi.org/10.1016/j.addr.2007.03.015] [PMID: 17482310]

[38]   Reyes DR, Iossifidis D, Auroux PA, Manz A. Micro total analysis systems. 1. Introduction, theory, and technology. Anal Chem 2002; 74(12): 2623-36.
       [http://dx.doi.org/10.1021/ac0202435] [PMID: 12090653]

[39]   Ma PX, Langer R. Morphology and mechanical function of long-term *in vitro* engineered cartilage. J Biomed Mater Res 1999; 44(2): 217-21.
       [http://dx.doi.org/10.1002/(SICI)1097-4636(199902)44:2<217::AID-JBM12>3.0.CO;2-6]   [PMID: 10397923]

[40]   Sachlos E, Czernuszka JT. Making tissue engineering scaffolds work. Review: the application of solid freeform fabrication technology to the production of tissue engineering scaffolds. Eur Cell Mater 2003; 5(29): 29-39.
       [http://dx.doi.org/10.22203/eCM.v005a03] [PMID: 14562270]

[41]   Ikada Y. Challenges in tissue engineering. J R Soc Interface 2006; 3(10): 589-601.
       [http://dx.doi.org/10.1098/rsif.2006.0124] [PMID: 16971328]

[42]   Fisher JP, Jo S, Mikos AG, Reddi AH. Thermoreversible hydrogel scaffolds for articular cartilage engineering. J Biomed Mater Res A 2004; 71(2): 268-74.
       [http://dx.doi.org/10.1002/jbm.a.30148] [PMID: 15368220]

[43]   Smith LE, Rimmer S, MacNeil S. Examination of the effects of poly(N-vinylpyrrolidinone) hydrogels in direct and indirect contact with cells. Biomaterials 2006; 27(14): 2806-12.
       [http://dx.doi.org/10.1016/j.biomaterials.2005.12.018] [PMID: 16426677]

[44]   Karamian E, Khandan A, Eslami M, Gheisari H, Rafiaei N. Investigation of HA nanocrystallite size crystallographic characterizations in NHA, BHA and HA pure powders and their influence on biodegradation of HA. InAdvanced Materials Research 2014 Jan 13; 829: 314-8.

[45]   Heydary HA, Karamian E, Poorazizi E, Khandan A, Heydaripour J. A Novel Nano-Fiber of Iranian Gum Tragacanth-Polyvinyl alcohol/Nanoclay Composite for Wound Healing Applications. Procedia Materials Science 2015; 11: 176-82.
       [http://dx.doi.org/10.1016/j.mspro.2015.11.079]

[46]   Zarkoob S, Eby RK, Reneker DH, Hudson SD, Ertley D, Adams WW. Structure and morphology of electrospun silk nanofibers. Polymer (Guildf) 2004; 45(11): 3973-7.
       [http://dx.doi.org/10.1016/j.polymer.2003.10.102]

[47]   Matthews JA, Wnek GE, Simpson DG, Bowlin GL. Electrospinning of collagen nanofibers. Biomacromolecules 2002; 3(2): 232-8.
       [http://dx.doi.org/10.1021/bm015533u] [PMID: 11888306]

[48]   Ohkawa K, Cha D, Kim H, Nishida A, Yamamoto H. Electrospinning of chitosan. Macromol Rapid Commun 2004; 25(18): 1600-5.
       [http://dx.doi.org/10.1002/marc.200400253]

[49]   Reneker DH, Chun I. Nanometre diameter fibres of polymer, produced by electrospinning. Nanotechnology 1996; 7(3): 216.
       [http://dx.doi.org/10.1088/0957-4484/7/3/009]

[50]   Liang D, Hsiao BS, Chu B. Functional electrospun nanofibrous scaffolds for biomedical applications. Adv Drug Deliv Rev 2007; 59(14): 1392-412.
       [http://dx.doi.org/10.1016/j.addr.2007.04.021] [PMID: 17884240]

[51]   Nazarov R, Jin HJ, Kaplan DL. Porous 3-D scaffolds from regenerated silk fibroin. Biomacromolecules 2004; 5(3): 718-26.
       [http://dx.doi.org/10.1021/bm034327e] [PMID: 15132652]

[52] Mikos AG, Sarakinos G, Leite SM, Vacanti JP, Langer R. Laminated three-dimensional biodegradable foams for use in tissue engineering. Biomaterials 1993; 14(5): 323-30.
[http://dx.doi.org/10.1016/0142-9612(93)90049-8] [PMID: 8507774]

[53] Mano JF, Silva GA, Azevedo HS, *et al.* Natural origin biodegradable systems in tissue engineering and regenerative medicine: present status and some moving trends. J R Soc Interface 2007; 4(17): 999-1030.
[http://dx.doi.org/10.1098/rsif.2007.0220] [PMID: 17412675]

[54] Moore MJ, Jabbari E, Ritman EL, *et al.* Quantitative analysis of interconnectivity of porous biodegradable scaffolds with micro-computed tomography. J Biomed Mater Res A 2004; 71(2): 258-67.
[http://dx.doi.org/10.1002/jbm.a.30138] [PMID: 15376269]

[55] Martins A, Pinho ED, Faria S, *et al.* Surface modification of electrospun polycaprolactone nanofiber meshes by plasma treatment to enhance biological performance. Small 2009; 5(10): 1195-206.
[PMID: 19242938]

[56] Chen G, Ushida T, Tateishi T. Scaffold design for tissue engineering. Macromol Biosci 2002; 2(2): 67-77.
[http://dx.doi.org/10.1002/1616-5195(20020201)2:2<67::AID-MABI67>3.0.CO;2-F]

[57] Eberli D, Freitas Filho L, Atala A, Yoo JJ. Composite scaffolds for the engineering of hollow organs and tissues. Methods 2009; 47(2): 109-15.
[http://dx.doi.org/10.1016/j.ymeth.2008.10.014] [PMID: 18952175]

[58] Mooney DJ, Mazzoni CL, Breuer C, *et al.* Stabilized polyglycolic acid fibre-based tubes for tissue engineering. Biomaterials 1996; 17(2): 115-24.
[http://dx.doi.org/10.1016/0142-9612(96)85756-5] [PMID: 8624388]

[59] Moroni L, Schotel R, Hamann D, de Wijn JR, van Blitterswijk CA. 3D Fiber☐Deposited Electrospun Integrated Scaffolds Enhance Cartilage Tissue Formation. Adv Funct Mater 2008; 18(1): 53-60.
[http://dx.doi.org/10.1002/adfm.200601158]

[60] Zhao X, Zhang S. Molecular designer self-assembling peptides. Chem Soc Rev 2006; 35(11): 1105-10.
[http://dx.doi.org/10.1039/b511336a] [PMID: 17057839]

[61] Liu HK, Sun WY, Tang WX, Yamamoto T, Ueyama N. Self-assembly of the first copper (ii) infinite 2d network with large cavities formed between the two adjacent layers. Inorg Chem 1999; 38(26): 6313-6.
[http://dx.doi.org/10.1021/ic9907563] [PMID: 11671351]

[62] Lin J, Landay JA. Employing patterns and layers for early-stage design and prototyping of cross-device user interfaces.
[http://dx.doi.org/10.1145/1357054.1357260]

[63] Hutmacher DW. Scaffolds in tissue engineering bone and cartilage. Biomaterials 2000; 21(24): 2529-43.
[http://dx.doi.org/10.1016/S0142-9612(00)00121-6] [PMID: 11071603]

[64] Thomson RC, Wake MC, Yaszemski MJ, Mikos AG. Biodegradable polymer scaffolds to regenerate organs. InBiopolymers Ii 1995 Jan 1; 245-74. Springer Berlin Heidelberg.
[http://dx.doi.org/10.1007/3540587888_18]

[65] Maquet V, Jerome R. Design of macroporous biodegradable polymer scaffolds for cell transplantation. InMaterials Science Forum 1997 Sep 11; 250: 15-42.
[http://dx.doi.org/10.4028/www.scientific.net/MSF.250.15]

[66] Whang K, Thomas CH, Healy KE, Nuber G. A novel method to fabricate bioabsorbable scaffolds. Polymer (Guildf) 1995; 36(4): 837-42.
[http://dx.doi.org/10.1016/0032-3861(95)93115-3]

[67]   Mandal BB, Kundu SC. Cell proliferation and migration in silk fibroin 3D scaffolds. Biomaterials 2009; 30(15): 2956-65.
[http://dx.doi.org/10.1016/j.biomaterials.2009.02.006] [PMID: 19249094]

[68]   Altman GH, Diaz F, Jakuba C, *et al.* Silk-based biomaterials. Biomaterials 2003; 24(3): 401-16.
[http://dx.doi.org/10.1016/S0142-9612(02)00353-8] [PMID: 12423595]

[69]   Karadağ E, Saraydin D, Çetinkaya S, Güven O. *In vitro* swelling studies and preliminary biocompatibility evaluation of acrylamide-based hydrogels. Biomaterials 1996; 17(1): 67-70.
[http://dx.doi.org/10.1016/0142-9612(96)80757-5] [PMID: 8962950]

[70]   Stevenson WT, Sefton MV. The equilibrium water content of some thermoplastic hydroxyalkyl methacrylate polymers. J Appl Polym Sci 1988; 36(7): 1541-53.
[http://dx.doi.org/10.1002/app.1988.070360703]

[71]   Roorda WE, Boddé HE, De Boer AG, Bouwstra JA, Junginer HE. Synthetic hydrogels as drug delivery systems. Pharm Weekbl Sci 1986; 8(3): 165-89.
[PMID: 3526277]

[72]   Knapczyk J, Krowczynski L, Krzck J, *et al.* Requirements of chitosan for pharmaceutical and biomedical applications Chitin and Chitosan: Sources, Chemistry, Biochemistry, Physical Properties and Applications. London: Elsevier 1989; pp. 657-63.

[73]   Hirano S, Seino H, Akiyama Y, Nonaka I. Chitosan: a biocompatible material for oral and intravenous administrations. InProgress in biomedical polymers 1990 Jan 1; 283-90.
[http://dx.doi.org/10.1007/978-1-4899-0768-4_28]

[74]   Machida Y, Nagai T, Abe M, Sannan T. Use of chitosan and hydroxypropylchitosan in drug formulations to effect sustained release. Drug Des Deliv 1986; 1(2): 119-30.
[PMID: 3509325]

[75]   Hirano S, Tsuchida H, Nagao N. N-acetylation in chitosan and the rate of its enzymic hydrolysis. Biomaterials 1989; 10(8): 574-6.
[http://dx.doi.org/10.1016/0142-9612(89)90066-5] [PMID: 2605289]

[76]   Aiba S. Studies on chitosan: 4. Lysozymic hydrolysis of partially N-acetylated chitosans. Int J Biol Macromol 1992; 14(4): 225-8.
[http://dx.doi.org/10.1016/S0141-8130(05)80032-7] [PMID: 1504044]

[77]   Molinaro G, Leroux JC, Damas J, Adam A. Biocompatibility of thermosensitive chitosan-based hydrogels: an *in vivo* experimental approach to injectable biomaterials. Biomaterials 2002; 23(13): 2717-22.
[http://dx.doi.org/10.1016/S0142-9612(02)00004-2] [PMID: 12059021]

[78]   Bhattarai N, Gunn J, Zhang M. Chitosan-based hydrogels for controlled, localized drug delivery. Adv Drug Deliv Rev 2010; 62(1): 83-99.
[http://dx.doi.org/10.1016/j.addr.2009.07.019] [PMID: 19799949]

[79]   Chen JP, Cheng TH. Thermo-responsive chitosan-graft-poly(N-isopropylacrylamide) injectable hydrogel for cultivation of chondrocytes and meniscus cells. Macromol Biosci 2006; 6(12): 1026-39.
[http://dx.doi.org/10.1002/mabi.200600142] [PMID: 17128421]

[80]   Berger J, Reist M, Mayer JM, Felt O, Peppas NA, Gurny R. Structure and interactions in covalently and ionically crosslinked chitosan hydrogels for biomedical applications. Eur J Pharm Biopharm 2004; 57(1): 19-34.
[http://dx.doi.org/10.1016/S0939-6411(03)00161-9] [PMID: 14729078]

[81]   Jin J, Song M, Hourston DJ. Novel chitosan-based films cross-linked by genipin with improved physical properties. Biomacromolecules 2004; 5(1): 162-8.
[http://dx.doi.org/10.1021/bm034286m] [PMID: 14715022]

[82]   Wu Z, Sheng Z, Sun T, *et al.* Preparation of collagen-based materials for wound dressing. Chin Med J

(Engl) 2003; 116(3): 419-23.
[PMID: 12781050]

[83] Shigemasa Y, Minami S. Applications of chitin and chitosan for biomaterials. Biotechnol Genet Eng Rev 1996; 13(1): 383-420.
[http://dx.doi.org/10.1080/02648725.1996.10647935] [PMID: 8948118]

[84] Rao SB, Sharma CP. Use of chitosan as a biomaterial: studies on its safety and hemostatic potential. J Biomed Mater Res 1997; 34(1): 21-8.
[http://dx.doi.org/10.1002/(SICI)1097-4636(199701)34:1<21::AID-JBM4>3.0.CO;2-P]   [PMID: 8978649]

[85] Draye JP, Delaey B, Van de Voorde A, Van Den Bulcke A, De Reu B, Schacht E. *In vitro* and *in vivo* biocompatibility of dextran dialdehyde cross-linked gelatin hydrogel films. Biomaterials 1998; 19(18): 1677-87.
[http://dx.doi.org/10.1016/S0142-9612(98)00049-0] [PMID: 9840003]

[86] Dover R, Otto WR, Nanchahal J, Riches DJ. Toxicity testing of wound dressing materials *in vitro*. Br J Plast Surg 1995; 48(4): 230-5.
[http://dx.doi.org/10.1016/0007-1226(95)90007-1] [PMID: 7640856]

[87] Rosdy M, Clauss LC. Cytotoxicity testing of wound dressings using normal human keratinocytes in culture. J Biomed Mater Res 1990; 24(3): 363-77.
[http://dx.doi.org/10.1002/jbm.820240308] [PMID: 2318900]

[88] Cima LG, Vacanti JP, Vacanti C, Ingber D, Mooney D, Langer R. Tissue engineering by cell transplantation using degradable polymer substrates. J Biomech Eng 1991; 113(2): 143-51.
[http://dx.doi.org/10.1115/1.2891228] [PMID: 1652042]

[89] Karande T, Agrawal C. Function and Requirement of Synthetic Scaffolds in Tissue Engineering. Boca Raton, FL: CRC Press 2008.

[90] Karamian E, Motamedi MR, Khandan A, Soltani P, Maghsoudi S. An *in vitro* evaluation of novel NHA/zircon plasma coating on 316L stainless steel dental implant. Progress in Natural Science: Materials International 2014; 24(2): 150-6.
[http://dx.doi.org/10.1016/j.pnsc.2014.04.001]

[91] Khandan A, Abdellahi M, Barenji RV, Ozada N, Karamian E. Introducing natural hydroxyapatite-diopside (NHA-Di) nano-bioceramic coating. Ceram Int 2015; 41(9): 12355-63.
[http://dx.doi.org/10.1016/j.ceramint.2015.06.065]

[92] Karamian E, Khandan A, Kalantar Motamedi MR, Mirmohammadi H. Surface characteristics and bioactivity of a novel natural HA/zircon nanocomposite coated on dental implants. BioMed research international 2014 Apr 16; 2014

[93] Khandan A, Karamian E, Bonakdarchian M. Mechanochemical synthesis evaluation of nanocrystalline bone-derived bioceramic powder using for bone tissue engineering. Dent Hypotheses 2014; 5(4): 155.
[http://dx.doi.org/10.4103/2155-8213.140606]

[94] Heydary HA, Karamian E, Poorazizi E, Heydaripour J, Khandan A. Electrospun of polymer/bioceramic nanocomposite as a new soft tissue for biomedical applications. Journal of Asian Ceramic Societies 2015; 3(4): 417-25.
[http://dx.doi.org/10.1016/j.jascer.2015.09.003]

[95] Khandan A, Abdellahi M, Ozada N, Ghayour H. Study of the bioactivity, wettability and hardness behaviour of the bovine hydroxyapatite-diopside bio-nanocomposite coating. Journal of the Taiwan Institute of Chemical Engineers 2015 Oct 26.

[96] Khandan A, Ozada N, Karamian E. Novel microstructure mechanical activated nano composites for tissue engineering applications. J Bioeng Biomed Sci 2015; 5(143): 2.

[97] Yazdimamaghani M, Razavi M, Vashaee D, Tayebi L. Development and degradation behavior of magnesium scaffolds coated with polycaprolactone for bone tissue engineering. Mater Lett 2014; 132:

106-10.
[http://dx.doi.org/10.1016/j.matlet.2014.06.036]

[98] Yazdimamaghani M, Razavi M, Vashaee D, Tayebi L. Microstructural and mechanical study of PCL coated Mg scaffolds. Surf Eng 2014; 30(12): 920-6.
[http://dx.doi.org/10.1179/1743294414Y.0000000307]

[99] Yazdimamaghani M, Razavi M, Vashaee D, Tayebi L. Surface modification of biodegradable porous Mg bone scaffold using polycaprolactone/bioactive glass composite. Mater Sci Eng C 2015; 49: 436-44.
[http://dx.doi.org/10.1016/j.msec.2015.01.041] [PMID: 25686970]

[100] Yazdimamaghani M, Razavi M, Mozafari M, Vashaee D, Kotturi H, Tayebi L. Biomineralization and biocompatibility studies of bone conductive scaffolds containing poly(3,4-ethylenedioxythiophene):poly(4-styrene sulfonate) (PEDOT:PSS). J Mater Sci Mater Med 2015; 26(12): 274.
[http://dx.doi.org/10.1007/s10856-015-5599-8] [PMID: 26543020]

[101] Razavi M, Fathi M, Savabi O, Vashaee D, Tayebi L. *In vivo* assessments of bioabsorbable AZ91 magnesium implants coated with nanostructured fluoridated hydroxyapatite by MAO/EPD technique for biomedical applications. Mater Sci Eng C 2015; 48: 21-7.
[http://dx.doi.org/10.1016/j.msec.2014.11.020] [PMID: 25579892]

[102] Kazemi A, Abdellahi M, Khajeh-Sharafabadi A, Khandan A, Ozada N. Study of *in vitro* bioactivity and mechanical properties of diopside nano-bioceramic synthesized by a facile method using eggshell as raw material. Mater Sci Eng C 2017; 71: 604-10.
[http://dx.doi.org/10.1016/j.msec.2016.10.044] [PMID: 27987751]

[103] Razavi M, Fathi M, Savabi O, Vashaee D, Tayebi L. *In vitro* study of nanostructured diopside coating on Mg alloy orthopedic implants. Mater Sci Eng C 2014; 41: 168-77.
[http://dx.doi.org/10.1016/j.msec.2014.04.039] [PMID: 24907750]

[104] Subia B, Kundu J, Kundu SC. Biomaterial scaffold fabrication techniques for potential tissue engineering applications. INTECH Open Access Publisher 2010.
[http://dx.doi.org/10.5772/8581]

[105] Medberry CJ, Crapo PM, Siu BF, *et al.* Hydrogels derived from central nervous system extracellular matrix. Biomaterials 2013; 34(4): 1033-40.
[http://dx.doi.org/10.1016/j.biomaterials.2012.10.062] [PMID: 23158935]

[106] Pati F, Jang J, Ha DH, *et al.* Printing three-dimensional tissue analogues with decellularized extracellular matrix bioink. Nat Commun 2014; 5: 3935.
[http://dx.doi.org/10.1038/ncomms4935] [PMID: 24887553]

[107] Najafinezhad A, Abdellahi M, Ghayour H, Soheily A, Chami A, Khandan A. A comparative study on the synthesis mechanism, bioactivity and mechanical properties of three silicate bioceramics. Mater Sci Eng C 2017; 72: 259-67.
[http://dx.doi.org/10.1016/j.msec.2016.11.084] [PMID: 28024584]

[108] Sharafabadi AK, Abdellahi M, Kazemi A, Khandan A, Ozada N. A novel and economical route for synthesizing akermanite (Ca2MgSi2O7) nano-bioceramic. Mater Sci Eng C 2017; 71: 1072-8.
[http://dx.doi.org/10.1016/j.msec.2016.11.021] [PMID: 27987661]

CHAPTER 5

Metallic Scaffolds

Mehdi Razavi[1,*]

[1] *Department of Radiology, School of Medicine, Stanford University, Palo Alto, California 94304, USA*

Abstract: The focus of hard tissue engineering is mostly on osteo and dental clinical applications. Whereas hard tissues are usually under the load, biomaterials used for this purpose must have sufficient mechanical properties as well as corrosion resistance, enough wear resistance and biocompatibility. A lot of amazing researches are in process throughout the world in an attempt to develop new scaffolds for tissue engineering. Today, most research efforts are made to develop scaffolds through using the natural and synthetic polymers for soft tissue engineering; however, metallic scaffolds have also been the interest of *in vitro* and *in vivo* research for hard tissue engineering. With regard to the excellent mechanical behavior of metals rather than polymers and ceramics, metallic scaffolds have been preferred for bone tissue engineering applications in which the tissue is under the load. Up to now, numerous biocompatible metallic biomaterials have been utilized as implants in dental and orthopaedic surgery in order to repair damaged bones and to provide support for bone healing. In this article, efforts have been made to review the applications of titanium, tantalum, nitinol and magnesium in scaffolds.

Keywords: Magnesium, Metallic biomaterials, Nitinol, Tantalum, Titanium.

INTRODUCTION

Metals and their alloys have been extensively utilized in orthopaedic systems such as the head of the femoral component of a total hip joint replacement (THJR) (Co–Cr– Mo alloy), the stem of a total shoulder joint replacement (Ti–6Al–4V alloy), the tibial tray in a total knee joint replacement (TKJR) (Ti–6Al–4V alloy), and a spinal fusion cage (Ti) [1 - 4]. The development of porous metals and coatings for osseointegration has revolutionized the field of orthopaedics, particularly total joint reconstruction. Several new highly porous metals have been recently introduced to improve the biomaterial properties of these traditional metals, namely porosity, surface coefficient, and modulus of elasticity [5 - 7].

* **Corresponding author Mehdi Razavi:** Department of Radiology, School of Medicine, Stanford University, Palo Alto, California 94304, USA; Tel: +16504847293; E-mails: merazavi@stanford.edu; mrazavi2659@gmail.com

Mehdi Razavi (Ed.)

These new biomaterials all share a microscopic characteristic appearance similar to cancellous bone which have been mainly used for osteo and dental applications include acetabular cups, femoral stems and total knee arthroplasty components, and tibial component for total knee replacement, stem for revision hip arthroplasty, Tantalum rods implanted for avascular necrosis of the hip [8].

High biocompatibility, low uniform *in vivo* corrosion rate, and high specific strength in Ti-based alloys are among the reasons for the selection of this kind of materials. However, one major problem is the high probability of aseptic implant loosening due to three phenomena. One of the phenomena is bone resorption that is caused by stress shielding which is because of the mismatch in the elastic modulus of material and the tissue. The second and the third phenomena are the weak interfacial bonding between the implant and the bone (poor osseo-integration) and lack of biological anchorage for tissue in-growth, which are both the results of the difference in the morphologies of the bone and the implant metal/alloy [1]. To deal with the modulus mismatch issue, many research and development programs have been put into practice in order to produce and characterize metallic materials which their mechanical properties are close to those of trabecular bone [9, 10]. Such materials, called metallic scaffolds, have three-dimensional interconnected porous structures, typical pore sizes in the range of 200-500 μm with the total porosity of 50–75 vol/vol% [11]. Furthermore, porous scaffolds have been introduced in order to improve the biological fixation [12 - 16]. The bonding between the implant and the bone is obtained when the tissue grows into the pores of a metallic implant. Substantial interconnectivity of pores in metallic implants allows the bio-fluid to move through the pores, which can stimulate the bone tissue ingrowth, and thus, result in the development of highly porous metallic scaffolds that could be utilized as in bone tissue engineering [12].

Many methods such as the gas foaming, space holder method, laser engineered net-shaping process, and selective electron beam method have been employed to develop these metals/alloys, and the first one is, undoubtedly, the most popular method [1]. One of the feasible techniques for making metallic scaffolds is considered the space holder method in which temporary powder particles, space holders, are devised as pore formers for scaffolds [17]. The whole process of scaffold production using the space holder technique can be divided into four main steps including mixing the metal matrix powder and space-holding particles, pressing the granular materials, removing the space-holding particles, and sintering the porous scaffold. As a powder metallurgy route, powder sintering has been in wide use due to its straightforwardness in making the scaffolds [17]. In this technique, particles of metal powder are pressed and then sintered. However, the formation of pores from the spaces in powder particle arrangements is inevitable [18]. In this chapter, some properties, advantages, drawbacks, recent researches and future research trends of common metallic scaffolds are to be presented.

TITANIUM

Titanium is well tolerated and almost an inert biomaterial in the body. In an optimal situation, it results in osseo integration with bone [19, 20]. Additionally, it forms an extremely stable protective layer of TiO_2 providing excellent biocompatibility. Even if this layer is damaged, it is quickly rebuilt. In titanium, the nature of the oxide film protecting the metal substrate from corrosion is particularly important, and its physicochemical properties like crystallinity, impurity segregation, *etc.*, are quite relevant. Compared to stainless steels and cobalt-based alloys, Titanium alloys show superior biocompatibility. Since alloys of Titanium-aluminium-vanadium (ASTM F136, ASTM F1108 and ASTMF1472) have better mechanical properties compared to commercially pure titanium (cpTi) (ASTM F67, they are utilized more extensively in total joint implants. However, since elements like vanadium are toxic in the elemental state, there are still some concerns regarding the existence of long-term Ti-6Al-4V implants in the body. Such concerns have resulted in the fabrication of beta type titanium alloys with nontoxic alloying elements such as Ta, Nb, Zr [21]. Currently, significant research have been carried out to develop new titanium alloys with lower moduli, particularly prepared for biomaterials applications. Such alloys are Ti–12Mo–6Zr–2Fe (TMZF), Ti–15Mo–5Zr–3Al, Ti–15Zr–4Nb–2Ta–0.2Pd, Ti–15Sn–4Nb–2Ta–0.2Pd, Ti–13Nb–13Zr, new β-type biomedical Ti–29Nb–13Ta–4.6Zr,11 and Ti–35Nb–5Ta–7Zr alloys [22]. However, the Young moduli of all developed titanium alloys are still more than that of the cancellous bone [22, 23]. Recently, this new generation of Ti alloys is under research, and it seems that it has not yet been commercialized.

Porous titanium alloys have shown good biocompatibility. During the past twenty years, bioactive titanium meshes have been utilized in spine fusion surgery very successfully [24]. The titanium mesh cage contoured into cylindrical shape has been successfully employed for anterior lumbar interbody fusion (ALIF). They were also utilized with autografts to graft bones in spinal fusion; however, this is limited by factors such as complications and second site morbidity [24]. One strategy to deal with this concern is to use hydroxyapatite to give the required bioactivity to the titanium mesh cage with a porous network to stimulate osteo-conduction [25]. In addition, in spite of great advances made in complete tissue-engineered oral and maxillofacial structures, the current standard for load-bearing applications such as maxilla, mandible, and craniofacial reconstruction remains in titanium meshes and titanium 3D scaffolds. Since Ti and its alloys are not ferromagnetic, they do not harm the patient in magnetic resonance imaging (MRI) units. Potentially, by loading the scaffold with specific growth factors, Titanium osseo-integration can be improved. In applications in which there are gaps, like craniofacial reconstruction or augmentation of bone or peri-implant defects, stimulation of bone regeneration has usually been accompanied by delivering TGF and BMP-2 through titanium scaffold [26]. The latter growth factors are capable of eliciting specific cellular responses, which result in the rapid formation of new tissue. Moreover, stem cells have been cultured onto titanium scaffolds [27] in an attempt to encourage the calcified nodules formation so that the development of mineralized extracellular matrix (ECM) onto the cells/scaffold complexes is enhanced. As permanent load-bearing bone implants, porous titanium and titanium alloys apparently possess excellent mechanical properties [28]. Many basic scientific pre-clinical and clinical researches carried out so far support the usefulness of Ti scaffolds. As far as marginal bone defects and bone growth are concerned, Ti foams allow for bone in-growth through interconnected pores [29]. On the other hand, as a clinical tool for bone reconstructive surgery, titanium fibre-mesh is a useful scaffold material warranting further investigations. *In vitro*, titanium fibre-mesh scaffold is utilized for the adhesion and osteoblastic differentiation of progenitor cells [30], but it reveals to be osteo-conductive *in vivo*, showing encouraging results [31]. The results obtained in these pre-clinical researches confirm that bone healing is possible by using biochemically modified Ti scaffolds, particularly by using growth factors and osteo-progenitor cells. Nevertheless, the assessment of the potential for using these biochemically-modified Ti scaffolds for clinical applications in the future depends on the ability of the studies to display outstanding long-term results. Clinically, cylindrical titanium meshes have had consistently good results for the reconstruction of large anterior column defects. From a biomechanical standpoint, it seems that implanting synthetic cages into the anterior column offers immediately effective segmental stability, restoration of the anterior vertebral support, and correction of the sagittal plane deformity. Such anterior interbody cages have an acceptable axial load-bearing ability; thus, morcellized autograft can fill the inside of the cage [32].

There are numerous publication reporting the clinical outcomes of titanium scaffolds; hence, longer follow-up and a larger sample group of patients are required in order to obtain consistent clinical success rates.

Several techniques, such as compression and sintering of fibres and beads, electron beam melting, combustion synthesis, solid-state foaming by expansion of argon-filled pores and polymeric sponge replication, have been employed to introduce a degree of porosity in titanium scaffolds [33]. Rapid prototyping (RP) techniques can be utilized as a viable substitute to achieve extensive and a detailed control over scaffold architecture with a combination of computer-aided design (CAD) and computer-aided manufacturing (CAM) [34]. RP enables us to build objects with predefined microstructures and macrostructures, and provides the potential for making scaffolds that have controlled hierarchical structures [35].

In a study, porous titanium scaffolds were developed, with heterogeneous distribution of pores with the pore sizes of up to 600 μm in diameter and a total porosity of up to 75% [12]. In this research, high permeability was seen for samples with the highest values of porosity. Compared to cast titanium, porous titanium had low resistance to corrosion. Nevertheless, the mechanical parameters of the studied samples were similar to those for cancellous bone [12].

Ryan *et al.* [33] developed a multi-stage rapid prototyping technique, which fabricates porous titanium scaffolds with interconnected pores, and reproducible pore size and porosity. The porous characteristics of the scaffold were governed by a sacrificial wax template, which was produced by using a 3D-printer. Powder metallurgy routes were utilized in order to produce the titanium scaffolds by filling around the wax template with titanium slurry. Pore sizes ranging from 200 to 400 μm were achieved by changing the wax design template. Scaffolds with 66.8% porosities indicated compression strengths of 104.4 MPa and 23.5 MPa in axial and transverse directions, respectively, which revealed their anisotropic nature. 3D reconstruction paved the way for the main architectural parameters like pore size, level of anisotropy, interconnecting porosity and level of structural disorder to be measured. Furthermore, the experiments showed that the osteoblasts preserve their metabolic activity on the surface of titanium scaffolds [33].

In another work, titanium scaffolds were developed from TiH_2 slurry by replication sponge reactive sintering technique, and they were coated with hydroxyapatite [36]. The scaffolds show a 3D interconnected porous structure, mechanically and morphologically similar to trabecular bone. The bioactivity of such scaffolds suggests a potential for osseo-integration. Moreover, interconnected pores in the size range of 100–600 μm related to 75% porosity were obtained, which led to compressive strength and elastic modulus of 23.72 MPa of 0.30 GPa, respectively [36].

A research analysed the performance of titanium alloy scaffolds *in vivo* through using 3D fibre deposition, a rapid prototyping technique that allows the development of porous implants with accurately controlled structural properties, and the investigation of the effect of structural parameters on the *in vivo* biomaterials' behaviour [37]. The titanium alloy scaffolds with different structural properties, *e.g.* pore size, porosity and interconnecting pore size, were implanted on the decorticated transverse processes of 10 goats' posterior lumbar spines. *In vivo* results indicated that an enhance in porosity and pore size, and accordingly enhance in permeability of titanium alloy implants positively affected their osteo-conductive behaviour [37].

TANTALUM

As a transition metal tantalum with atomic number of 73 and atomic weight of 180.05, is inert *in vivo*. Since mid-1900s, multiple medical devices such as pacemaker electrodes, foil and mesh for nerve repairs, radiopaque markers, and cranioplasty plates have been made that use this material [38, 39]. Tantalum, as an elemental material, is highly resistant to chemical attack in body fluid, and has been extensively explored as a biomaterial [40, 41]. Moreover, its elastic modulus is similar to that of bone, which minimizes stress shielding. In the solid state, tantalum has an elastic modulus of about 185 GPa, which is far beyond that of bone (0.8–15 GPa). Tantalum-based implants have had an extraordinary biocompatibility and safety record in orthopaedic, cranio-facial, and dentistry literature [42]. Bermudez et al. [43] have demonstrated its excellent corrosion–erosion resistance in highly acidic environments, with no remarkable changes in weight or roughness compared to titanium and stainless steel implants. Good biocompatibility of tantalum has been displayed in a canine joint replacement model at long term follow-up [44]. Dental implants with tantalum-based components utilized for osseous anchorage have had excellent 8-year follow-up [45]. The oxide layer that is formed on the surface of tantalum implants *in vivo* is quite stable in a wide range of pH and potential ranges [42]. Johansson *et al.* [46] have indicated outstanding biocompatibility of tantalum and titanium with only slight differences in interfacial tissue reactions between these metals. As revealed in high-resolution examination, titanium had no multi-nucleated macrophages in the tissue which surrounded the metallic implant, whereas tantalum implants showed an occasional macrophage around the implant. Having implanted tantalum wire into soft tissues and a rat's femora to measure the reactions of soft and hard tissue to this metal, Matsuno *et al.* [47] found tantalum to have appropriate biocompatibility with no surrounding inflammatory responses. After 4 weeks of implantation, there was outstanding corrosion resistance but no dissolution of tantalum was noticed. The results are supported by several researches in which histological analysis was employed to reveal any evidence of inflammatory reaction or giant cells in tissue that surrounded porous tantalum implants [45]. This metal is highly ductile forming a stable oxide component (Ta_2O_5) on its surface [39].

The extremely high melting temperature of Ta (3017 °C) and its high affinity towards oxygen makes it too difficult, if not impossible, to process Ta structures through conventional processing methods. In spite of the fact that Trabecular Metal™ is commercially available, the relatively high cost of manufacture and failure to produce a modular tantalum implant has restricted its extensive use [48].

Inherent properties and proven biocompatibility of porous tantalum make it fascinating for designing and manufacturing bone graft substitute, cementless components for total joint arthroplasty, or a scaffold for potential cartilage resurfacing. Porous tantalum implants can be made from the pyrolysis of thermosetting polymer foam. This foam, in turn, creates a low-density vitreous carbon skeleton (98% porosity) with an array of regular pores with twelve sides. Then, pure tantalum is deposited onto this interconnected vitreous carbon scaffold by using chemical vapour deposition or infiltration [45]. By introducing pores, Implex Corp. and Zimmer have made a material that has a bonelike modulus and that preserves the material characteristics, which have introduced bulk tantalum as a versatile biomaterial. Trabecular Metal™ scaffolds have an open cell architecture, which is made of polyhedral (12–14-sided) pores. This unique shape is formed by the deposition of chemical vapour of tantalum onto a skeleton of vitreous carbon. The vitreous carbon template is covered with tantalum, and results in an open cell structure. Unlike solid tantalum, a scarcity of published data exists for porous tantalum scaffolds. A number of clinical studies have investigated the *in vivo* integration potential of porous tantalum with tissues around it. According to these studies, porous tantalum scaffolds make bone formation easier and integrate well with hard [45] and soft tissue types [49]. Moreover, *in vitro* material and mechanical characterizations of porous tantalum scaffolds have also been performed, which have yielded valuable radiographic [50], compressive, tensile, and bending data [51].

Tantalum is more corrosion resistant compared to titanium. Its bioactivity is similar to that of titanium. The main limitations of porous tantalum scaffolds could be the very high costs of production and problems with machining, together with lack of long-term clinical data [12].

Porous tantalum is sufficiently strong to allow physiological load-carrying applications, and can be used as an alternative metal for primary and revision of total knee arthroplasty (TKA) with several unique properties. Bobyn and colleagues [45] presented basic data supporting the use of this material, which is a trabecular metal made of a carbon substrate with elemental tantalum deposited on its surface and is highly biocompatible in animal models. Researches have shown substantial cortical bone ingrowth between the trabecular network and high levels of bone growth onto the scaffold. Initial stability of the trabecular metal is also higher than that of standard materials like cobalt chrome. In addition, this new material has better osteo-conduction than other technologies that are used for biological fixation [19]. Bobyn *et al.* [45] implanted porous tantalum cylinders with subsequent mechanical and histological testing at interval follow-up by using a transcortical canine model. Two different pore sizes were evaluated including cylinders averaging 430 µm and another group averaging 650 µm. In the small pore model, new bone occupied 42% of the pores in 1 month, 63% in 4 months, and 80% in 1 year. The large pore model occupied 13% in 2 weeks, 53% in 1 month, and 70% in 4 and 1 year and 1 month on the average. Histological studies showed increasing regions of bone–implant contact as time passed, and there was an evidence of Haversian remodelling within the pores. Mechanical testing revealed minimum shear fixation strength of 18.5MPa in 1 month, which is far higher than CoCr sintered beads (9.3 MPa) and several other porous tantalum components and augments currently available to use in both primary and revision THA (Total hip arthroplasty (THA)). A great variety of implants ranging from amonoblock acetabular component for primary THA to custom augments to be used in reconstituting bone stock in complex revision cases have been offered. These components have high surface frictional characteristics, a low modulus of elasticity, and outstanding osseo-integration behaviour such as bioactivity, biocompatibility, and bone in-growth properties [45]. A porous tantalum implant has been designed to treat osteonecrosis of the femoral head in its early stages. The implant aims to provide subchondral support of cartilage on the surface while the avascular lesion reconstitutes itself inside the femoral head. Lab researches have confirmed the efficiency of this implant in supporting a subchondral plate in a model simulating a necrotic femoral head. Porous tantalum implants are also used in revision and primary TKA (Total knee arthroplasty); they have been investigated to find out if they can be used for cervical and lumbar spinal arthrodeses in animal models. Having used porous tantalum blocks with and without recombinant bone morphogenic protein (rhBMP-)-2 in a goat model, Sidhu *et al.* [52] found improved bone in-growth with rhBMP-2 and porous tantalum blocks for anterior cervical inter body fusion, though the number of animals was too few to measure a statistical difference. In the same way, Zou *et al.* reported bone in-growth and successful lumbar spinal fusion by employing porous tantalum rings/cages [53].

NICKEL-TITANIUM ALLOY (NITINOL)

The near-equi-atomic nickel–titanium alloy (NiTi or Nitinol) has unusual mechanical properties (*e.g.*, the super-elasticity and shape-memory effects related to a thermo-elastic phase transformation near ambient temperature, martensite twinning and prevention of slip by fine Ni4Ti3 precipitates) making multifunctional applications involving high recovery strain, high strength and a relatively low Young's modulus possible [54]. Nitinol has numerous applications because it has a mixture of properties, even in a porous state, such as enhanced biocompatibility, shape memory effect, super-plasticity, and high damping properties [55]. Porous nickel titanium is a promising bone substitute because the near-equi-atomic NiTi shape memory alloy has the same super-elastic biomechanical properties as some human hard tissues like bones and tendons, low elastic modulus, the unique shape memory effect, high strength, outstanding biocompatibility, and new bone-ingrowth ability and vascularization [56]. Since the elastic modulus of the Nitinol foams (~2.3 GPa) and the compressive strength (~ 208 MPa) are close to those of human bone and due to its biocompatibility, porous NiTi is used in making intramedullary nails and spinal intervertebral spacers, which are utilized in the treatment of scoliosis [57]. Compared to other porous metals for implants (*e.g.*, Co and stainless steel), an additional advantage of porous NiTi is NiTi's excellent compatibility for computer tomography scanning and magnetic resonance imaging [58]. With regard to the unique collection of mechanical, magnetic imaging and biological properties of porous NiTi, further biomedical applications are expected to be developed in the future [54]. Vast *in vivo* testing and preclinical experience illustrate that Nitinol is more biocompatible than stainless steels [57]. Furthermore, as reported, it exhibits good biocompatibility on surface modified NiTi [59]. Nitinol's biocompatibility, its physical properties and shape memory effects indicate that this alloy may have many applications in the orthopaedic field. These gains are about creating scaffolds that change shape after implantation because of Nitinol's shape memory (SME) which can be initiated at 37 degrees Celsius. However, the release of Ni ions creates allergy and toxicity in NiTi alloys. This concern and potential carcinogenicity of Ni have limited the use of NiTi alloys in Europe and the US. Surface modifications like oxidation treatment of NiTi in order to obtain a Ni-free surface [59] and several alternative Ni-free shape memory alloys, mainly Nb-based, are recently in process in order to deal with this problem though their long-term biological performance are yet to be assessed [60]. Most research activities in this area are focused on how to improve the manufacturing processes, surface biocompatibility, and general mechanical properties [56].

A porous form of NiTi was introduced a few years after the discovery of the unusual shape memory properties of NiTi. Because of additional benefits common to other porous or foamed metals including low density, high surface area, and high permeability, porous NiTi was suggested in many applications such as bone implants, energy absorption, light-weight actuators and hydrogen isotope separation [54]. Porous nickel–titanium (nitinol) has already been investigated as an orthopaedic implant material for craniofacial applications [61]. Porous nitinol has the benefit of interfacial porosity and a permanent structural framework for the long-term replacement of bone defects [62]. Biomedical applications remain the main aim for NiTi with open porosity with regard to its good biocompatibility that can be compared with conventional porous stainless steel and titanium implant materials [63]. Furthermore, a combination of high strength, low stiffness, high toughness, and shape-recovery behaviour facilitates implant insertion and ensures mechanical integrity inside the host tissue [54]. NiTi is a superior alloy in monolithic, non-porous form for many bone implant applications due to its biocompatibility and unusual mechanical properties. The applications consist of cervical and lumbar vertebral replacements, maxillofacial and dental implants, bone plates, joint replacements, spine fracture fixation, bone tissue engineering, anchorage and repair [64]. In addition, nitinol's shape-memory characteristics pave the way for *in situ* recovery of implant shape after any injury to the implant or surrounding hard tissue [62]. Since Nitinol is low in corrosion due to the formation of a natural passive oxide layer, it has been extensively utilized in maxillofacial surgeries [62]. In a study, it was found that nitinol provided substantial bone ingrowth and apposition in rabbits by 6 and 12 weeks post-implantation [61].

Porous nitinol has been employed in maxillofacial and a number of orthopaedic surgeries in Russia and China for about 15 years [65]. As an interbody fusion bone scaffold, it has also aroused interest in intervertebral disc pathologies [66]. However, so far, not many preclinical trials using animal models and very scarce clinical trials have been conducted, and more research is needed to find out the biological performance of porous nitinol better. Most clinical studies using nitinol meshes are restricted to thoracic and cardiovascular surgery in which nitinol finds applications, particularly in self-expanded metallic stents. Nevertheless, continual follow-up is required to determine the clinical long-term success of these porous nitinol constructs [19]. Production techniques for porous NiTi have so far been restricted to powder-metallurgy techniques, as reviewed by Ryan *et al.* [67] for porous metals (including NiTi) for orthopaedic applications since it has a high melting point (1310 °C). Porous NiTi has been made from elemental Ni and Ti powders by self-propagating high-temperature synthesis (SHS) [68], hot isostatic pressing (HIP) with argon expansion [69], spark plasma sintering (SPS) [70], capsule-free HIP (CF-HIP) [71] and conventional sintering (CS) [72]. NiTi implant materials design originally focused on minimizing the host tissue response to make "bio-inert" implants. The second stage of implant technology tried to make "bioactive" implants that would extract a desired response from the host tissue. This technique may have coating surfaces with apatite mineral to promote bone bonding or apposition on the implant surface. Currently, a "third generation" of NiTi implants with surfaces that are molecularly designed to induce bone regeneration on implant surfaces is under investigation [54].

In a systematic and comparative research, porous NiTi, porous Ti, dense NiTi, and dense Ti were implanted into 5 mm diameter holes in the distal part of the femur/tibia of rabbits for 15 weeks. The porous NiTi materials proved to bond well to newly formed bone tissues and the highest average strength of 357 N and the best ductility were reached from the porous NiTi materials. The bonding curve, which is obtained from the NiTi scaffold, indicates similar super-elasticity to natural bones, hence shielding new bone tissues from large load stress. That seems to be why new bone tissues can infiltrate deeply into the porous NiTi scaffold when they are compared to the one made of porous Ti. Regarding the good cyto-compatibility, the super-elastic biomechanical properties of the porous NiTi scaffold show good signs of fast formation and ingrowth of new bones [56].

In vitro cell culture tests have been performed on different NiTi foams. Prymak *et al.* [55] indicated immediate adherence of peripheral blood leukocytes to porous NiTi surfaces, and rapid viability within 24 h. Short-term *in vitro* tests (8 days) revealed no immediate cytotoxicity from porous NiTi, and surface deposition of mice osteoblast cells disregarding the type of surface treatment [73]. It seems that nickel release levels affect the adherence of osteoblast cells and their proliferation on porous NiTi surface. This is in agreement with the findings of Gu *et al.* [74], where no cell attachment was noticed on porous NiTi surfaces, which contained unreacted, elemental Ni left from an incomplete SHS process, whereas fast proliferation and differentiation was found after surface treatment. Assad *et al.* [75] confirmed a low adverse potential at the *in vitro* cellular level by using cyto-compatibility testing and three standard genotoxicity tests. It was determined that porous NiTi's short-term biocompatibility was comparable to that of dense NiTi. In addition, *in vivo* standard allergy potential evaluation revealed that porous NiTi cannot produce systemic toxicity reactions, irritation, and sensitization in animal models [76]. Porous NiTi also had excellent bone implant contact and a high level of bone ingrowth in rabbits and rats without signs of getting loose [77]. Intervertebral fusion devices are among recently identified applications for porous NiTi in spine surgery, with one product commercially available since 2002 under the trade-name ActiporeTM (from Biorthex, Canada) for lumbar and cervical interbody devices.

MAGNESIUM

Metallic biomaterials are permanent *in vivo*, and in the case of plates, screws and pins which are utilized to secure serious fractures, a second surgical procedure must be done to remove the implant after the tissue healing [78 - 80]. However, second operation enhances the costs to the health care system and further morbidity to the patient [81, 82]. Magnesium (Mg), an exceptionally lightweight metal [78], is largely found in bone tissue, is an essential element to human body, and its presence is useful for bone growth and strength [83 - 85] and also Mg is a co-factor for many enzymes and acts as stabilizer of DNA and RNA structures [86]. It is the fourth most abundant cation in the human body with approximately

12.5 g stored in bone tissue. The level of Mg ranges between 0.7 and 1.05 mmol/L in the extracellular fluid, and the intestine and kidneys maintain its homeostasis [83]. Because of efficient excretion of the element in the urine, hyper-Mg is rare [83]. Mg and its alloys are very lightweight metals with densities ranging from 1.74 to 2.0 g/cm^3, which is less than that of Ti alloys (4.4–4.5 g/cm^3) and is near bone density (1.8–2.1 g/cm^3) [78]. They have a wide range of elongation and tensile strengths from 3% to 21.8% and from 86.8 to 280MPa, respectively [87]. Compared to the fracture toughness of ceramic biomaterials, Mg has greater fracture toughness, and compared to other metals, its elastic modulus (41–45 GPa) is closer to that of bone [88, 89]. This property could have an important role in keeping away from the stress shielding effect [90 - 92]. Mg's ductility is better than synthetic hydroxyapatite and its strength is higher than existing biodegradable polymers [93]. Pure Mg's elastic modulus is closer to that of cortical and cancellous bones, and this is a superior feature for bone scaffolds [94]. The major disadvantage of Mg in many engineering applications, its low corrosion resistance, especially in electrolytic, aqueous environments, is an interesting property as a biodegradable implant for biomedical applications [95 - 98]. Here, the *in vivo* corrosion of the magnesium-based implant involves the formation of a soluble, non-toxic oxide harmlessly excreted in the urine [99]. In physiological saline environment, Mg alloys degrade through the below electrochemical reactions [78, 100, 101]:

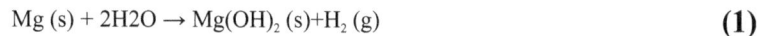

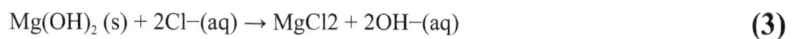

$$Mg\ (s) + 2H2O \rightarrow Mg(OH)_2\ (s) + H_2\ (g) \tag{1}$$

$$Mg\ (s) + 2Cl^-(aq) \rightarrow MgCl_2 \tag{2}$$

$$Mg(OH)_2\ (s) + 2Cl^-(aq) \rightarrow MgCl2 + 2OH^-(aq) \tag{3}$$

In the first reaction, a grey Mg(OH)$_2$ film is developed on the surface of Mg when it reacts with water, and hydrogen bubbles are produced; moreover, Mg can also directly react with chloride ions to form Mg chloride (2). This highly soluble MgCl$_2$ is also formed in the reaction between Mg(OH)$_2$ and chloride ions, as shown in (3) [85, 102, 103]. Mg implant may lose its mechanical integrity due to its high corrosion before the tissue is completely healed. In addition, its corrosion reaction produces so much hydrogen gas that it is too high to be dealt with by the host tissue [104 - 106]. With advances in the technology of Mg processing, Mg alloys have undergone many improvements with regard to their corrosion resistance and mechanical properties. Mg's mechanical properties can be improved through alloying and thermomechanical processes. Adding alloying elements like aluminium, indium, silver, tin, silicon, zinc, and zirconium could improve the strength and elongation of Mg alloys [107]. A renewed interest is also noticed in employing this material in biomedical applications, *e.g.* for coronary stents [108]; and recently, researchers have paid more attention to the application of magnesium-rare-earth alloys with new elements such as cerium, neodymium and praseodymium for bone fixation devices [104] for osteo-applications. As biodegradable biomaterials, Mg-Ca alloys have recently been produced and evaluated *in vitro* and *in vivo* for orthopaedic applications [109].

There are several possibilities to adapt the corrosion rate of magnesium by using alloying elements and surface coatings, processes that must result in a non-toxic, biocompatible material [78]. Moreover, some manufacturing processes like hot extruding, hot rolling, and equal-channel angular pressing (ECAP) could also improve the strength of Mg alloys and, in some cases, their ductility [107]. Although concerns about the toxicity of dissolved Mg have been raised, it has been proved that the excess of Mg is excreted from the body in urine [83]. Moreover, concern does remain about using pure Mg as the dissolution rate in physiological conditions is rapid. Potentially it leads to hyper-magnesia although a number of potential routes have been proposed to control the corrosion rate; especially providing it with a ceramic coating [110], titanium coating [111] or through the use of Mg alloys, including AZ31, AZ91, WE43, LAE442 and Mg-Mn-Zn alloys [104].

Many studies introduce Mg as osteo-conductive and a bone growth stimulator. A substantial enhance in bone area has been observed in Mg-based implants in comparison to those based on PLA [104]. The corrosion layer around Mg implants contains calcium phosphates, which appears to be in direct contact with the surrounding bone [104]. Xu *et al.* [112] have indicated new bone formation around Mg-Mn-Zn implants in their *in vivo* degradation in rats. Witte *et al.* [113] observed that 3 months after the operation, open porous Mg scaffolds which were implanted in rabbits were degraded to a large extent, foreign body giant cells destroying the remaining corrosion products were rare, and no osteolytic changes could be noticed around the implant site. Porous Mg has indicated to have a better degradation behaviour with regard to lower pH change, slower hydrogen evolution, and slower decrease in compressive yield strength in simulated body fluid (SBF) immersion tests [114]. Zreiqat *et al.* [115] reported an increasing bone cell adhesion on Mg-enriched alumina which was expressed by enhanced level of a5b1 integrin receptor and collagen extracellular matrix protein. By using Mg-enriched apatites or collagen materials, two researches showed good biocompatibility on tissue growth and bone cell attachment [116, 117].

Confined long-term survival data are available for Mg or Mg alloys porous scaffolds; however, the material seems favourable for certain bone ingrowth applications like trabecular bone regeneration [19]. In biodegradable scaffolds, it is desirable for the scaffold materials to be completely biodegraded in a human body after an appropriate period. Some surface treatments have been devised for porous Mg constructs to control the rate of degradation and to improve the biocompatibility [118, 119]. So far, only *in vitro* [118] and preclinical studies which use animal models have proposed employing Mg scaffolds as degradable ones for bone substitute applications. Actually, works regarding the *in vivo* behaviour of porous magnesium at the preclinical level are still insufficient [19]. In spite of the fact that porosity will decrease the bulk properties of a material, porous Mg still possesses the strength and stiffness close to that of native bone. The porosity and pore size has influence on the yield, compressive, and flexural strength whereas Young's modulus has reduced with the pore volume and size. Pore morphology, volume and size can also affect the mechanical properties of porous Mg materials [120], but this is not critical for Mg scaffolds because their mechanical properties can still be compared with bone. The lower limit of bone strength is about 3MPa, while the compressive strength of cancellous bone is 0.2–80MPa and Young's modulus is 0.01–2GPa [94]. Therefore, Mg scaffolds may achieve the range of bone stiffness and strength by modulating their porosity and pore sizes. Moreover, porosity finally decreases porous Mg's corrosion resistance, which is also noteworthy. Random cellular Mg can be made through low-pressure casting, powder or chip sintering (laser assisted, conventional, or spark plasma), or removable spacer methods. These production techniques generate a random cell structure, wide distributions of cell sizes, and morphology that result in unpredictable material properties in the range of hundred microns [121]. Major processes used to make Mg with topologically ordered open cell structure consist of space holder method (Fig. **1**), solid free-form process, replication, leaching method, electrodeposition, and vapour deposition.

Magnesium scaffolds, adjustable to mechanical properties comparable to human cancellous bone, are made from cast magnesium alloys in a negative salt-pattern moulding process. In a study, open porous scaffolds, made of the magnesium alloy AZ91D and implanted into the distal femur condyle of rabbits, were compared to autologous bone, transplanted into the contralateral condyle in a 3 and 6 months follow-up group. In 3 months, magnesium scaffolds were largely degraded, and most of the original magnesium alloy disappeared. At the same time, a fibrous capsule surrounded the operation site. Histological analysis showed that magnesium scaffolds inflicted no significant harm on their adjacent tissues. According to this study, even fast degrading magnesium scaffolds have a good biocompatibility and react *in vivo* with a suitable inflammatory host response [113]. In another study, a powder metallurgy route was utilized to generate Mg scaffolds; and then they were coated with polycaprolactone (PCL) and bioactive glass (BaG). After that, gelatine (Gel)-Bioactive glass (BaG) was coated on the PCL-BaG by using freeze-drying process. According to the results obtained from the *in vitro* bioactivity evaluation, Mg scaffold/PCL-BaG showed better bioactivity by forming bioactive minerals in the cauliflower-like structure on the surface. Mg scaffold and Mg scaffold/PCL-BaG were completely degraded after 3 and 7 days, respectively, while about 87% of Mg scaffold/PCL-BaG/Gel-BaG remained after 2 weeks [122].

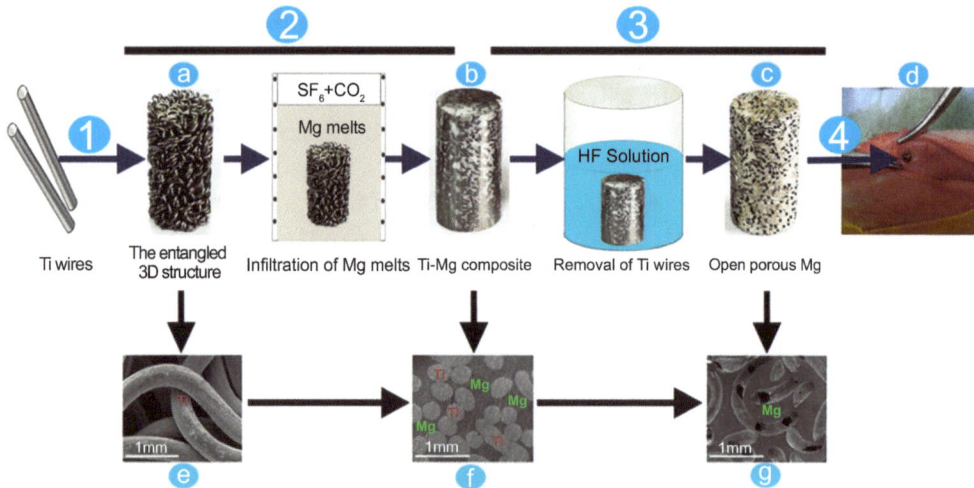

Fig. (1). Illustration of preparation process of the open-porous magnesium scaffold and *in vivo* animal model. Step1: the 3D entangled titanium wire material (a,e) was prepared with Ti wires. Step2: the Ti-Mg composite (b,f) was prepared with high purity Mg melts. Step3: Ti wires were removed by HF solution and open-porous magnesium scaffold (c,g) was successful manufactured.Step4:open-porous magnesium scaffolds were implanted into the lateral epicondyle of rabbits (d) [123].

CONCLUDING REMARKS

In tissue engineering, porous metallic scaffolds are used to replace damaged hard tissues in an attempt to restore its functionality. Such structural scaffolds have an imposed pore structure and interconnectivity, and are designed so that they maintain their shape and strength by repairing the injured bone. Porous metallic scaffolds offer interfacial porosity and permanent structural framework for the long-term replacement of bone defects and they can be made by different processes (*e.g.* decomposition of foaming agents, powder metallurgy, rapid prototyping technologies, replication, *etc.*). Great progress has been made in developing metallic scaffolds by rapid prototyping techniques; hence, many researchers and surgeons are of the opinion that biochemically-modified porous metallic scaffolds are more suitable than biodegradable scaffolds for the development of implants for load-bearing applications. Nowadays, there are a number of *in vivo* and *in vitro* tissue-culturing methods for bone repair by employing metallic scaffolds with macro-porous structure. Porous metallic structures have been tested as bone-engineered constructs by employing cell-based and the growth-factor-based strategies. The aim is to find a functional replacement for the injured hard tissue in a process, which avoids bone harvesting. With regard to all parameters in fabrication, a metallic scaffold with porosity of about 55% maybe the best to be made with the space holder method. Among many favourable techniques of making metal scaffolds, solid free form is presently regarded as the best method for the fabrication of metal scaffolds with optimized pore morphology for cell growth and cell proliferation. This method permits the design and materialization of topologically ordered porous metal with periodic structure for improved mechanical output and function of a porous scaffold. Porous metals such as tantalum, titanium, nitinol and magnesium are in their early stages of evolution; however, the initial clinical data and preclinical studies support their use as alternatives to traditional orthopaedic implant materials.

FUTURE PERSPECTIVES

More work should be done to determine properties that have received limited attention, *e.g.* permeability (k), surface roughness, fracture toughness, and corrosion resistance, or no attention, *e.g.* fatigue crack growth (FCG) rate *vs* stress intensity range. There is a need for extensive parametric studies for each production method; especially, studies should be carried out for the influence of each process variable on a host of properties. For a certain production method, a large number of results should be used in order to develop a relationship between a certain property and all process variables, which could be used to identify a collection of these variables' values that will result in a desired value of that property. Desired values should be values of cancellous bone like mean pore size on the order of 1 mm in diameter, compressive strength =10 MPa, and E = 6–8 GPa. The challenge is how to put all the values of these process variables together, for a certain production method, to obtain all the desirable metal properties at the same time. There is a scope for the development of international standards—under the auspices of ASTM or the International Standardization Organization—to determine the mechanical properties of porous metals, especially the compressive strength and fracture toughness. More work should be done to produce porous variants of other metals/alloys such as Co–Cr–Mo alloy used in orthopaedic applications. Fabrication of nanostructured porous metals and their detailed characterization including the determination of *in vitro* biocompatibility, and the use of newly introduced and emerging additive-manufacturing methods (*e.g.* solid ground curing, a combination of SLS, hot isostatic pressing, cold isostatic pressing, a combination of 3D printing and sintering by using sintering conditions like temperature, gas flow rate, holding time, high-speed laser additive manufacturing, and direct metal laser sintering) can lead to the fabrication of patient-specific orthopaedic implants. Long-term experimental and clinical researches will be needed to determine the advantages and results of porous metals. Although the study of porous NiTi has developed quickly in the past few years, biological studies are still in their initial stage in comparison to other porous Ti and Ti–6Al–4V alloys and to dense NiTi. More comprehensive studies are required regarding biological performance to develop the biomedical applications of porous NiTi. To do this, optimization and long term *in vivo* studies regarding surface-modified systems are still required. More investigations are required in the solid free-form fabrication method to make a scaffold having properties, which have especially been tailored for cell regeneration and tissue growth. Using biodegradable metals to develop tissue-engineering scaffold is in its early stages. Little work has already been done and much work is yet to be done. The directions could be towards finding suitable processes for making porous structures from all prospective biodegradable metals, understanding the effect of porous structure on mechanical and degradation properties, and understanding the cell regeneration and degradation product transport in the porous structure. Another interesting direction to explore could be integrating biodegradable polymers or ceramics and drugs. Development, performance and integration with bone tissue of porous magnesium-based implants are also issues, which need more research. Future research in this area will probably focus on the efficient combinations of osteo-inductive materials, osteo-inductive growth factors and cell-based tissue regeneration approach by employing composite constructs carriers to reconstruct and repair hard tissues. Hence, there is a need for a perfectly controlled hybrid scaffold to be developed in the future.

CONFLICT OF INTEREST

The author declares no conflict of interest, financial or otherwise.

ACKNOWLEDGEMENTS

Declared none.

REFERENCES

[1]   Lewis G. Properties of open-cell porous metals and alloys for orthopaedic applications. J Mater Sci Mater Med 2013; 24(10): 2293-325.
[http://dx.doi.org/10.1007/s10856-013-4998-y] [PMID: 23851927]

[2]   Khodaei M, Meratian M, Shaltooki M, Hashemibeni B, Savabi O, Razavi M. Surface modification of Ti6Al4 V implants by heat, H2O2, and alkali treatments. Surf Eng 2016; 32
[http://dx.doi.org/10.1080/02670844.2016.1159818]

[3]   Khodaei M, Meratian M, Savabi O, Razavi M. The effect of pore structure on the mechanical properties of titanium scaffolds. Mater Lett 2016; 171
[http://dx.doi.org/10.1016/j.matlet.2016.02.101]

[4]   Jazayeri HE, Tahriri M, Razavi M, *et al.* A current overview of materials and strategies for potential use in maxillofacial tissue regeneration. Mater Sci Eng C 2017; 70(Pt 1): 913-29.
[http://dx.doi.org/10.1016/j.msec.2016.08.055] [PMID: 27770969]

[5]   Yazdimamaghani M, Razavi M, Vashaee D, Tayebi L. Surface modification of biodegradable porous Mg bone scaffold using polycaprolactone/bioactive glass composite. Mater Sci Eng C 2015; 49: 436-44.
[http://dx.doi.org/10.1016/j.msec.2015.01.041] [PMID: 25686970]

[6]   Yazdimamaghani M, Razavi M, Vashaee D, Tayebi L. Development and degradation behavior of magnesium scaffolds coated with polycaprolactone for bone tissue engineering. Mater Lett 2014; 132
[http://dx.doi.org/10.1016/j.matlet.2014.06.036]

[7]   Yazdimamaghani M, Razavi M, Vashaee D, Moharamzadeh K, Boccaccini AR, Tayebi L. Porous magnesium-based scaffolds for tissue engineering. Mater Sci Eng C 2017; 71: 1253-66.
[http://dx.doi.org/10.1016/j.msec.2016.11.027] [PMID: 27987682]

[8]   Matassi F, Botti A, Sirleo L, Carulli C, Innocenti M. Porous metal for orthopedics implants. Clin Cases Miner Bone Metab 2013; 10(2): 111-5.
[http://dx.doi.org/10.11138/ccmbm/2013.10.2.111] [PMID: 24133527]

[9]   Yazdimamaghani M, Razavi M, Vashaee D, Tayebi L. Microstructural and mechanical study of PCL coated Mg scaffolds. Surf Eng 2014; 30
[http://dx.doi.org/10.1179/1743294414Y.0000000307]

[10]   Razavi M, Fathi M, Savabi O, Boroni M. A review of degradation properties of Mg based biodegradable implants. Res Rev Mater Sci Chem 2012; 1: 15-58.

[11]   Levine B. A new era in porous metals: Applications in orthopaedics. Adv Eng Mater 2008; 10: 788-92.
[http://dx.doi.org/10.1002/adem.200800215]

[12]   Dabrowski B, Swieszkowski W, Godlinski D, Kurzydlowski KJ. Highly porous titanium scaffolds for orthopaedic applications. J Biomed Mater Res B Appl Biomater 2010; 95(1): 53-61.
[http://dx.doi.org/10.1002/jbm.b.31682] [PMID: 20690174]

[13]   Heidari F, Razavi M. M. E.bahrololoom, R. Bazargan-Lari, D. Vashaee, H. Kotturi, L. Tayebi, Mechanical properties of natural chitosan/hydroxyapatite/magnetite nanocomposites for tissue engineering applications. Mater Sci Eng C 2016; 65
[http://dx.doi.org/10.1016/j.msec.2016.04.039]

[14]   Yazdimamaghani M, Razavi M, Mozafari M, Vashaee D, Kotturi H, Tayebi L. Biomineralization and biocompatibility studies of bone conductive scaffolds containing poly(3,4-ethylenedioxythiophene):poly(4-styrene sulfonate) (PEDOT:PSS). J Mater Sci Mater Med 2015; 26(12): 274.
[http://dx.doi.org/10.1007/s10856-015-5599-8] [PMID: 26543020]

[15]   Fahmy MD, Jazayeri HE, Razavi M, Masri R, Tayebi L. Three-dimensional bioprinting materials with potential application in preprosthetic surgery. J Prosthodont 2016; 25(4): 310-8.
[http://dx.doi.org/10.1111/jopr.12431] [PMID: 26855004]

[16]   Jazayeri HE, Fahmy MD, Razavi M, *et al.* Dental applications of natural-origin polymers in hard and soft tissue engineering. J Prosthodont 2016; 25(6): 510-7.
[http://dx.doi.org/10.1111/jopr.12465] [PMID: 27003096]

[17]   Arifvianto B, Zhou J. Fabrication of metallic biomedical scaffolds with the space holder method: A review. Materials (Basel) 2014; 7: 3588-622.
[http://dx.doi.org/10.3390/ma7053588]

[18]   Dunand DC. Processing of Titanium Foams. Adv Eng Mater 2004; 6: 369-76.
[http://dx.doi.org/10.1002/adem.200405576]

[19]   Alvarez K, Nakajima H. Metallic scaffolds for bone regeneration. Materials (Basel) 2009; 2: 790-832.
[http://dx.doi.org/10.3390/ma2030790]

[20]   Davies JE. Bone bonding at natural and biomaterial surfaces. Biomaterials 2007; 28(34): 5058-67.
[http://dx.doi.org/10.1016/j.biomaterials.2007.07.049] [PMID: 17697711]

[21]   Okazaki Y. A New Ti–15Zr–4Nb–4Ta alloy for medical applications. Curr Opin Solid State Mater Sci 2001; 5: 45-53.
[http://dx.doi.org/10.1016/S1359-0286(00)00025-5]

[22]   Wen CE, Yamada Y, Shimojima K, Chino Y, Hosokawa H, Mabuchi M. Novel titanium foam for bone tissue engineering. J Mater Res 2002; 17: 2633-9.
[http://dx.doi.org/10.1557/JMR.2002.0382]

[23]   Burugapalli K, Razavi M, Zhou L, Huang Y. *In vitro* Cytocompatibility Study of a Medical β-Type Ti-35.5Nb-5.7Ta Titanium Alloy. J Biomater Tissue Eng 2016; 6: 141-8.
[http://dx.doi.org/10.1166/jbt.2016.1424]

[24]   Zdeblick TA, Phillips FM. Interbody cage devices. Spine 2003; 28(15) (Suppl.): S2-7.
[http://dx.doi.org/10.1097/01.BRS.0000076841.93570.78] [PMID: 12897467]

[25]   Niu CC, Chen LH, Lai PL, Fu TS, Chen WJ. Trapezoidal titanium cage in anterior cervical interbody fusion: a clinical experience. Chang Gung Med J 2005; 28(4): 212-21.
[PMID: 16013340]

[26]   Jansen JA, Vehof JW, Ruhé PQ, *et al.* Growth factor-loaded scaffolds for bone engineering. J Control Release 2005; 101(1-3): 127-36.
[http://dx.doi.org/10.1016/j.jconrel.2004.07.005] [PMID: 15588899]

[27]   Zhang W, Walboomers XF, van Kuppevelt TH, Daamen WF, Bian Z, Jansen JA. The performance of human dental pulp stem cells on different three-dimensional scaffold materials. Biomaterials 2006; 27(33): 5658-68.
[http://dx.doi.org/10.1016/j.biomaterials.2006.07.013] [PMID: 16916542]

[28]   Crowninshield RD. Mechanical properties of porous metal total hip prostheses. Instr Course Lect 1986; 35: 144-8.
[PMID: 3819401]

[29]   Faria PE, Carvalho AL, Felipucci DN, Wen C, Sennerby L, Salata LA. Bone formation following implantation of titanium sponge rods into humeral osteotomies in dogs: a histological and histometrical study. Clin Implant Dent Relat Res 2010; 12(1): 72-9.
[http://dx.doi.org/10.1111/j.1708-8208.2008.00132.x] [PMID: 19076179]

[30]   van den Dolder J, Jansen JA. Titanium fiber mesh: A nondegradable scaffold material. Eng Funct Skelet Tissues 2007; 69-80.

[31]   van den Dolder J, Farber E, Spauwen PH, Jansen JA. Bone tissue reconstruction using titanium fiber mesh combined with rat bone marrow stromal cells. Biomaterials 2003; 24(10): 1745-50.
[http://dx.doi.org/10.1016/S0142-9612(02)00537-9] [PMID: 12593956]

[32]   Eck KR, Bridwell KH, Ungacta FF, Lapp MA, Lenke LG, Riew KD. Analysis of titanium mesh cages in adults with minimum two-year follow-up. Spine 2000; 25(18): 2407-15.
[http://dx.doi.org/10.1097/00007632-200009150-00023] [PMID: 10984797]

[33]   Ryan GE, Pandit AS, Apatsidis DP. Porous titanium scaffolds fabricated using a rapid prototyping and powder metallurgy technique. Biomaterials 2008; 29(27): 3625-35.
[http://dx.doi.org/10.1016/j.biomaterials.2008.05.032] [PMID: 18556060]

[34]   Yeong WY, Chua CK, Leong KF, Chandrasekaran M. Rapid prototyping in tissue engineering: challenges and potential. Trends Biotechnol 2004; 22(12): 643-52.
[http://dx.doi.org/10.1016/j.tibtech.2004.10.004] [PMID: 15542155]

[35]   Sun W, Darling A, Starly B, Nam J. Computer-aided tissue engineering: overview, scope and

challenges. Biotechnol Appl Biochem 2004; 39(Pt 1): 29-47.
[http://dx.doi.org/10.1042/BA20030108] [PMID: 14563211]

[36]   Cachinho SC, Correia RN. Titanium scaffolds for osteointegration: mechanical, *in vitro* and corrosion behaviour. J Mater Sci Mater Med 2008; 19(1): 451-7.
[http://dx.doi.org/10.1007/s10856-006-0052-7] [PMID: 17607517]

[37]   Li JP, Habibovic P, van den Doel M, *et al.* Bone ingrowth in porous titanium implants produced by 3D fiber deposition. Biomaterials 2007; 28(18): 2810-20.
[http://dx.doi.org/10.1016/j.biomaterials.2007.02.020] [PMID: 17367852]

[38]   Levine BR, Sporer S, Poggie RA, Della Valle CJ, Jacobs JJ. Experimental and clinical performance of porous tantalum in orthopedic surgery. Biomaterials 2006; 27(27): 4671-81.
[http://dx.doi.org/10.1016/j.biomaterials.2006.04.041] [PMID: 16737737]

[39]   Black J. Biological performance of tantalum. Clin Mater 1994; 16(3): 167-73.
[http://dx.doi.org/10.1016/0267-6605(94)90113-9] [PMID: 10172264]

[40]   Shimko DA, Shimko VF, Sander EA, Dickson KF, Nauman EA. Effect of porosity on the fluid flow characteristics and mechanical properties of tantalum scaffolds. J Biomed Mater Res B Appl Biomater 2005; 73(2): 315-24.
[http://dx.doi.org/10.1002/jbm.b.30229] [PMID: 15736288]

[41]   Findlay DM, Welldon K, Atkins GJ, Howie DW, Zannettino AC, Bobyn D. The proliferation and phenotypic expression of human osteoblasts on tantalum metal. Biomaterials 2004; 25(12): 2215-27.
[http://dx.doi.org/10.1016/j.biomaterials.2003.09.005] [PMID: 14741587]

[42]   Kato H, Nakamura T, Nishiguchi S, *et al.* Bonding of alkali- and heat-treated tantalum implants to bone. J Biomed Mater Res 2000; 53(1): 28-35.
[http://dx.doi.org/10.1002/(SICI)1097-4636(2000)53:1<28::AID-JBM4>3.0.CO;2-F]   [PMID: 10634949]

[43]   Bermúdez MD, Carrión FJ, Martínez-Nicolás G, López R. Erosion-corrosion of stainless steels, titanium, tantalum and zirconium. Wear 2005; 258: 693-700.
[http://dx.doi.org/10.1016/j.wear.2004.09.023]

[44]   Bobyn JD, Toh KK, Hacking SA, Tanzer M, Krygier JJ. Tissue response to porous tantalum acetabular cups: a canine model. J Arthroplasty 1999; 14(3): 347-54.
[http://dx.doi.org/10.1016/S0883-5403(99)90062-1] [PMID: 10220190]

[45]   Bobyn JD, Stackpool GJ, Hacking SA, Tanzer M, Krygier JJ. Characteristics of bone ingrowth and interface mechanics of a new porous tantalum biomaterial. J Bone Joint Surg Br 1999; 81(5): 907-14.
[http://dx.doi.org/10.1302/0301-620X.81B5.9283] [PMID: 10530861]

[46]   Johansson CB, Hansson HA, Albrektsson T. Qualitative interfacial study between bone and tantalum, niobium or commercially pure titanium. Biomaterials 1990; 11(4): 277-80.
[http://dx.doi.org/10.1016/0142-9612(90)90010-N] [PMID: 2383624]

[47]   Matsuno H, Yokoyama A, Watari F, Uo M, Kawasaki T. Biocompatibility and osteogenesis of refractory metal implants, titanium, hafnium, niobium, tantalum and rhenium. Biomaterials 2001; 22(11): 1253-62.
[http://dx.doi.org/10.1016/S0142-9612(00)00275-1] [PMID: 11336297]

[48]   Balla VK, Bodhak S, Bose S, Bandyopadhyay A. Porous tantalum structures for bone implants: fabrication, mechanical and *in vitro* biological properties. Acta Biomater 2010; 6(8): 3349-59.
[http://dx.doi.org/10.1016/j.actbio.2010.01.046] [PMID: 20132912]

[49]   Hacking SA, Bobyn JD, Toh K, Tanzer M, Krygier JJ. Fibrous tissue ingrowth and attachment to porous tantalum. J Biomed Mater Res 2000; 52(4): 631-8.
[http://dx.doi.org/10.1002/1097-4636(20001215)52:4<631::AID-JBM7>3.0.CO;2-6]   [PMID: 11033545]

[50]   Wang JC, Yu WD, Sandhu HS, Tam V, Delamarter RB. A comparison of magnetic resonance and

computed tomographic image quality after the implantation of tantalum and titanium spinal instrumentation. Spine 1998; 23(15): 1684-8.
[http://dx.doi.org/10.1097/00007632-199808010-00014] [PMID: 9704376]

[51]   Zardiackas LD, Parsell DE, Dillon LD, Mitchell DW, Nunnery LA, Poggie R. Structure, metallurgy, and mechanical properties of a porous tantalum foam. J Biomed Mater Res 2001; 58(2): 180-7.
[http://dx.doi.org/10.1002/1097-4636(2001)58:2<180::AID-JBM1005>3.0.CO;2-5]   [PMID: 11241337]

[52]   Sidhu KS, Prochnow TD, Schmitt P, Fischgrund J, Weisbrode S, Herkowitz HN. Anterior cervical interbody fusion with rhBMP-2 and tantalum in a goat model. Spine J 2001; 1(5): 331-40.
[http://dx.doi.org/10.1016/S1529-9430(01)00113-9] [PMID: 14588311]

[53]   Zou X, Li H, Teng X, *et al.* Pedicle screw fixation enhances anterior lumbar interbody fusion with porous tantalum cages: an experimental study in pigs. Spine 2005; 30(14): E392-9.
[http://dx.doi.org/10.1097/01.brs.0000170588.80377.3f] [PMID: 16025015]

[54]   Bansiddhi A, Sargeant TD, Stupp SI, Dunand DC. Porous NiTi for bone implants: a review. Acta Biomater 2008; 4(4): 773-82.
[http://dx.doi.org/10.1016/j.actbio.2008.02.009] [PMID: 18348912]

[55]   Prymak O, Bogdanski D, Köller M, *et al.* Morphological characterization and *in vitro* biocompatibility of a porous nickel-titanium alloy. Biomaterials 2005; 26(29): 5801-7.
[http://dx.doi.org/10.1016/j.biomaterials.2005.02.029] [PMID: 15949545]

[56]   Liu X, Wu S, Yeung KW, *et al.* Relationship between osseointegration and superelastic biomechanics in porous NiTi scaffolds. Biomaterials 2011; 32(2): 330-8.
[http://dx.doi.org/10.1016/j.biomaterials.2010.08.102] [PMID: 20869110]

[57]   Tarniţă D, Tarniţă DN, Bîzdoacă N, Mîndrilă I, Vasilescu M. Properties and medical applications of shape memory alloys. Rom J Morphol Embryol 2009; 50(1): 15-21.
[PMID: 19221641]

[58]   Holton A, Walsh E, Anayiotos A, Pohost G, Venugopalan R. Comparative MRI compatibility of 316 L stainless steel alloy and nickel-titanium alloy stents. J Cardiovasc Magn Reson 2002; 4(4): 423-30.
[http://dx.doi.org/10.1081/JCMR-120016381] [PMID: 12549230]

[59]   Michiardi A, Aparicio C, Planell JA, Gil FJ. New oxidation treatment of NiTi shape memory alloys to obtain Ni-free surfaces and to improve biocompatibility. J Biomed Mater Res B Appl Biomater 2006; 77(2): 249-56.
[http://dx.doi.org/10.1002/jbm.b.30441] [PMID: 16245290]

[60]   Suzuki A, Kanetaka H, Shimizu Y, *et al.* Orthodontic buccal tooth movement by nickel-free titanium-based shape memory and superelastic alloy wire. Angle Orthod 2006; 76(6): 1041-6.
[http://dx.doi.org/10.2319/083105-306] [PMID: 17090162]

[61]   Simske SJ, Sachdeva R. Cranial bone apposition and ingrowth in a porous nickel-titanium implant. J Biomed Mater Res 1995; 29(4): 527-33.
[http://dx.doi.org/10.1002/jbm.820290413] [PMID: 7622538]

[62]   Ayers RA, Simske SJ, Bateman TA, Petkus A, Sachdeva RL, Gyunter VE. Effect of nitinol implant porosity on cranial bone ingrowth and apposition after 6 weeks. J Biomed Mater Res 1999; 45(1): 42-7.
[http://dx.doi.org/10.1002/(SICI)1097-4636(199904)45:1<42::AID-JBM6>3.0.CO;2-Q]   [PMID: 10397956]

[63]   Thierry B, Merhi Y, Bilodeau L, Trépanier C, Tabrizian M. Nitinol *versus* stainless steel stents: acute thrombogenicity study in an *ex vivo* porcine model. Biomaterials 2002; 23(14): 2997-3005.
[http://dx.doi.org/10.1016/S0142-9612(02)00030-3] [PMID: 12069342]

[64]   Itin VI, Gyunter VE, Shabalovskaya Sa, Sachdeva RL. Mechanical properties and shape memory of porous nitinol. Mater Charact 1994; 32: 179-87.

[http://dx.doi.org/10.1016/1044-5803(94)90087-6]

[65]   Dai K, Chu Y. Studies and applications of NiTi shape memory alloys in the medical field in China. Biomed Mater Eng 1996; 6(4): 233-40.
[PMID: 8980832]

[66]   Likibi F, Chabot G, Assad M, Rivard CH. Influence of orthopedic implant structure on adjacent bone density and on stability. Am J Orthop 2008; 37(4): E78-83.
[PMID: 18535685]

[67]   Ryan G, Pandit A, Apatsidis DP. Fabrication methods of porous metals for use in orthopaedic applications. Biomaterials 2006; 27(13): 2651-70.
[http://dx.doi.org/10.1016/j.biomaterials.2005.12.002] [PMID: 16423390]

[68]   Jiang HC, Rong LJ. Ways to lower transformation temperatures of porous NiTi shape memory alloy fabricated by self-propagating high-temperature synthesis. Mater Sci Eng A 2006; 438–440: 883-6.
[http://dx.doi.org/10.1016/j.msea.2006.01.103]

[69]   Lagoudas DC, Vandygriff EL. Processing and characterization of NiTi porous SMA by elevated pressure sintering-not use. J Intell Mater Syst Struct 2002; 13: 837-50.
[http://dx.doi.org/10.1177/1045389X02013012009]

[70]   Zhao Y, Taya M, Kang Y, Kawasaki A. Compression behavior of porous NiTi shape memory alloy. Acta Mater 2005; 53: 337-43.
[http://dx.doi.org/10.1016/j.actamat.2004.09.029]

[71]   Yuan B, Zhang XP, Chung CY, Zhu M. The effect of porosity on phase transformation behavior of porous Ti-50.8 at.% Ni shape memory alloys prepared by capsule-free hot isostatic pressing. Mater Sci Eng A 2006; 438–440: 585-8.
[http://dx.doi.org/10.1016/j.msea.2006.02.141]

[72]   Bertheville B. Porous single-phase NiTi processed under Ca reducing vapor for use as a bone graft substitute. Biomaterials 2006; 27(8): 1246-50.
[http://dx.doi.org/10.1016/j.biomaterials.2005.09.014] [PMID: 16174525]

[73]   Wu S, Liu X, Chan YL, *et al.* Nickel release behavior, cytocompatibility, and superelasticity of oxidized porous single-phase NiTi. J Biomed Mater Res A 2007; 81(4): 948-55.
[http://dx.doi.org/10.1002/jbm.a.31115] [PMID: 17252548]

[74]   Gu YW, Li H, Tay BY, Lim CS, Yong MS, Khor KA. *In vitro* bioactivity and osteoblast response of porous NiTi synthesized by SHS using nanocrystalline Ni-Ti reaction agent. J Biomed Mater Res A 2006; 78(2): 316-23.
[http://dx.doi.org/10.1002/jbm.a.30743] [PMID: 16637041]

[75]   Assad M, Chernyshov A, Leroux MA, Rivard C-H. A new porous titanium-nickel alloy: Part 1. Cytotoxicity and genotoxicity evaluation. Biomed Mater Eng 2002; 12(3): 225-37.
[PMID: 12446938]

[76]   Assad M, Chernyshov A, Leroux MA, Rivard CH. A new porous titanium-nickel alloy: part 2. Sensitization, irritation and acute systemic toxicity evaluation. Biomed Mater Eng 2002; 12(4): 339-46.
[PMID: 12652028]

[77]   Kujala S, Ryhänen J, Danilov A, Tuukkanen J. Effect of porosity on the osteointegration and bone ingrowth of a weight-bearing nickel-titanium bone graft substitute. Biomaterials 2003; 24(25): 4691-7.
[http://dx.doi.org/10.1016/S0142-9612(03)00359-4] [PMID: 12951012]

[78]   Staiger MP, Pietak AM, Huadmai J, Dias G. Magnesium and its alloys as orthopedic biomaterials: a review. Biomaterials 2006; 27(9): 1728-34.
[http://dx.doi.org/10.1016/j.biomaterials.2005.10.003] [PMID: 16246414]

[79]   Kheirkhah M, Fathi M, Salimijazi HR, Razavi M. Surface modification of stainless steel implants using nanostructured forsterite (Mg2SiO4) coating for biomaterial applications. Surf Coat Tech 2015;

276
[http://dx.doi.org/10.1016/j.surfcoat.2015.06.012]

[80] Razavi M, Fathi M, Savabi O, Vashaee D, Tayebi L. *In vitro* analysis of electrophoretic deposited fluoridated hydroxyapatite coating on micro-arc oxidized AZ91 magnesium alloy for biomaterials applications. Metall Mater Trans, A Phys Metall Mater Sci 2014; 46
[http://dx.doi.org/10.1007/s11661-014-2694-2]

[81] Razavi M, Fathi MH, Savabi O, Vashaee D, Tayebi L. Biodegradation, bioactivity and *in vivo* biocompatibility analysis of plasma electrolytic oxidized (PEO) biodegradable Mg implants. Phys Sci Int J 2014; 4: 708-22.
[http://dx.doi.org/10.9734/PSIJ/2014/9265]

[82] Razavi M, Fathi MH, Savabi O, Vashaee D, Tayebi L. Micro-arc oxidation and electrophoretic deposition of nano-grain merwinite (Ca3MgSi2O8) surface coating on magnesium alloy as biodegradable metallic implant. Surf Interface Anal 2014.
[http://dx.doi.org/10.1002/sia.5465]

[83] Saris N-E, Mervaala E, Karppanen H, Khawaja JA, Lewenstam A. Magnesium. An update on physiological, clinical and analytical aspects. Clin Chim Acta 2000; 294(1-2): 1-26.
[http://dx.doi.org/10.1016/S0009-8981(99)00258-2] [PMID: 10727669]

[84] Razavi M, Fathi M, Savabi O, Vashaee D, Tayebi L. *In vivo* study of nanostructured akermanite/PEO coating on biodegradable magnesium alloy for biomedical applications, J. Biomed. Mater. Res - Part A 2015; 103
[http://dx.doi.org/10.1002/jbm.a.35324]

[85] Razavi M, Fathi M, Savabi O, Vashaee D, Tayebi L. Improvement of biodegradability, bioactivity, mechanical integrity and cytocompatibility behavior of biodegradable mg based orthopedic implants using nanostructured Bredigite (Ca7MgSi 4O 16) bioceramic coated *via* ASD/EPD technique. Ann Biomed Eng 2014; 42(12): 2537-50.
[http://dx.doi.org/10.1007/s10439-014-1084-7] [PMID: 25118669]

[86] Hartwig A. Role of magnesium in genomic stability. Mutat Res 2001; 475(1-2): 113-21.
[http://dx.doi.org/10.1016/S0027-5107(01)00074-4] [PMID: 11295157]

[87] Razavi M, Fathi MH, Meratian M. Microstructure, mechanical properties and bio-corrosion evaluation of biodegradable AZ91-FA nanocomposites for biomedical applications. Mater Sci Eng A 2010; 527
[http://dx.doi.org/10.1016/j.msea.2010.07.063]

[88] Razavi M, Fathi M, Savabi O, *et al.* Controlling the degradation rate of bioactive magnesium implants by electrophoretic deposition of akermanite coating. Ceram Int 2013; 40: 3865-72.
[http://dx.doi.org/10.1016/j.ceramint.2013.08.027]

[89] Razavi M, Fathi MH, Meratian M. Fabrication and characterization of magnesium-fluorapatite nanocomposite for biomedical applications. Mater Charact 2010; 61
[http://dx.doi.org/10.1016/j.matchar.2010.09.008]

[90] Razavi M, Fathi M, Savabi O, *et al.* Coating of biodegradable magnesium alloy bone implants using nanostructured diopside (CaMgSi 2 O 6). Appl Surf Sci 2014; 288: 130-7.
[http://dx.doi.org/10.1016/j.apsusc.2013.09.160]

[91] Razavi M, Fathi M, Savabi O, Vashaee D, Tayebi L. *In vitro* study of nanostructured diopside coating on Mg alloy orthopedic implants. Mater Sci Eng C 2014; 41: 168-77.
[http://dx.doi.org/10.1016/j.msec.2014.04.039] [PMID: 24907750]

[92] Razavi M, Fathi M, Savabi O, Hashemi Beni B, Vashaee D, Tayebi L. Nanostructured merwinite bioceramic coating on Mg alloy deposited by electrophoretic deposition. Ceram Int 2014; 40
[http://dx.doi.org/10.1016/j.ceramint.2014.02.020]

[93] Gu XN, Zheng YF. A review on magnesium alloys as biodegradable materials. Front Mater Sci China 2010; 4: 111-5.

[http://dx.doi.org/10.1007/s11706-010-0024-1]

[94]   Yusop AH, Bakir AA, Shaharom NA, Abdul Kadir MR, Hermawan H. Porous biodegradable metals for hard tissue scaffolds: a review. Int J Biomater 2012; 2012: 641430.
[http://dx.doi.org/10.1155/2012/641430] [PMID: 22919393]

[95]   Razavi M, Fathi M, Savabi O, Hashemi Beni B, Vashaee D, Tayebi L. Surface microstructure and *in vitro* analysis of nanostructured akermanite (Ca2MgSi2O7) coating on biodegradable magnesium alloy for biomedical applications. Colloids Surf B Biointerfaces 2014; 117: 432-40.
[http://dx.doi.org/10.1016/j.colsurfb.2013.12.011] [PMID: 24721316]

[96]   Razavi M, Fathi MH, Meratian M. Bio-corrosion behavior of magnesium-fluorapatite nanocomposite for biomedical applications. Mater Lett 2010; 64
[http://dx.doi.org/10.1016/j.matlet.2010.07.079]

[97]   Fathi MH, Meratian M, Razavi M. Novel magnesium-nanofluorapatite metal matrix nanocomposite with improved biodegradation behavior. J Biomed Nanotechnol 2011; 7(3): 441-5.
[http://dx.doi.org/10.1166/jbn.2011.1310] [PMID: 21830486]

[98]   Razavi M, Fathi MH, Savabi O, Vashaee D, Tayebi L. *In vitro* evaluations of anodic spark deposited AZ91 alloy as biodegradable metallic orthopedic implant. Annu Res Rev Biol 2014.

[99]   Zreiqat H, Howlett CR, Zannettino A, *et al.* Mechanisms of magnesium-stimulated adhesion of osteoblastic cells to commonly used orthopaedic implants. J Biomed Mater Res 2002; 62(2): 175-84.
[http://dx.doi.org/10.1002/jbm.10270] [PMID: 12209937]

[100]   Razavi M, Fathi M, Savabi O, Vashaee D, Tayebi L. *In vivo* assessments of bioabsorbable AZ91 magnesium implants coated with nanostructured fluoridated hydroxyapatite by MAO/EPD technique for biomedical applications. Mater Sci Eng C 2015; 48: 21-7.
[http://dx.doi.org/10.1016/j.msec.2014.11.020] [PMID: 25579892]

[101]   Razavi M, Fathi M, Savabi O, *et al.* *In vivo* study of nanostructured diopside (CaMgSi2O6) coating on magnesium alloy as biodegradable orthopedic implants. Appl Surf Sci 2014.

[102]   Cramer SD, Covino BS. ASM Handbook Vol. 13a: Corrosion - Fundamentals, Testing, and Protection. Asm 2003; 13: 1135.
[http://dx.doi.org/10.1002/jbm.b.31896]

[103]   Razavi M, Fathi M, Savabi O, *et al.* Surface modification of magnesium alloy implants by nanostructured bredigite coating. Mater Lett 2013; 113
[http://dx.doi.org/10.1016/j.matlet.2013.09.068]

[104]   Witte F, Kaese V, Haferkamp H, *et al.* *In vivo* corrosion of four magnesium alloys and the associated bone response. Biomaterials 2005; 26(17): 3557-63.
[http://dx.doi.org/10.1016/j.biomaterials.2004.09.049] [PMID: 15621246]

[105]   Razavi M, Fathi M, Savabi O, Vashaee D, Tayebi L. Regenerative influence of nanostructured bredigite (Ca7MgSi4O16)/anodic spark coating on biodegradable AZ91 magnesium alloy implants for bone healing. Mater Lett 2015; 155
[http://dx.doi.org/10.1016/j.matlet.2015.04.129]

[106]   Razavi M, Fathi M, Savabi O, Vashaee D, Tayebi L. *In vivo* biocompatibility of Mg implants surface modified by nanostructured merwinite/PEO. J Mater Sci Mater Med 2015; 26(5): 184.
[http://dx.doi.org/10.1007/s10856-015-5514-3] [PMID: 25893390]

[107]   Gu X, Zheng Y, Cheng Y, Zhong S, Xi T. *In vitro* corrosion and biocompatibility of binary magnesium alloys. Biomaterials 2009; 30(4): 484-98.
[http://dx.doi.org/10.1016/j.biomaterials.2008.10.021] [PMID: 19000636]

[108]   Heublein B, Rohde R, Kaese V, Niemeyer M, Hartung W, Haverich A. Biocorrosion of magnesium alloys: a new principle in cardiovascular implant technology? Heart 2003; 89(6): 651-6.
[http://dx.doi.org/10.1136/heart.89.6.651] [PMID: 12748224]

[109] Li Z, Gu X, Lou S, Zheng Y. The development of binary Mg-Ca alloys for use as biodegradable materials within bone. Biomaterials 2008; 29(10): 1329-44.
[http://dx.doi.org/10.1016/j.biomaterials.2007.12.021] [PMID: 18191191]

[110] Li L, Gao J, Wang Y. Evaluation of cyto-toxicity and corrosion behavior of alkali-heat-treated magnesium in simulated body fluid. Surf Coat Tech 2004; 185: 92-8.
[http://dx.doi.org/10.1016/j.surfcoat.2004.01.004]

[111] Zhang E, Xu L, Yang K. Formation by ion plating of Ti-coating on pure Mg for biomedical applications. Scr Mater 2005; 53: 523-7.
[http://dx.doi.org/10.1016/j.scriptamat.2005.05.009]

[112] Xu L, Yu G, Zhang E, Pan F, Yang K. *In vivo* corrosion behavior of Mg-Mn-Zn alloy for bone implant application. J Biomed Mater Res A 2007; 83(3): 703-11.
[http://dx.doi.org/10.1002/jbm.a.31273] [PMID: 17549695]

[113] Witte F, Ulrich H, Rudert M, Willbold E. Biodegradable magnesium scaffolds: Part 1: appropriate inflammatory response. J Biomed Mater Res A 2007; 81(3): 748-56.
[http://dx.doi.org/10.1002/jbm.a.31170] [PMID: 17390368]

[114] Gu XN, Zhou WR, Zheng YF, Liu Y, Li YX. Degradation and cytotoxicity of lotus-type porous pure magnesium as potential tissue engineering scaffold material. Mater Lett 2010; 64: 1871-4.
[http://dx.doi.org/10.1016/j.matlet.2010.06.015]

[115] Zreiqat H, Howlett CR, Zannettino A, *et al.* Mechanisms of magnesium-stimulated adhesion of osteoblastic cells to commonly used orthopaedic implants. J Biomed Mater Res 2002; 62(2): 175-84.
[http://dx.doi.org/10.1002/jbm.10270] [PMID: 12209937]

[116] Yamasaki Y, Yoshida Y, Okazaki M, *et al.* Synthesis of functionally graded MgCO3 apatite accelerating osteoblast adhesion. J Biomed Mater Res 2002; 62(1): 99-105.
[http://dx.doi.org/10.1002/jbm.10220] [PMID: 12124791]

[117] Yamasaki Y, Yoshida Y, Okazaki M, *et al.* Action of FGMgCO3Ap-collagen composite in promoting bone formation. Biomaterials 2003; 24(27): 4913-20.
[http://dx.doi.org/10.1016/S0142-9612(03)00414-9] [PMID: 14559004]

[118] Geng F, Tan L, Zhang B, *et al.* Study on beta-TCP coated porous Mg as a bone tissue engineering scaffold material. J Mater Sci Technol 2009; 25: 123-9.

[119] Yazdimamaghani M, Razavi M, Vashaee D, *et al.* *In vitro* analysis of Mg scaffolds coated with polymer/hydrogel/ceramic composite layers. Surf Coat Tech 2016; 301
[http://dx.doi.org/10.1016/j.surfcoat.2016.01.017]

[120] Wen CE, Yamada Y, Shimojima K, Chino Y, Hosokawa H, Mabuchi M. Compressibility of porous magnesium foam: dependency on porosity and pore size. Mater Lett 2004; 58: 357-60.
[http://dx.doi.org/10.1016/S0167-577X(03)00500-7]

[121] Adachi T, Osako Y, Tanaka M, Hojo M, Hollister SJ. Framework for optimal design of porous scaffold microstructure by computational simulation of bone regeneration. Biomaterials 2006; 27(21): 3964-72.
[http://dx.doi.org/10.1016/j.biomaterials.2006.02.039] [PMID: 16584771]

[122] Yazdimamaghani M, Razavi M, Vashaee D, Pothineni VR, Rajadas J, Tayebi L. Significant degradability enhancement in multilayer coating of polycaprolactone-bioactive glass/gelatin-bioactive glass on magnesium scaffold for tissue engineering applications. Appl Surf Sci 2015; 338: 137-45.
[http://dx.doi.org/10.1016/j.apsusc.2015.02.120]

[123] Cheng MQ, Wahafu T, Jiang GF, *et al.* A novel open-porous magnesium scaffold with controllable microstructures and properties for bone regeneration. Sci Rep 2016; 6: 24134.
[http://dx.doi.org/10.1038/srep24134] [PMID: 27071777]

CHAPTER 6

Gradient Fabrication

Nasim Kiaie[1,*] and **Mehdi Razavi**[2]

[1] *Department of Biomedical Engineering, Amirkabir University of Technology, Tehran,15875, Iran*

[2] *Department of Radiology, School of Medicine, Stanford University, Palo Alto, California 94304, USA*

Abstract: The importance of applying the (physical, mechanical or chemical) gradient for the development of porous scaffolds is undeniable in tissue engineering. Gradient scaffolds enable us to engineer heterogeneous interfacial tissues, to mimic the natural microenvironment of cells, Extra Cellular Matrix (ECM) alignment and clustering the cells. Therefore, they can properly realize the biomimetic approach. Such scaffolds are suitable to create functional tissues through the incorporation of physical and chemical signal gradients. Additionally, using the gradient structures, high throughput screening of cell-scaffold interactions becomes possible for optimization of scaffold design parameters and prevention of errors during the experiments. Thus, in this chapter, we aim to first introduce different types of gradients and then discuss the production techniques of the gradient scaffolds.

Keywords: Bioactive agent release, Fibrous scaffold, Gradient, Mechanical properties, Porosity, Pore size, Surface treatment.

INTRODUCTION

The human body is a complex system containing various types of tissues different in terms of materials, physical, mechanical, electrical and optical properties [1, 2] and hence the different types of gradations interfaces between these tissues.

Gradient scaffolds are the structures which can imitate the interfaces tissues in the body to lessen the invasiveness of grafting techniques. These scaffolds sometimes referred to "next generation scaffolds". Some strategies are employed to reach the repeatable gradients in these structures with the aim of mimicking natural tissues. It is known that with the introduction of the gradient, the cell behaviors (adhesion, spreading, migration, survival, and differentiation) will change. Gradients in

---
[*] **Corresponding author Nasim Kiaie:** Department of Biomedical Engineering, Amirkabir University of Technology, Tehran, Iran; Tel: +98 912 7238387; Fax: +98 21 66468186; E-mail: nasim.kiaie@aut.ac.ir

hydrophilicity and protein absorption can influence cell behaviors on these scaffolds. Stem cells differentiation and mobilization are also under the effect of physical and chemical gradients [3 - 5].

Gradient-based strategies have been applied in some areas such as electrophoresis, chromatography, drug discovery, and catalysts, as well as in the design of orthopedic and orthodontic implants (*e.g.* maxillofacial, hip or knee replacements). Such graded metallic and ceramic implants have been created in order to simulate the natural bone architecture with low porosity cortical and high porosity cancellous areas [6], to prevent stress-shielding phenomenon and to match the stiffness of the implant to that of the bone. Surface treatment methods of metallic implants in a gradient manner are also available with the goal of preventing the release of metal ions, leading to improvement of the biocompatibility and enhancement of the corrosion resistance [7]. Although above-mentioned applications of the gradient are not the focus of this chapter, the methods of creating a gradient in them could be used in the field of fabricating gradient scaffolds.

In this chapter, at first we review some properties of the scaffold in which gradient could be applied. These features include porosity and pore size, mechanical properties and stiffness, physicochemical features of the surface, concentration and density of bioactive molecules embedded into scaffolds as chemical signals and finally, diameter and composition of fibers in fibrous scaffolds. Then, we discuss a number of methods for fabrication of scaffolds with the mentioned gradients.

GRADIENT IN DIFFERENT PARAMETERS OF THE SCAFFOLD

Clearly, the behaviors of cells into scaffolds depend greatly on the features of the scaffold [8, 9]. Cell migration is one of the most important processes of the body which could occur in three forms: (a) chemotaxis: in this process, the migration of cells is done in response to chemical stimuli. In fact, the existence of gradient in the concentration of a certain soluble agent or chemoattractant in the environment surrounding the cell directs its movement toward higher or lower concentrations; (b) haptotaxis: in this process what stimulate cells to migrate is a gradient in chemoattractants which is expressed on the surface or is substrate bounded, it is not in the soluble form; (c) durotaxis or mechanotaxis: a process in which migration of cells takes place in response to a mechanical cue [5, 10]. All these types of gradients, such as gradient in pores of scaffold or gradient in mechanical properties described here are regarded as mechanical stimuli for induction of durotaxis, which will be discussed with more details.

Gradient in Pores of Scaffold

Contact guidance theory suggests that the existence of pores in a scaffold is necessary for the cell viability. Based on this theory, binding and then spreading of cells require adequate contact with the substrate. Pore size, porosity, interconnectivity of pores and even pore shape play an important role in intracellular signaling, mass transport of nutrients and metabolites, cellular organization and even angiogenesis *in vivo* [11 - 13].

Making the gradient in pores of a scaffold was first applied for bone substitutes. Graded bone implants with two regions of poor and rich porosity can best mimic the natural cancellous bone [6, 14]. The gradient in pores for supporting the hard tissues generation has been successfully produced [6, 15]. In tissue engineering scaffolds, the gradient in pore size is important in designing a scaffold for tendon-bone interface [16, 17]. Moreover, graded pores are applicable in co-culture of two different cell types [18] or engineering of small intestine tissue [19].

Gradient in Mechanical Properties of Scaffold

A tissue designed through a biomimetic approach might have the same type of gradients of some tissues in the body, such as osteochondral tissue, intervertebral discs, skin layers, and walls of blood vessels. In the temporomandibular joint, higher stiffness is evident in anteroposterior as compared to the mediolateral direction [20].

Mechanical properties of the scaffold affect the cell response [21, 22]. In fact, morphology and function of each cell type depend heavily on threshold values of stiffness. The recent researches show that stiffer scaffolds cause more contact of cells with biomaterial surface which is preferable for cell migration. "Mechanotaxis" is a term referred to a phenomenon based on which migration of cells occurs from softer regions of the scaffold to the stiffer parts [5, 20]. Additionally, different studies confirm that each cell type prefers a specific value of surface stiffness, for example, neurons more efficiently extent and differentiate on the soft materials [4] and it has been shown that the morphology and spreading of smooth muscle cells depend on the module of the surfaces [23].

Gradient Surface Treatment

The surface of biomaterials is very important since it is the first part of the scaffold which is exposed to the biological system, determining interactions with protein and cells [24 - 26]. Since then, many efforts have been devoted to tailor the surface characteristics of biomaterials [27 - 30] such as charge, wettability, roughness, and crystallinity which play a critical role in cell behaviors [3].The surface of scaffold could be altered by insertion of the different functional groups on its surface to impart a specific feature, increase or decrease cell attachment [28]; For example, reducing the cell attachment is essential for implants which are in direct contact with blood to prevent thrombosis and clot formation, while ameliorating cell attachment is preferable for tissue engineering applications.

The gradient substrates could be induced by patterning the surface [31]. Through patterning, some areas of scaffold surface become more reactive to the cells as compared to other parts. Patterned surfaces affect site-specific biomaterial interactions. This matter is very important for differentiation of stem cell into specific tissue [32].

The surface of scaffold could be modified by grafting different functional groups. For example, applying the amine functional groups is a straightforward method to change the surface chemistry, influencing wettability of the surface. It is known that protein adsorption on the surfaces and consequently cell attachment is under the influence of amine functionalization [33] and a gradient in these functional groups can influence cell attachment in a gradient manner and the subsequent proceedings, such as cell proliferation and differentiation could be influenced [34]. In the case of amine functionalization, differentiation of human adipose derived stem cells was under the effect of the gradient in amine functional groups. In another work, the density of RGD peptide grafted on a silicon bed was altered and the behavior of mesenchymal stem cells during the culture on this substrate was shown to change greatly [35].

The gradient in the topography of surface is important in determining the behavior of cells on a scaffold [22]. A gradient in surface nano-topography was created in silicon materials to investigate its effect on the response of mesenchymal stem cells [35].

In order to achieve gradient in surface properties, the surface could be coated with different materials, where different thicknesses and compositions of these coatings not only change the surface chemistry and consequently the cell behavior but also cause a transition in degradation rate or mechanical properties of the surface. To achieve such graded coatings, electrophoretic deposition (EPD) [36 - 39] and electrolytic deposition (ELD) methods are exploitable [40].

Gradient Bioactive Molecules

Several processes in the body are under the influence of endogenous bioactive signal molecules gradients. Some of the processes such as repair and wound healing, immunity, morphogenesis, angiogenesis, axonal guidance, cellular migration, and differentiation are governed by "signaling pathways". For example, in the wound healing, the gradient in chemotactic factors secreted by macrophages induce migration of fibroblasts into the wound region [41].

The gradient in chemical factors such as chemokines, hormones, proteins and growth factors has attracted the attention of researchers in the field of tissue engineering [42]. Controlled release of bioactive molecules as chemical signals from scaffolds is an idea to be tested in biomimetic approach which is useful for engineering microenvironment of the cells [22]. Biomimetic approach has been investigated in many studies including axon and nerve regeneration [43], angiogenesis induction [1], investigating migration of different cells in response to a factor [10] and study of chemotaxis [44]. Additionally, in order to prevent necrotic zones in scaffolds, survival factors can be fixed at the center of the scaffold. In this manner, a radial gradient in chemical factors from the center to the edges is achieved [45]. Another key area that may benefit from gradients of bioactive signals is interfacial tissue engineering, for example, co-culture of osteoblast and fibroblast in a single scaffold as a bone-tendon interface through gradient delivery of genes [46]. Additionally, in scaffolds seeded with stem cells, encapsulating different agents in scaffold and release of them in a gradient manner can enhance differentiation of stem cells to a certain lineage [47].

The gradient in the chemical signals could be introduced by two procedures: first, creating concentration gradient via control of the release of soluble factors. Spatial and temporal release of growth factors and cell adhesion molecules (CAMs) from particulate carriers is under the area of biomimetic tissue engineering [22]. With this purpose, combining drug delivery systems with gradient strategies become important especially when scaffold is made of microspheres [1, 47 - 49]. Second, immobilizing these factors into the scaffold with varying surface densities. As a case in point, immobilizing RGD-containing peptide influences the alignment of the fibroblasts which is applicable in tendon-bone tissue engineering [35].

Gradient Fibers into Fibrous Scaffolds

Fibrous scaffolds have been the center of many studies in the recent years because they give the best biomimicry to the natural ECM. These scaffolds are mostly prepared via electrospinning method, therefore, changing setup and parameters of electrospinning equipment enable us to prepare scaffolds with a gradient in diameter of fibers and their alignment or even some types of the gradient in composition of the scaffold. In this method, the composition of different scaffold regions can be controlled by using two syringes in electrospinning where each one contains a specific polymer. For example, a polymer solution (*e.g.* PCL) can be electrospun with a composite solution (PCL + nano-calcium phosphate particles) to mimic tissues with a gradient in mineral content such as tendon or ligament [50, 51]. Furthermore, other types of gradient could be applied in the fibrous scaffolds. For example, it is possible to create a gradient in the release of bioactive molecules by incorporating the desired factor into fibers and then control the amount of these fibers into scaffold [52]. The gradient can also be created in fiber bound agents. The work done by Sundararaghavan and Burdick is an example. They prepared two solutions of high RGD bound and low RGD bound hyaluronic acid and spun them into fibers on a single collector. The resulting fibrous scaffold with varying densities of RGD achieved for desirable cell infiltration [53]

STRATEGIES TO CREATE GRADIENT SCAFFOLD

In this section, we presented common methods used for fabrication of scaffolds with different types of gradients.

Methods of Creating Gradient in Pores

Many different techniques have been developed to create graded pores in biomaterials [54]. The goal of this chapter is to seek methods in creating graded pores in the scaffolds. Considering the fact that most of the scaffolds are polymeric and biodegradable, methods of fabricating graded pores in such materials may be divided into 6 categories as discussed below.

3D Printing

This technique is a subset of Solid Free Form Fabrication Methods. These methods are superior in terms of resolution compared to other methods. Solid free-form methods, sometimes referred to as rapid prototyping, make it possible to precisely control the shape of the scaffold. Apart from 3D printing, fused deposition modeling (FDM), ink-jet printing and indirect casting (IC), stereolithography (SL) and selective laser sintering (SLS) are other solid free-form fabrication methods which are widely used in biomedical engineering [55]. In 3D printing, powders of material are printed layer by layer on each other and a binder or a solvent is ejected from another jet to join layers. With the help of 3D printing, many complex shapes with the desired patterns and pores are created. For example, titanium scaffold with graded interconnected porosities for bone tissue engineering has been manufactured via 3D printing [6, 56].

Phase Separation Methods

Phase separation is an old method in creating porous scaffolds. Wessling M. team was among the first who developed phase separation micro-molding method to create gradient pores [57]. Based on this method, polymer solution is cast onto a mold in which patterns are created. Lowering the solution temperature initiates separation of phases, and porous scaffold could be achieved. In this method, there are two limitations: (1) control over pore size and pore distribution is not feasible owing to the instability of this thermodynamic process and (2), the amount of solvent used in this method is high which is not environment-friendly. However, phase separation methods are followed by freeze drying to remove the solvent and, therefore, the second limitation could be solved to some extent. In order to manage size and distribution of pores to solve the first mentioned problem, in situ co-continuous polymer blends could be utilized. These types of blends have an inter-winding and interpenetrating phase structure owing to their unique thermal flow behavior and initiate coarsening at high temperatures. In this method, temperature distribution changes in a controlled manner leading to a controllable gradient in phase structure. Finally, the phase which is poor of polymers will be dissolved and the desired porous structure remains [17].

Another method reported for fabrication of a graded porous structure is combining non-solvent phase separation with block copolymer self-assembly methods. This way, a surface layer with a thickness of 100 nm composed of uniform mesopores attained, while underlay is a macroporous sponge. This porous structure was designed with the objective of ultrafiltration of water, but the method of its fabrication can find applications in tissue engineering scaffolds [58].

Centrifugation Methods

These methods are used for creating a gradient along the rotation radius in cylindrical geometries. As it is shown in Fig. (**1**). centrifugation force could be used to separate particles of a material in powder state or suspension. After spinning, separated particles join together by freeze-drying or heat-sintering. Harley *et al.* used this approach to create graded porosity in scaffolds through spinning collagen suspension in acetic acid [44].

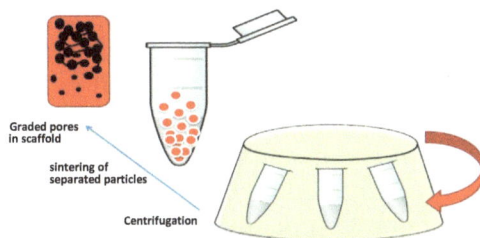

Fig. (1). Schematic for centrifugation method to create a gradient in pores of the scaffold. Centrifugation force separate particles of different weight in a suspension. After sintering, heavy particles are more close to each other and the distance between them is smaller as compared to light particles. Finally, a gradient in pores is created.

Lamination Method

It seems that the simplest method for inducing the gradient in pores is fabricating distinct layers and then joining them together. Interconnectivity of pores is the main concern in this method. Layers of scaffolds with specific porosities form separately and then assembling these layers onto each other forms the final structure (Fig. **2**). Multi-layered scaffolds have been applied for engineering interfacial tissues which gradient in porosity is required for them such as tendon to bone interfaces [16, 59]. Each layer could be produced with one of the traditional methods of fabricating porous scaffolds such as freeze drying. Application of multilayered scaffolds is investigated especially in the orthopedic and musculoskeletal tissue engineering [60].

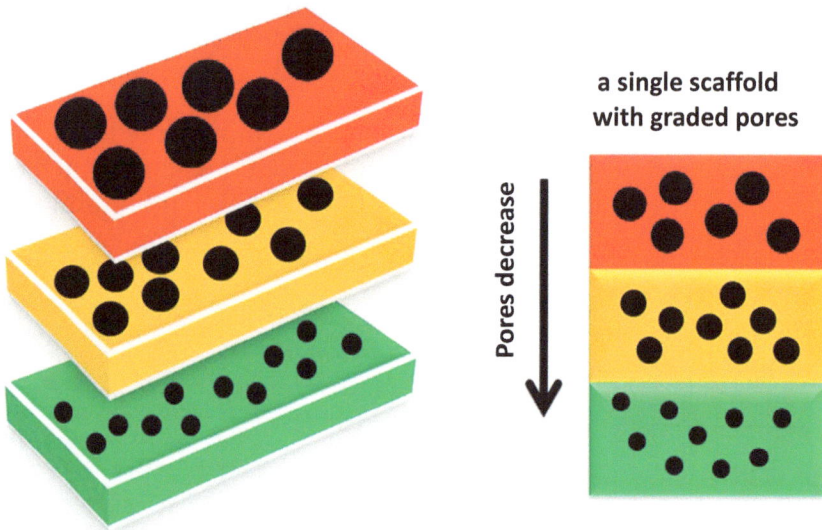

Fig. (2). A schematic for three distinct layers with specific pores which are compressed to make a unique gradient scaffold.

This method has been successfully applied for small intestine tissue engineering in a way that tubular structure with dimensions of rat small intestine fabricated with solvent-cast and particulate-leached technique. Compression was used in order to make adherence of layers and to achieve final thickness [19]. In another study, melted polymers were mixed together and then particle leaching was done to create pores. Three layers with distinct porosities were achieved *via* different ratios of porogen mixing. Finally, three layers were compressed after molding to make final scaffold [18]. Moreover, different sizes and diameters of powders or fibers can be employed for preparing the layered materials with different porosities [14, 17].

Microsphere Scaffolds

Microspheres demonstrated promise in making gradient porous scaffolds [54]. From one side, microsphere could take the place of porogen in the processing of scaffolds. It means that while small pores can be created during scaffold fabrication process, larger pores could be created as a result of leaching of incorporated microsphere [61]. On the other side, microsphere of two different sizes can be sintered in a way that the shape of microspheres retains and spaces between these microspheres create pores with two different sizes distribution [62]. Sintering of microspheres could be done by different solvents, such as ethanol or through a liquid or gaseous CO_2. The basis for the later approach is the same as gas foaming method. In this technique, low-pressure CO_2 followed by depressurization joins microspheres together without total plasticization of them. In comparison to liquid CO_2 or ethanol, this is an inexpensive and relatively mild process and is done in low temperatures which are preferable for scaffold preparation in the presence of cells. Besides, it is possible to import porogen salts into the microspheres during the preparation of microsphere. Hence, another type of gradient in porosity could be achieved by changing the amount of porogen in two different sizes of microspheres [61].

Methods of Creating Gradient in Mechanical Properties

Making gradient in mechanical features of the scaffold is important to make these structures similar to that of the natural tissues. The gradient in mechanical properties exists in some tissues, such as bone and tooth. All of the aforementioned methods for the preparation of graded pores can be used to produce graded mechanical properties because porosity has a direct link with the mechanical feature. Specifically, there are two main methods to fabricate such graded materials as below.

Gradient in Cross-linking Density

Making gradient in mechanical properties of scaffold leads to structures akin to some natural tissues in the body, such as bone substitutes [63]. In order to have scaffolds with different regions of modules and stiffness, the simplest adopted method is cross-linking of desired parts of scaffold more than other parts [63]. Generally, polymeric scaffolds cross-link *via* two main ways; first is the chemical crosslinkers [63] and the second is photo or UV irradiation, referred to as photo-masking [64]. In the second approach, mechanical properties including elastic modules could be tuned via control of irradiation intensity and time of exposure. The gradient in crosslinking density can be induced by means of Microfluidic Devices. Microfluidic is an interesting area where its application in tissue engineering has attracted much attention. Microfluidic devices are generally fabricated by soft lithographic techniques mainly on PDMS substrates. Such devices have a wide range of applications. For example, in a study, a 3D collagen gel with graded mechanical properties was fabricated with the help of an H-shaped microfluidic device. In this design, cells are located in a cross-channel in which a gradient of peptide grafted collagen exists in such a way that source channel contains genipin and the sink channel is filled with collagen solution. A gradient in genipin concentration as the crosslinker is generated in the cross-channel. This gradient is immobilized when collagen gel assembled into the 3D fibrillar state [65].

Mixing Chambers

An approach that enables us to change the composition of the scaffold in a controlled gradient manner would result in a gradient in mechanical properties. For this aim, researchers invented "gradient making apparatus" which can produce composition gradient in micrometer scale [66]. A schematic of such equipment is shown in Fig. (3).

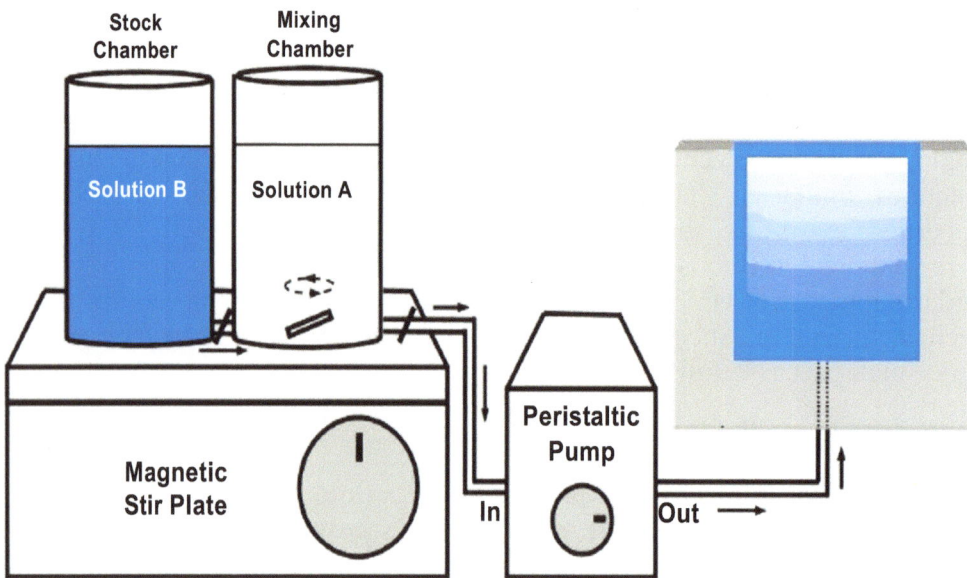

Fig. (3). A schematic for mixing chamber. Polymer B enters the mixing chamber with a determined flow rate diluting the polymer A solution. As a result, a gradient from polymer A to B is achieved.

In another approach, the solution of two different polymers is mixed. Then freezing in liquid nitrogen and finally gas foaming process is done to produce porous scaffolds. In fact, the gradient in composition and subsequently mechanical properties has been induced in mixing step. In this step, solutions of two polymers are loaded into two different syringes with a pump installed on each one. The first pump is programmed to increase the flow rate of polymer A and the second one to decrease the flow rate of polymer B. Two polymers are mixed in a static mixer and deposited on a substrate or into a mold. The result is a scaffold with two ends, one rich in polymer A and other rich in polymer B and in the middle of the scaffold, a gradient from polymer A to B started to appear [67].

Methods of Creating Gradient in Surface Treatment

In order to induce gradient in surface chemistry, a number of methods have been suggested by researchers. In a number of reviews, methods of surface modification to create gradient are discussed and categorized as physical and chemical treatments or deposition of a material onto the substrate [68, 69]. We gathered all these methods and put them into 5 major categories as follows.

Making Gradient in Density of Polymer Graft or Functional Groups

In order to have a gradient in the density of polymer graft, the process of polymerization should be controlled by the concentration of initiator. Gradient can be made feasible by diffusion of initiator into the scaffold or immersion of scaffold in initiator solution with different rates. Depletion of the monomer solution is another technique [69]. On the other hand, initiators could be bound to self-assembled monolayers (SAMs) such as silane groups. Control of the initiator amount is done via altering silane density on the surface when covering the surface with SAMs. Photolithographic method process is a process through which monolayers from desired sections of the surface are removed via oxidation with oxygen radicals [70]. A similar concept is used to change the density of polymers grafted onto the substrate. Electrochemical attachment is the application of a gradient electrical field with various current densities to control the density of grafted polymers [35]. In this method, porous silicon is prepared through anodization process and then electro-grafting is performed in which changing the current density leads to changes in surface oxidation and consequently functional group attachment.

Making a gradient in molecular weight of polymeric chains is possible in cases when polymerization is done on the surface. This gradient can be created by pumping a solution of monomer over the surface with controllable contact time.

In terms of functional groups, the most valid method of creating gradient is through applying plasma (such as nitrogen, ammonia, oxygen and sulfur dioxide) to introduce amino, carboxyl, hydroxyl groups and sulphonic acid groups on the surface [71]. With controlling parameters related to the plasma, such as its concentration, different types of the gradients in surface functionalities could be created. For example, a chemoattractant surface is created through gradient polymerizing poly pyrol on a substrate with the help of plasma [72]. Another approach of creating graded functional groups is the control of polymeric surface degradation with the help of a reactive solution [71].

Coating Surface with a Distinct Layer

Scaffolds could be coated with another material to induce desired properties in their surface without changing the bulk properties [73, 74]. The process of coating is done generally via spin-coating apparatus. The simplest method of coating the scaffold is immersion in the solution of coating molecules to allow absorption of such molecules onto the surface. In this way, the gradient in thickness and density of coating could be achieved by altering the immersion time [70] or a gradual decrease in the coating solution levels [71].

Plasma polymerization is another method to make thin layers of coating. In this method, electrical excitation of monomer molecules in vapor state produces a plasma phase which could be deposited upon contact with the surface. A gradient in plasma polymer is achieved using the valves controlling monomer entrance into the chamber. Furthermore, some functional groups remain in the plasma deposit and gradient in these groups could be created [75].

Making Gradient in Surface Wettability and Surface Energy

Wettability and surface energy have a direct relationship with each other. Hydrophilic surfaces owing to having high surface energy tend to absorb water. Therefore, when wettability of surface increase, surface energy increase, and the surface will be more reactive. Wettability of surface can be increased if hydrophilic functional groups containing oxygen atoms exist on the surface. Hence, etching surfaces with chemical and physical methods can produce peroxide moieties on the surface. Generally, oxidation of surface is completed through etching via UV or photo exposure, gas plasma discharge and immersion in NaOH. These peroxides and other hydrophilic functional groups created from this process can be further used for grafting other polymers on the different regions of the surface. To reduce the hydrophilicity, applying a plasma containing fluoride gas molecules is favorable [71].

To alter the wettability of glass or silica surfaces, a photolithography method is suitable. In this method, the surface could be covered with self-assembled monolayers of silanes (SAMs). At the first step, a gradient in SAMs is created by a series of methods. Microcontact printing, degradation of SAMs in a determined pattern through photocatalytic oxidation, low-energy electrons or a focused X-ray beam are some examples [70]. At next step, a gradient in hydrophilic functional groups has been prepared by diffusion through solvents [71].

Wettability and surface energy can change by imparting ions on the surface via ion deposition methods. The gradient can be induced by control of ion beam [76].

Making Gradient in Nanostructure of Surface (Including nano-topography, Roughness, and Crystallinity)

There exist many methods to alter surface roughness. Most of these methods use a high energy source (such as plasma and UV) to impact the chemical composition and then roughness of the surface. Making gradient with these methods is achieved by controlling the distance between the surface and the source. For example, in UV-based methods moving the photomask under a UV lamp can create gradients. To change the roughness of the surface, the most widely used method is polishing surface.

This could be done by a chemical solution. A gradient temperature can cause a gradient in crystallinity and roughness of surfaces. In this approach, annealing of a polymeric superficial layer is done with varying temperatures [70]. Another way to induce gradient in surface topography is using a graded electrical field. With control of current density during the process of anodization, surface pores change and different zones with variable topographies achieve [35].

Thin film casting followed by UV treatment or temperature gradient annealing is another way for having the gradient in topography. A thin film is a cast on the substrate and then specific parts on this covering can crosslink in response to UV or temperature raise [77].

Making Gradient in Density of Nanoparticles/Microspheres on Surface

This type of gradient could be achieved through immersing a determined section of a charged surface onto suspension of particles with opposite charges. Electrostatic interactions are responsible for deposition of particles onto the surface [78]. Sometimes nanoparticles are fixed on the surface *via* covalent bonds. Another approach described by Roth *et al.* [79] was depositing gold particles onto a polymeric substrate. In his work, a thin layer of gold forms on the substrate after thermal evaporation of this metal in a vacuum chamber. Then, because of stronger metal-metal interactions compared to polymer-metal interactions, gold atoms tend to form clusters on the surface and with the help of a blocking mask, gradient in the density of these clusters would be achieved.

Methods of Creating Gradient in Bioactive Molecules Embedded into Scaffold

The gradient in chemical factors effect cell behaviors. This type of gradient was first applied to the culture medium of cells via Boyden chamber (as well as Zigmond and Dunn chambers) [80]. Laminar flow-based microfluidic devices were then utilized. These methods were limited to 2D cell cultures. Therefore, researchers tried to induce the chemical factor gradient in 3D scaffolds with different approaches. Here, two main approaches including concentration gradient (controlled release of bioactive agent from scaffold) and density gradient (immobilizing bioactive agent into the scaffold in a gradient manner) are discussed.

Controlled Delivery of Bioactive Factors from the Scaffold

Bioactive signaling molecules can be embedded into the scaffold and release upon contact with the human body fluids. In this regard, microsphere scaffolds matter a lot because of their high surface area, causing the controllable release of bioactive agent. Microspheres loaded with different bioactive molecules could be incorporated into different scaffolds. Microspheres loaded with factors not only could be incorporated into the scaffold but could themselves make the entire scaffold. As an example of incorporation of such microspheres in scaffolds attention could be directed towards a study in which microspheres can be prepared by electrospraying between two layers of a fibrous scaffold [49]. Methods of creating a gradient in these scaffolds are as previously discussed in "microsphere scaffold" in pore formation strategies [62]. Release of bioactive molecules from scaffold could be done without the use of microspheres. In some scaffolds, bioactive factor is dispersed into the scaffolds in two different compartments known as "sink" and "source" and a gradient between these compartments is created [43].

Immobilizing Bioactive Molecules into Scaffold

As previously mentioned, the second approach for creating gradient bioactive molecules is immobilizing these agents into scaffold with varying densities. This could be achieved by adsorption or covalent binding. Solution of factor flows through the scaffold with a capillary of gravity forces and is absorbed into the pores. In this state, diffusion is the dominant mechanism. An example is a work done by Tamamoto *et al.* [81] in their work a simple diffusion-based method was used to immobilize amine-containing molecules into a 3D gel. Polyacrylamide disk exposed to NaOH solution from one side and PBS from the other side and concentration gradients of carboxyl groups then generated into gel. This gradient carboxyl funcionalized gel is ready to couple with amine groups. Conjugation of protein and peptides within a 3D gel can be done *via* covalent binding. For example, to create a gradient of bioactive peptide fragments immobilized within 3D collagen gel, the microfluidic device described before could be used. In this device, source channel filled with a collagen solution and sink channel filled with peptide grafted collagen solution. Therefore, a gradient in bioactive peptide sequence as an adhesive ligand is generated in cross-channel. When collagen gel assembles into a 3D fibrillar gel, these gradients are immobilized [82].

Methods of Creating Fiber Gradient Scaffolds

Making gradient in fibers is done with utilizing an electrospinning apparatus in which two spinnerets exist. With the help of this equipment not only gradient in composition of fibers achieved, but also the gradient in diameter and distribution of fibers is created [50, 52]. As it is shown in Fig. (**4**). the polymer solution ejected from each spinneret is collected on a single drum and resulted in scaffold with a gradient in fibers.

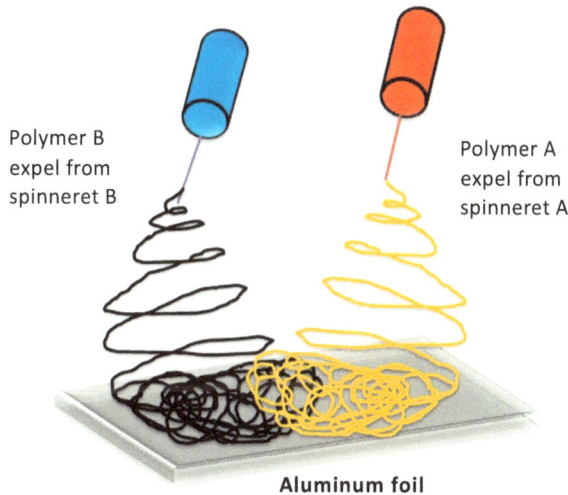

Polymer B expel from spinneret B

Polymer A expel from spinneret A

Aluminum foil

Fig. (4). A schematic of two spinneret apparatuses and gradient created from polymer A to B. In this design, three different zones are created, one is rich in polymer A and the opposite side is rich in polymer B. The interface of two polymers has a bit of both polymers.

CONCLUDING REMARKS

With attention to the significance of gradient in scaffolds, different types of gradients and their fabrication method are discussed in this chapter. It was shown that gradient in parameters of scaffold include porosity and pore size, mechanical strength, properties of the surface, loaded bioactive molecules into scaffold and gradient in fibers of scaffolds made by electrospinning determine cell fate, such as attachment, migration, proliferation, and differentiation. Therefore, with the help of methods described in this chapter, we would be able to make "next generation scaffolds" with the ability to simulate properties of natural tissues and cell microenvironment. This enables us to engineer scaffolds for complex and interfacial tissues.

FUTURE RESEARCH

Regarding the importance of gradient scaffolds in creating structures with gradients in properties with the goal of mimicking natural interfaces in the tissues, finding new gradient scaffolds would probably be the focus of researchers in the future in the field of tissue engineering. Albeit, exploring new techniques for making 2D and even 3D gradients in the scaffolds to have different independent types of gradients in different dimensions would be the main concern in such researches. As it is evident from the most recent studies in this field, preparing scaffolds with three or more component gradients would be an interesting approach.

CONFLICT OF INTEREST

The authors declare no conflict of interest, financial or otherwise.

ACKNOWLEDGEMENTS

Declared none.

REFERENCES

[1]   Akar B, Jiang B, Somo SI, *et al.* Biomaterials with persistent growth factor gradients *in vivo* accelerate vascularized tissue formation. Biomaterials 2015; 72: 61-73.
[http://dx.doi.org/10.1016/j.biomaterials.2015.08.049] [PMID: 26344364]

[2]   Glasser A, Campbell MC. Biometric, optical and physical changes in the isolated human crystalline lens with age in relation to presbyopia. Vision Res 1999; 39(11): 1991-2015.
[http://dx.doi.org/10.1016/S0042-6989(98)00283-1] [PMID: 10343784]

[3]   Conserva E, Lanuti A, Menini M. Cell behavior related to implant surfaces with different microstructure and chemical composition: an *in vitro* analysis. Int J Oral Maxillofac Implants 2010; 25(6): 1099-107.
[PMID: 21197485]

[4]   Wang N. Stem cells go soft: pliant substrate surfaces enhance motor neuron differentiation. Cell Stem Cell 2014; 14(6): 701-3.
[http://dx.doi.org/10.1016/j.stem.2014.05.007] [PMID: 24905160]

[5]   Wrighton KH. Cell migration: the mechanics of group travel. Nat Rev Mol Cell Biol 2012; 13(12): 753-3.
[http://dx.doi.org/10.1038/nrm3481] [PMID: 23175279]

[6]   Maleksaeedi S, Wang JK, El-Hajje A, *et al.* Toward 3D printed bioactive titanium scaffolds with bimodal pore size distribution for bone ingrowth. Procedia CIRP 2013; 5: 158-63.
[http://dx.doi.org/10.1016/j.procir.2013.01.032]

[7] Saiz E, Tomsia AP, Gomez-Vega JM, Fujino S. Graded coatings for metallic implant alloys, advances in joining of ceramics. John Wiley & Sons, Inc. 2006; pp. 159-72.

[8] Yazdimamaghani M, Razavi M, Mozafari M, Vashaee D, Kotturi H, Tayebi L. Biomineralization and biocompatibility studies of bone conductive scaffolds containing poly(3,4-ethylenedioxythiophene):poly(4-styrene sulfonate) (PEDOT:PSS). J Mater Sci Mater Med 2015; 26(12): 274.
[http://dx.doi.org/10.1007/s10856-015-5599-8] [PMID: 26543020]

[9] Jazayeri HE, Fahmy MD, Razavi M, *et al.* Dental applications of natural-origin polymers in hard and soft tissue engineering. J Prosthodont 2016; 25(6): 510-7.
[http://dx.doi.org/10.1111/jopr.12465] [PMID: 27003096]

[10] Hale NA, Yang Y, Rajagopalan P. Cell migration at the interface of a dual chemical-mechanical gradient. ACS Appl Mater Interfaces 2010; 2(8): 2317-24.
[http://dx.doi.org/10.1021/am100346k] [PMID: 20735103]

[11] Loh QL, Choong C. Three-dimensional scaffolds for tissue engineering applications: role of porosity and pore size. Tissue Eng Part B Rev 2013; 19(6): 485-502.
[http://dx.doi.org/10.1089/ten.teb.2012.0437] [PMID: 23672709]

[12] Yazdimamaghani M, Razavi M, Vashaee D, Moharamzadeh K, Boccaccini AR, Tayebi L. Porous magnesium-based scaffolds for tissue engineering. Mater Sci Eng C 2017; 71: 1253-66.
[http://dx.doi.org/10.1016/j.msec.2016.11.027] [PMID: 27987682]

[13] Jazayeri HE, Tahriri M, Razavi M, *et al.* A current overview of materials and strategies for potential use in maxillofacial tissue regeneration. Mater Sci Eng C 2017; 70(Pt 1): 913-29.
[http://dx.doi.org/10.1016/j.msec.2016.08.055] [PMID: 27770969]

[14] Wang Q, Wang Q, Wan C. Preparation and evaluation of a biomimetic scaffold with porosity gradients *in vitro*. An Acad Bras Cienc 2012; 84(1): 9-16.
[http://dx.doi.org/10.1590/S0001-37652012005000003] [PMID: 22441592]

[15] Hadi Miyanaji LY, Zhang Shanshan, Zandinejad Amirali. A preliminary study of the graded dental porcelain ceramic structures fabricated *via* binder jetting 3D printing. 2014.

[16] Kim BS, Kim EJ, Choi JS, Jeong JH, Jo CH, Cho YW. Human collagen-based multilayer scaffolds for tendon-to-bone interface tissue engineering. J Biomed Mater Res A 2014; 102(11): 4044-54.
[http://dx.doi.org/10.1002/jbm.a.35057] [PMID: 24327550]

[17] Zhang W. Controllable growth of porous structures from co-continuous polymer blend. 2011.

[18] Scaffaro R, Lopresti F, Botta L, Rigogliuso S, Ghersi G. Melt processed pcl/peg scaffold with discrete pore size gradient for selective cellular infiltration, macromolecular materials and engineering. 2015.

[19] Knight T, Basu J, Rivera EA, Spencer T, Jain D, Payne R. Fabrication of a multi-layer three-dimensional scaffold with controlled porous micro-architecture for application in small intestine tissue engineering. Cell Adhes Migr 2013; 7(3): 267-74.
[http://dx.doi.org/10.4161/cam.24351] [PMID: 23563499]

[20] Singh M. Osteochondral tissue engineering for the TMJ condyle using a novel gradient scaffold 2008.

[21] Mason B, Califano J, Reinhart-King C. Matrix Stiffness: A Regulator of Cellular Behavior and Tissue Formation. In: Bhatia SK, Ed. Engineering Biomaterials for Regenerative Medicine. Springer New York 2012; pp. 19-37.
[http://dx.doi.org/10.1007/978-1-4614-1080-5_2]

[22] Barthes J, Özçelik H, Hindié M, Ndreu-Halili A, Hasan A, Vrana NE. Cell microenvironment engineering and monitoring for tissue engineering and regenerative medicine: the recent advances. BioMed Res Int 2014; 2014: 921905.
[http://dx.doi.org/10.1155/2014/921905] [PMID: 25143954]

[23] Isenberg BC, Dimilla PA, Walker M, Kim S, Wong JY. Vascular smooth muscle cell durotaxis

depends on substrate stiffness gradient strength. Biophys J 2009; 97(5): 1313-22.
[http://dx.doi.org/10.1016/j.bpj.2009.06.021] [PMID: 19720019]

[24]   Yazdimamaghani M, Razavi M, Vashaee D, *et al*. *in vitro* analysis of Mg scaffolds coated with polymer/hydrogel/ceramic composite layers. Surf Coat Tech 2016; 301: 126-32.
[http://dx.doi.org/10.1016/j.surfcoat.2016.01.017]

[25]   Yazdimamaghani M, Razavi M, Vashaee D, Tayebi L. Surface modification of biodegradable porous Mg bone scaffold using polycaprolactone/bioactive glass composite. Mater Sci Eng C 2015; 49: 436-44.
[http://dx.doi.org/10.1016/j.msec.2015.01.041] [PMID: 25686970]

[26]   Yazdimamaghani M, Razavi M, Vashaee D, Tayebi L. Development and degradation behavior of magnesium scaffolds coated with polycaprolactone for bone tissue engineering. Mater Lett 2014; 132: 106-10.
[http://dx.doi.org/10.1016/j.matlet.2014.06.036]

[27]   Vladkova TG. Surface engineered polymeric biomaterials with improved biocontact properties, International Journal of Polymer Science 2010. 2010.

[28]   Wu G, Li P, Feng H, Zhang X, Chu PK. Engineering and functionalization of biomaterials via surface modification. J Mater Chem B Mater Biol Med 2015; 3(10): 2024-42.
[http://dx.doi.org/10.1039/C4TB01934B]

[29]   Razavi M, Fathi MH, Savabi O, Vashaee D, Tayebi L. Biodegradation, bioactivity and *in vivo* biocompatibility analysis of plasma electrolytic oxidized (PEO) biodegradable Mg implants. Physical Science International Journal 2014; 4(5): 708.
[http://dx.doi.org/10.9734/PSIJ/2014/9265]

[30]   Razavi M, Fathi M, Savabi O, Boroni M. A review of degradation properties of Mg based biodegradable implants. Res Rev Mater Sci Chem 2012; 1: 15-58.

[31]   Hasirci V, Pepe-Mooney BJ. Understanding the cell behavior on nano-/micro-patterned surfaces. Nanomedicine (Lond) 2012; 7(9): 1375-89.
[http://dx.doi.org/10.2217/nnm.12.7] [PMID: 22812706]

[32]   Hosseinkhani M, Shirazi R, Rajaei F, Mahmoudi M, Mohammadi N, Abbasi M. Engineering of the embryonic and adult stem cell niches. Iran Red Crescent Med J 2013; 15(2): 83-92.
[http://dx.doi.org/10.5812/ircmj.7541] [PMID: 23682319]

[33]   Arima Y, Iwata H. Effects of surface functional groups on protein adsorption and subsequent cell adhesion using self-assembled monolayers. J Mater Chem 2007; 17(38): 4079-87.
[http://dx.doi.org/10.1039/b708099a]

[34]   Liu X, Shi S, Feng Q, *et al*. Surface chemical gradient affects the differentiation of human adipose-derived stem cells via ERK1/2 signaling pathway. ACS Appl Mater Interfaces 2015; 7(33): 18473-82.
[http://dx.doi.org/10.1021/acsami.5b04635] [PMID: 26237746]

[35]   Clements LR, Wang P-Y, Tsai W-B, Thissen H, Voelcker NH. Electrochemistry-enabled fabrication of orthogonal nanotopography and surface chemistry gradients for high-throughput screening. Lab Chip 2012; 12(8): 1480-6.
[http://dx.doi.org/10.1039/c2lc20732j] [PMID: 22395420]

[36]   Razavi M, Fathi M, Savabi O, Vashaee D, Tayebi L. Micro-arc oxidation and electrophoretic deposition of nano-grain merwinite ($Ca_3MgSi_2O_8$) surface coating on magnesium alloy as biodegradable metallic implant. Surf Interface Anal 2014; 46(6): 387-92.
[http://dx.doi.org/10.1002/sia.5465]

[37]   Razavi M, Fathi M, Savabi O, Vashaee D, Tayebi L. Biodegradable magnesium alloy coated by fluoridated hydroxyapatite using MAO/EPD technique. Surf Eng 2014; 30(8): 545-51.
[http://dx.doi.org/10.1179/1743294414Y.0000000284]

[38]   Razavi M, Fathi M, Savabi O, Vashaee D, Tayebi L. *In vivo* study of nanostructured akermanite/PEO

coating on biodegradable magnesium alloy for biomedical applications. J Biomed Mater Res A 2015; 103(5): 1798-808.
[http://dx.doi.org/10.1002/jbm.a.35324] [PMID: 25203515]

[39]   Razavi M, Fathi M, Savabi O, Vashaee D, Tayebi L. Improvement of biodegradability, bioactivity, mechanical integrity and cytocompatibility behavior of biodegradable mg based orthopedic implants using nanostructured Bredigite (Ca7MgSi 4O 16) bioceramic coated via ASD/EPD technique. Ann Biomed Eng 2014; 42(12): 2537-50.
[http://dx.doi.org/10.1007/s10439-014-1084-7] [PMID: 25118669]

[40]   Boccaccini AR, Keim S, Ma R, Li Y, Zhitomirsky I. Electrophoretic deposition of biomaterials. J R Soc Interface 2010; 7 (Suppl. 5): S581-613.
[http://dx.doi.org/10.1098/rsif.2010.0156.focus] [PMID: 20504802]

[41]   Stefonek-Puccinelli TJ, Masters KS. Co-immobilization of gradient-patterned growth factors for directed cell migration. Ann Biomed Eng 2008; 36(12): 2121-33.
[http://dx.doi.org/10.1007/s10439-008-9581-1] [PMID: 18850272]

[42]   Singh M, Berkland C, Detamore MS. Strategies and applications for incorporating physical and chemical signal gradients in tissue engineering. Tissue Eng Part B Rev 2008; 14(4): 341-66.
[http://dx.doi.org/10.1089/ten.teb.2008.0304] [PMID: 18803499]

[43]   Cao X, Shoichet MS. Defining the concentration gradient of nerve growth factor for guided neurite outgrowth. Neuroscience 2001; 103(3): 831-40.
[http://dx.doi.org/10.1016/S0306-4522(01)00029-X] [PMID: 11274797]

[44]   Park JS, Rhau B, Hermann A, *et al.* Synthetic control of mammalian-cell motility by engineering chemotaxis to an orthogonal bioinert chemical signal. Proc Natl Acad Sci USA 2014; 111(16): 5896-901.
[http://dx.doi.org/10.1073/pnas.1402087111] [PMID: 24711398]

[45]   Odedra D, Chiu LL, Shoichet M, Radisic M. Endothelial cells guided by immobilized gradients of vascular endothelial growth factor on porous collagen scaffolds. Acta Biomater 2011; 7(8): 3027-35.
[http://dx.doi.org/10.1016/j.actbio.2011.05.002] [PMID: 21601017]

[46]   Lattermann C, Zelle BA, Whalen JD, *et al.* Gene transfer to the tendon-bone insertion site. Knee Surg Sports Traumatol Arthrosc 2004; 12(5): 510-5.
[http://dx.doi.org/10.1007/s00167-003-0482-4] [PMID: 15014945]

[47]   Gupta V MN, Berkland CJ, Detamore MS. Microsphere-based scaffolds carrying opposing gradients of chondroitin sulfate and tricalcium phosphate, Front. Bioeng Biotechnol 2015.

[48]   Huang W, Li X, Shi X, Lai C. Microsphere based scaffolds for bone regenerative applications. Biomater Sci 2014; 2(9): 1145-53.
[http://dx.doi.org/10.1039/C4BM00161C]

[49]   Tang G, Zhao Y, Yuan X. Preparation of fiber-microsphere scaffolds for loading bioactive substances in gradient amounts. Chin Sci Bull 2013; 58(27): 3415-21.
[http://dx.doi.org/10.1007/s11434-013-5974-0]

[50]   Ramalingam M, Young MF, Thomas V, *et al.* Nanofiber scaffold gradients for interfacial tissue engineering. J Biomater Appl 2013; 27(6): 695-705.
[http://dx.doi.org/10.1177/0885328211423783] [PMID: 22286209]

[51]   Wang X, Ding B, Li B. Biomimetic electrospun nanofibrous structures for tissue engineering. Mater Today (Kidlington) 2013; 16(6): 229-41.
[http://dx.doi.org/10.1016/j.mattod.2013.06.005] [PMID: 25125992]

[52]   Moffat KL. Biomimetic Nanofiber Scaffold Design for Tendon-to-Bone Interface Tissue Engineering. 2010, Page 264.

[53]   Sundararaghavan HG, Burdick JA. Gradients with depth in electrospun fibrous scaffolds for directed cell behavior. Biomacromolecules 2011; 12(6): 2344-50.

[http://dx.doi.org/10.1021/bm200415g] [PMID: 21528921]

[54]   Miao X, Sun D. Graded/Gradient Porous Biomaterials. Materials (Basel) 2009; 3(1): 26.
        [http://dx.doi.org/10.3390/ma3010026]

[55]   Chia HN, Wu BM. Recent advances in 3D printing of biomaterials. J Biol Eng 2015; 9(1): 4.
        [http://dx.doi.org/10.1186/s13036-015-0001-4] [PMID: 25866560]

[56]   Fahmy MD, Jazayeri HE, Razavi M, Masri R, Tayebi L. Three-Dimensional Bioprinting Materials
        with Potential Application in Preprosthetic Surgery. J Prosthodont 2016; 25(4): 310-8.
        [http://dx.doi.org/10.1111/jopr.12431] [PMID: 26855004]

[57]   Vogelaar JN, van Rijn CJ, Nijdam W. Matthias wessling, phase separation micromolding—PSµM.
        Adv Mater 2003; 15(16): 1385-9.
        [http://dx.doi.org/10.1002/adma.200304949]

[58]   Gu Y. Porous graded materials derived from block copolymer self-assembly for water and energy
        applications 2015.

[59]   Weisgerber D, Caliari S, Harley BC. Synthesis of layered, graded bioscaffolds. In: Thomopoulos S,
        Birman V, Genin GM, Eds. Structural Interfaces and Attachments in Biology. Springer New York
        2013; pp. 351-71.
        [http://dx.doi.org/10.1007/978-1-4614-3317-0_16]

[60]   Atesok K, Doral MN, Karlsson J, et al. Multilayer scaffolds in orthopaedic tissue engineering. Knee
        Surg Sports Traumatol Arthrosc 2014; •••: 1-9.
        [PMID: 25466277]

[61]   David M. Grant, Colin A. Scotchford, and Virginie Sottile, Porous chitosan constructs support bone
        marrow stem cells for osteochondral modelling. Eur Cell Mater 2014; 28: 70.

[62]   Singh M, Sandhu B, Scurto A, Berkland C, Detamore MS. Microsphere-based scaffolds for cartilage
        tissue engineering: using subcritical CO(2) as a sintering agent. Acta Biomater 2010; 6(1): 137-43.
        [http://dx.doi.org/10.1016/j.actbio.2009.07.042] [PMID: 19660579]

[63]   Jelen C, Mattei G, Montemurro F, De Maria C, Mattioli-Belmonte M, Vozzi G. Bone scaffolds with
        homogeneous and discrete gradient mechanical properties. Mater Sci Eng C 2013; 33(1): 28-36.
        [http://dx.doi.org/10.1016/j.msec.2012.07.046] [PMID: 25428038]

[64]   Patterson P. Creation of a mechanical gradient peg-collagen scaffold by photomasking techniques.
        2013.

[65]   Sundararaghavan HG, Monteiro GA, Firestein BL, Shreiber DI. Neurite growth in 3D collagen gels
        with gradients of mechanical properties. Biotechnol Bioeng 2009; 102(2): 632-43.
        [http://dx.doi.org/10.1002/bit.22074] [PMID: 18767187]

[66]   Bailey BM, Nail LN, Grunlan MA. Continuous gradient scaffolds for rapid screening of cell-material
        interactions and interfacial tissue regeneration. Acta Biomater 2013; 9(9): 8254-61.
        [http://dx.doi.org/10.1016/j.actbio.2013.05.012] [PMID: 23707502]

[67]   Chatterjee K, Kraigsley AM, Bolikal D, Kohn J, Simon CG. Gas-Foamed Scaffold Gradients for
        Combinatorial Screening in 3D. J Funct Biomater 2012; 3(1): 173-82.
        [http://dx.doi.org/10.3390/jfb3010173] [PMID: 24956523]

[68]   Moon Suk Kim GK, Hai BL. Gradient polymer surface for biomedical applications. Prog Polym Sci
        2008; 33(1): 138-64.
        [http://dx.doi.org/10.1016/j.progpolymsci.2007.06.001]

[69]   Genzer J, Bhat RR. Surface-bound soft matter gradients. Langmuir 2008; 24(6): 2294-317.
        [http://dx.doi.org/10.1021/la7033164] [PMID: 18220435]

[70]   Sara Morgenthaler CZ. Surface-chemical and -morphological gradients. Soft Matter 2008; 4: 419-34.
        [http://dx.doi.org/10.1039/b715466f]

[71]   Wu J, Mao Z, Tan H, Han L, Ren T, Gao C. Gradient biomaterials and their influences on cell migration. Interface Focus 2012; 2(3): 337-55.
[http://dx.doi.org/10.1098/rsfs.2011.0124] [PMID: 23741610]

[72]   Olayo OR. Plasma gradient modified scaffolds to generate a chemoattractant surface. Superf Vacio 2014; 27(1): 20-3.

[73]   Yazdimamaghani M, Razavi M, Vashaee D, Tayebi L. Microstructural and mechanical study of PCL coated Mg scaffolds. Surf Eng 2014; 30(12): 920-6.
[http://dx.doi.org/10.1179/1743294414Y.0000000307]

[74]   Yazdimamaghani M, Razavi M, Vashaee D, Pothineni VR, Rajadas J, Tayebi L. Significant degradability enhancement in multilayer coating of polycaprolactone-bioactive glass/gelatin-bioactive glass on magnesium scaffold for tissue engineering applications. Appl Surf Sci 2015; 338: 137-45.
[http://dx.doi.org/10.1016/j.apsusc.2015.02.120]

[75]   Michelmore A, Clements L, Steele DA, Voelcker NH, Szili EJ. Gradient technology for high-throughput screening of interactions between cells and nanostructured materials. J Nanomater 2012; 2012: 1-7.
[http://dx.doi.org/10.1155/2012/839053]

[76]   Savostikov VM, Potekaev AI, Tabachenko AN. Physical and technological principles of designing layer-gradient multicomponent surfaces by combining the methods of ion-diffusion saturation and magnetron- and vacuum-arc deposition. Russ Phys J 2011; 54(7): 756-64.
[http://dx.doi.org/10.1007/s11182-011-9680-6]

[77]   Sudeshna Roy NB, Ritopa Das G. Harikrishnan, rabibrata mukherjee, thermally tailored gradient topography surface on elastomeric thin films. ACS Appl Mater Interfaces 2014; 6(9)

[78]   Kunzler TP, Huwiler C, Drobek T, Vörös J, Spencer ND. Systematic study of osteoblast response to nanotopography by means of nanoparticle-density gradients. Biomaterials 2007; 28(33): 5000-6.
[http://dx.doi.org/10.1016/j.biomaterials.2007.08.009] [PMID: 17720241]

[79]   Roth S, Burghammer M, Riekel C, *et al.* Self-assembled gradient nanoparticle-polymer multilayers investigated by an advanced characterization method: microbeam grazing incidence x-ray scattering. Appl Phys Lett 2003; 82(12): 1935-7.
[http://dx.doi.org/10.1063/1.1563051]

[80]   Chen HC. Boyden chamber assay. Methods Mol Biol 2005; 294: 15-22.
[PMID: 15576901]

[81]   Yamamoto M, Yanase K, Tabata Y. Generation of type I collagen gradient in polyacrylamide hydrogels by a simple diffusion-controlled hydrolysis of amide groups. Materials (Basel) 2010; 3(4): 2393.
[http://dx.doi.org/10.3390/ma3042393]

[82]   Sundararaghavan HG, Masand SN, Shreiber DI. Microfluidic generation of haptotactic gradients through 3D collagen gels for enhanced neurite growth. J Neurotrauma 2011; 28(11): 2377-87.
[http://dx.doi.org/10.1089/neu.2010.1606] [PMID: 21473683]

CHAPTER 7

In Vivo and *In Vitro* Experiments for the Evaluation of Porous Biomaterials

Rabia Cakir-Koc[*], **Yasemin Budama-Kilinc, Burak Ozdemir, Zeynep Kaya, Mehtap Sert** and **Neslinur Ozcelik**

Faculty of Chemistry and Metallurgical, Department of Bioengineering, Yildiz Technical University, Davutpasa St. No.127, 34210 Esenler, Istanbul, Turkey

Abstract: Biomaterials used for medical application may cause some biological responses when applied to the body. Hence, biomaterials must be tested by various *in vivo* and *in vitro* test systems, before using on humans, according to different standardizations like ISO 19033. These tests are made to determine the biocompatibility of biomaterials and indicate their potential toxicity, irritation, and non-hemocompatibility. Furthermore, biomaterials must have similar mechanical properties as *natural* tissue has. For this reason, biomaterials are investigated in terms of mechanical properties such as tensile strength, elasticity and plastic deformation, viscoelasticity, failure, fracture, fatigue, and wear. This chapter seeks to elucidate certain principles and procedures of *in vivo* and *in vitro* test methods that determine biocompatibility and mechanical properties of biomaterials.

Keywords: Animal studies, Biocompatibility, Biomaterials toxicity, Cell culture, Hemocompatibility, *In vivo*, *In vitro*, Mechanical tests.

INTRODUCTION

Materials that make contact with tissue or blood come with potential health risks and may even cause negative reactions. Biocompatibility is the optimum physical, chemical, and biological compatibility of the materials with the body tissue and compliance to the mechanical behavior of the body. Biocompatible materials by definition do not have any adverse effects on the surrounding tissues or other parts of body, such as inflammation or coagulation [1]. *In vitro* and *in vivo* tests aim to show biomaterial compatibility in the body as well as the required properties of new developed materials before being applied to the body [2]. These tests should be done before the selection of desired and ideal biocompatible biomaterial [1].

[*] **Corresponding author Rabia Cakir-Koc:** Faculty of Chemistry and Metallurgical, Department of Bioengineering, Yildiz Technical University, Istanbul, Turkey; Tel: +902123834657; Fax: +902123834626; E-mail: rabiacakir@gmail.com

Mehdi Razavi (Ed.)

Generally, *in vivo* tests applied to experimental animals are used to measure the reaction to certain materials, revealing any toxicity, pyrogenicity, carcinogenicity, skin irritation, and immunogenicity. In contrast, *in vitro* tests study the effects of a given material on living organisms like cell cultures without using animals to provide preliminary knowledge for *in vivo* studies. Some *in vivo* tests completely replace with *in vitro* tests due to various disadvantages of *in vivo* studies. For example draize skin irritation test replaced with *in vitro* skin irritating test, teratogenity tests are replaced with *in vitro* embryotoxicity/ teratogenicity [3, 4].

Non-hemocompatibility is broadly defined as "materials and their extracts that lead to any adverse effect in blood," and is a key aspect that vitro tests aim to determine. The possible adverse effects of biomaterials in the blood have more than one mechanism. For this reason, a comprehensive and unique definition of hemocompatibility cannot be made [5, 6]. Non-hemocompatible biomaterials may cause some special side effects, such as thrombus, clot formation, emboli nucleation, destruction of blood components in the cardiovascular system, or activation of complement systems and specific immunological pathways [7]. Thus, hemocompatibility tests must be applied to biomaterials that are in potential contact with blood.

Nowadays standards are described by various organizations, such as the International Organization for Standardization (ISO) 1099315 test. In these standards, sample preparation and application methods of tests and test selections (*e.g.*, cytotoxicity, genotoxicity, carcinogenicity, implantation, irritation, sensitivity, and systemic toxicity) are determined. In addition to pre-clinic and clinic studies, certain standards are defined to analyze and evaluate any biological reaction risks. On the other hand, the effects of the body to mechanical properties of biomaterials are also important [3]. This chapter thus explores in-depth the *in vivo* and *vitro* tests used for biocompatibility and the identification of mechanical properties of biomaterials for medical purposes.

BIOCOMPATIBILITY

The clinical application of biomaterial and systems as catheters, contact lenses, dialysis membranes and extracorporeal systems contacted with body tissues has considerable importance in modern medicine [1]. One of the most important factors to consider for materials applied to the body is the possibility of harmful side effects when interacting with tissues. Biocompatibility means that there is no harm caused by materials around the tissue or whole body. Researchers have conducted studies to examine and improve the interactions between tissues and biomaterials for years. Many tissue-biomaterial combinations have been conducted in testing contexts that aim to demonstrate the best performance of medical devices [8].

IN VIVO EXPERIMENTS

Sensitization

In vivo skin sensitization tests are examined in two groups:

Guinea Pig Maximization Test (GPMT)

The guinea pig maximization test (GPMT) was developed by Magnusson and Kligman in 1969 and continues to be modified by different researchers even today. Albino guinea pigs weighing 300-500 g are used for this test. Young animals are used in this procedure due to the decrease in sensitivity of elderly animals. Generally, 25 animals are enough to comprise an experimental group, while 10 animals are sufficient for preliminary work. As seen in the table below, the GPMT consists of three stages (Table **1**) [9].

Table 1. Guinea pig maximization test procedure.

Stage 1	INTRADERMAL INJECTION	Allergen compounds with or without Freund's adjuvant are prepared by mixing an equal volume of water and then injected. -Three injections (adjuvant alone, allergen alone, and adjuvant and allergen together in emulsion form) are administered simultaneously in the dorsal area. - A closed patch exposure is conducted one week after the injections.
Stage 2	TOPICAL INJECTİON	Allergens are used at the highest non-inflammatory concentration. One week after the intradermal injection, the dorsal area is shaved and the test agent absorbed into the applied patch.
Stage 3	CHALLENGE	Animals are challenged after the topical induction with 2x2 cm patch. The challenge phase is evaluated 24 hours after the patch is removed. This helps determine any weak, slowly developing reactions after an additional 24 hours. Sensitivity to various agents is determined and recorded on a scale system (where 1 is poor and 5 is extreme) [9].

Local Lymph Node Assay (LLNA)

A local lymph node assay (LLNA) is a method used for the assessment of contact allergens according to the function of lymphocyte proliferative responses provoked in draining lymph nodes after exposure to test materials as an alternative to other skin sensitization test [10]. The purpose of this method is to identify any hazards of chemical activity. Allergen chemicals lead to an increase of three times the number of lymph node cells (Table **2**) [11].

Table 2. LLNA procedure [12].

Beginning of experiment	After 5 days	After 5 hours
3 injections of the test material to the dorsum of both ears.	Radioactive thymidine injection *via* tail vein of mice.	Draining auricular lymph nodes are excised and prepared cell suspension is subjected to scintillation counting.

Irritation Experiments

Novel substances must be tested for eye and skin irritation before using them on humans. Animal models make up an essential step for testing biomaterials before clinical use of those in humans. However in recent years, order to replace animal irritation testing, *in vitro* reconstructed organotypic skin equivalents are being used [13]. In a study, EPISKIN™ and EpiDerm™ was tested as a replacement for the rabbit skin irritation method and suggested as new *in vitro* toxicity alternative to animal testing [14].

Some of these irritation studies are as follows.

Ocular Irritation Test

New Zealand rabbits have been used in traditional eye irritation tests, due to their lack of ocular pigmentation, which allows for the reaction to be well evaluated. In this test procedure, the compound is applied in solution form (total volume of 0.1 ml) to only one eye of the rabbit (the other eye is used as a control) and observation continues for three days. Ocular reactions in eyes are recorded 1, 24, 48, and 72 hours after exposure. In some cases, repeat exposures and longer time frames may be suitable [15].

Draize Skin Irritation Test

The Draize Skin Irritation Test reveals any presence of edema and/or erythema in the experimental animals, such as guinea pigs, mice, rats, and rabbits. After shaving the skin, the compound is applied to the area and observed 1, 24, 48, and 72 hours after exposure. The results are evaluated according to a scoring system [16].

In Vivo Toxicity Experiments

Mechanical and chemical properties of biomaterials (surface area, extract of the materials, thickness and extraction volume) have a major role on the toxicity of material. Experimental animals like rabbits, mice, and rats are generally used in these tests with different exposure routes (*i.e.*, intravenous, intraperitoneal, subcutaneous, oral, dermal, and inhalation). Adverse effects may occur from systemic toxicity of biomaterials and its constituents on the tissue and organs away from the implantation area. Thus, systemic toxicity tests evaluate these effects of foreign materials on the body.

Acute Toxicity: Adverse effects can be seen within 24 hours after the administration of single or multiple doses.

Subacute Toxicity: Repeated dose toxicity, occurs following administration of the test specimen with 14-28 day periods.

Subchronic Toxicity: throughout life—usually not exceeding 90 days, but constitutes 10% of the animal's lifetime—after administration of single or multiple daily dosages of the test [17].

Pyrogenicity Tests

Pyrogen is a harmful compound that increases body temperature. Pyrogenic contamination of drugs and materials is significant due to their resistance to sterilization (heat) procedures. Pyrogenicity tests have been conducted by using rabbits since the 1940s [18]. A test dose is injected to the each animals at a max of 10 ml per kg. The temperature of each animal is recorded at a maximum of 30-minute intervals starting at 90 min before the injection to 180 min after the injection. Response to tests is calculated to reveal any difference between maximum temperatures and initial temperature. If this difference is negative, then the result is no response (*i.e.*, revealing no adverse effects) to the material [19].

Genotoxicity Tests

Genotoxicity is damage to genetic material by physical or chemical agents. This damage is stratified as single strand breaks, double strand breaks, alkali labile sites, and DNA adducts. Genotoxicity tests are mainly used for cancer prevention studies, investigating the effects of environmental factors (*e.g.*, UV radiation), industrial chemicals, toxicity, and reliability of drugs or biomaterials before their release on the market. These tests have been used since the 1970s, when many *in vivo* and *in vitro* genotoxicity tests were developed [20].

Chromosome Abnormalities Tests

Chromosomal abnormalities are differences in normal chromosome structure or numerical abnormalities as a result of spontaneous, chemically or induced radiation [21]. Genetic material consisting of such damage causes high chromosomal abnormalities frequency and shows increased cancer risks if it is not repaired. *In vivo* chromosomal abnormalities tests often uses bone marrow cells.

In vivo chromosomal abnormalities tests allow for the assessment of factors such as metabolism, pharmacokinetics, and DNA repair mechanisms, which may vary by type and tissue, especially for mutagenic damage determination. Experimental animals are injected with colchicine (-tubulin polymerization inhibitor- for inhibition of cell division in the metaphase stage) 2 to 4 hours before scarification. After that various structural and numerical abnormalities is detected in bone marrow cells [22].

Micronucleus (MN) Tests

Micronuclei (MN) that form during mitosis are derived from whole chromosome formations or acentric chromosome fragments. An increase in the number of MN is considered an indirect indicator of numerical and structural chromosome aberrations in cells caused by the various agents [23].

Carcinogenicity Experiments

Carcinogenicity refers to incorrect growth and division of a cell by changes in DNA. The carcinogenic potential of a substance is closely related to its mutagenic capacity [24]. *In vivo* carcinogenicity tests to determine the biocompatibility of chemical or biomaterials are usually performed on rats or mice younger than six weeks old. An animal is exposed to the chemicals between 2 to 5 years. The first six months is very important, and extra dosages of chemical exposure may be administered during this period. Test animals are examined for tumor development by using histopathological methods so that potential carcinogenicity risks in humans may be identified [25].

Immunogenicity Experiments

Immunocompatible means that the immune system tolerates the biomaterial, as biomaterial should not interfere with the immune system [26]. Potential immunological responses to the biomaterial may present as hypersensitivity (*e.g.*, anaphylactic, cytotoxicity, immune complex, or cell-mediated immunity), chronic inflammation, immune-suppression, immune-stimulation, autoimmunity, histopathological changes, humoral responses, host resistance, clinical symptoms, and cellular response (*e.g.*, T cells, natural killer cells, macrophages, granulocytes) [17]. A hypersensitivity test is a common method used to characterize the compatibility of immune materials. Redness, swelling, and pain may be observed in the implant area of biomaterials within 24 hours in the case of immediate hypersensitivity. In contrast, delayed hypersensitivity is observed 48 hours after the implantation. Antibody levels against foreign material are detected in the blood by the immunoassay methods after 14 days [26].

Histological Experiments

With the histological evaluation using microscopes, various biological responses to the material can be easily revealed. Responses include the number and distribution of inflammatory cells, fibrous capsule formation, and tissue ingrowths into the material, necrosis. Mice, rats, guinea pigs, and rabbits are widely used in short-term tests (12 weeks), while rats, guinea pigs, rabbits, dogs, pigs, sheep, goats, and other animals are used in long-term tests [17].

Teratogenicity Experiments

Certain chemical compounds produce teratogenic effects like congenital malformations -anatomical or structural abnormalities present at birth- in experimental animals [27]. A teratogenicity test is generally conducted on rats, mice, or rabbits [28]. Chick embryos are also used for embryological studies, but are not considered suitable for the routine screening of teratogenicity [29].

In Vitro Experiments

The aim of *in vitro* tests is to obtain some knowledge about the biofunctions and biocompatibility of materials at a lower cost and in less time than *in vivo* and other complex tests [30]. Tested material can be directly used for evaluation or extracted materials on cells can be assayed. The appropriate tests are selected according to the characteristics of the material, the suitability of the test, and data analysis of biocompatibility [17]. However, *in vitro* tests cannot provide information about whole physiological, inflammatory, and immune responses against materials, so they are not a substitute for *in vivo* tests. Instead, they provide preliminary data and can be used as a screening test [31].

More sophisticated and specific *in vitro* tests are under development in order to reduce the use of experimental animals for *in vivo* tests, decrease the cost of experiments, control the animal and species differences, and avoid the obligation of approval from animal ethics committees [30]. *In vitro* tests generally aim to assess the toxicological risk of biomaterials, a patient's potential exposure to toxic chemicals, and the dose–response relationship of chemicals; scientists then combine this information to characterize the risk [17]. Cytotoxicity is defined as toxic effects on the level of cells. *In vitro* tests may be used to investigate the viability and death of cells, change of cell permeability (membrane destruction), enzymatic inhibition, detection of cytosolic enzymes, decrease of metabolic rate, inhibition or reduction of protein synthesis, DNA synthesis or cell proliferation.

Cell Culture Experiments

In vitro biocompatibility tests evaluate cell responses against tested materials by using different methods [32]. The L929 mouse fibroblast cell line is one of the most common cell cultures for biocompatibility assays [33, 34]. The cultivation and maintenance of L929 cells is relatively simple, and L929 cells have high correlation with specific animal analysis. Cell lines can also be selected according to the specific properties of biomaterials. Other cell lines like HeLa, human cervical carcinoma cells [35], human cutaneous epithelial cells [36], human or animal dental pulp cells, THP1 monocytes, and immortalize mouse odontoblast cells are commonly used in cell toxicity tests [37 - 40]. The most basic way to evaluate toxicity is examining the viability and proliferation of a cell when in contact with the biomaterial [30]. For comparison of tests, number, growth cycle, type of cells, exposure time, properties related to tested biomaterials should be standardized [17].

Comparison of *In Vivo* and *In Vitro* Experiments

The ethics concerns and criticism about experimental animals can be partially avoided by cell culture methods. The "three R" rules about using experimental animals are defined by Declaration of Helsinki [41]. One of these rules is "replacement," which requires the use of cell and tissue cultures, mathematical and computational analysis, immature forms of vertebrates, or invertebrates, instead of experimental animals. Variations among animals in the test group (*e.g.,* sex, age, weight, or genetics) complicate the judgment of experiments in *in vivo* studies.

In vitro tests can be completed in a relatively short time frame, which makes them more cost effective than *in vivo* animal tests. Also, the maintenance of animals, training personnel, and advanced infrastructure cost necessities are some disadvantages of using animal tests [41]. Briefly, the advantages of *in vitro* tests include their ease of approval, lower costs, short time periods, and reproducibility of the experiments.

Despite of ethical concerns and disadvantages about animal testing, there is no adequate alternative to testing on a living, whole-body system and some testing should be conduct on animals. Because animals and humans are similar according to organ systems which perform the same functions with mechanisms. Cell cultures are sometimes useful but they doesn't provide the response of whole system.

Common *In Vitro* Experiments

In vitro cell viability tests are generally based on membrane permeability, cell functions, morphological assessments, and cell proliferations [39]. Direct contact tests, agar diffusion tests, and elution tests are some of common *in vitro* tests.

Direct Contact Test

Direct contact tests detect the cytotoxicity of materials in direct contact with cells by measuring the morphological change of the cells, particularly L929 cells [30]. During this type of test, L929 cells are maintained in 35-mm-diameter cell culture plates. The testing materials are carefully placed in the culture plate and incubated with cells. After exposure to materials, viable cells are adherent and stained with crystal violet in the culture plates, while dead cells detach from the surface of the culture plate and are removed during a fixation procedure. Any present toxic effects may be evaluated according to vacuolization, rounding due to decreased adherence to the culture plate, crenation, and swelling [42].

Agar Diffusion Test

The agar diffusion test is another cytotoxicity test of materials, which is based on staining live cells [29]. In this test, the L-929 cell culture is prepared in a 60-m--diameter plate with a culture medium containing 2% agar. The testing materials are placed on the surface of the culture plate and incubated for at least 24 hours. After the staining procedure with a vital color, the colorless zone (zone index) with unstained injured cells forms around the test material. The size of the area of the zone index is related to the toxicity of the material [29]. However, one limitation is that the selection of a proper agar for use in this assay continues to be a major problem of this test [17].

Elution Test

Elution tests measure the toxic effect of extracts of biomaterials. The extraction of material is prepared by using 0.9% sodium chloride or serum-free medium applied to the cell culture. The cell viability after exposure to the extract can be evaluated using histochemical methods or vital strains [17].

Cell Count Experiments

Cell counting is an important method for the cultivation and assessment of cells. There are different types of counting chambers, such as the Hemocytometer and Petroff-Hausser counting chambers [43]. Flow cytometry is a method for advanced cell count, and it has been relatively expensive. Flow cytometry helps determine the types of cells and well as the shape of the internal and external structure of the cells [44]. One of the direct microscopic count techniques is the Coulter counter. This technique measures the number of cells [43].

Morphological Experiments

In vitro biocompatibility tests involve the morphological assessment of cells in contact with materials, usually by light microscopy or scanning electron microscopy. Cells such as platelets can be assessed using light microscopy, fluorescent methods, scanning electron microscopy, or transmission electron microscopy [17]. Differences in the morphology of various cell types can be observed with these methods, and any dramatic changes in the morphology of the cells can be examined at the light microscope level or in more detail at the electron microscope level [43].

Dye Experiments

The main principal of dye tests is based on certain dye properties. Some dyes can be taken into living cells by active transport or other mechanisms, while other types of cell dyes can stain only damaged or dead cells. One of the major differences between living and dead cells is that the living cells maintain the function of membrane transport [45]. For example, trypan blue dye distinguishes damaged cells from living cells, since it diffuses and accumulates into the dead cells [46]. Cell counts should be done within 3 to 5 minutes, due to an increase in dyed cells [45]. The morphology of non-living cells is swollen, larger, and dark blue after exposure to trypan blue, whereas living cells are smaller, rounded, and unstained [47]. In contrast, fluorescent dyes can stain living or non-living cells according to the properties of the dye, and the dyed cells can be observed under a florescent microscope or using flow cytometry in time [48].

Metabolic Experiments

These tests distinguish cells according to their metabolic activity. One of the most common tests is the 3-(4,5-dimethylthiazol-2-yl)-2,5-diphenyltetrazolium bromide (MTT) test described by Mossman and modified by Alley *et al.* [49, 50]. This indirect MTT test is applied to the culture cells and measures the metabolic activity by colorimetric changes. Actively absorbed MTT dyes are reduced by mitochondrial dehydrogenases enzymes of the metabolically active living cells and converted into purple formazan crystals. DMSO or isopropanol is used to dissolve the formazan crystals and color change is measured in appropriate wavelength [51]. The total amount of purple caused by formazane indicate the activity of dehydrogenases enzyme and, indirectly, the cell viability [49, 50, 52].

In Vitro Skin Irritating Test

The *in vitro* skin irritating test was developed to reduce the number of experiments on animals. There are two types of *in vitro* tests employed on human skin models, the EPISKIN™ [53] and EpiDerm™ [54]. To predict skin irritancy, the EPISKIN SIT was approved as a full replacement of the *in vivo* rabbit test [55, 56].

In Vitro Embryotoxicity/Teratogenicity Experiments

In vitro teratogenicity tests also aim to reduce animal use. In this test, embryo cultures of invertebrates and vertebrates and cell and organ cultures are used. However, teratogens may have different effects than using embryonic cultures. Therefore, more than one *in vitro* test should be used for more accurate results.

In Vitro Genotoxicity Tests

The genetic differences of cells in direct contact with biomaterials are evaluated by this group of tests. Genotoxicity tests may be used *in vitro* or *in vivo*. Some examples of genotoxicity tests include the micronuclei test, comet test, chromosomal abnormality tests, and Sister Chromatid Exchange tests.

Hemocompatibility

Blood is a body fluid that contains cells in its structure and regularly flows in one direction through a closed circulating system. Blood generally consists of two components: blood cells, defined as shaped components; and plasma, in which cells move suspended. The shaped cells are divided into three categories: erythrocytes, leucocytes, and platelets. Erythrocytes are responsible for carrying oxygen with the help of hemoglobin molecules. There are many types of leucocytes, which are responsible for the immune responses. There are many types of leucocytes, which are responsible for the immune responses. Platelets are primarily responsible for coagulation. There are also vitamins, hormones, amino acids, lipoproteins and organic compounds of different origins in blood plasma [57 - 59].

While there are many definitions of hemocompatibility, these definitions are often complicated, as they contain multiple response mechanisms of the body against materials or devices. Some materials can induce multiple alternative response mechanisms as well as single response mechanisms. Ultimately, hemo-compatibility is a property of a device or material that does not show any adverse effect when in contact with blood [5, 6]. Hemocompatibility is one of the most critical parameters for deciding how or where implantable materials such as orthopedic implants or artificial blood vessels will be applied. These products are required to improve hemocompatibility by using certain techniques, such as surface modification [60, 61]. When non-hemocompatible materials come into contact with blood, they cause specific adverse effects, such as the formation of thrombus and coagulum, shedding or nucleation of emboli, destruction of blood components in cardiovascular system, or the activation of the complement system and specific immunological pathways. These adverse effects may be observed after some interaction between blood and the materials [7].

Interaction of Material and Blood

Blood-material interaction can be defined as the effects in blood and blood components, in tissue and organ contact with blood by vessels, with biomaterials. The outcomes of this interaction may led to the formation of undesirable clinical side effects and results (ISO/TC 194, 1991) [62, 63]. Blood-material interaction is a highly complex relationship with variable parameters [64]. When an interface forms between certain material and blood, a series of interactions are recognized. These processes have been described in four steps, which may occur singularly or simultaneously [64, 65].

1. Adsorption of plasma proteins in the material surface
2. Adsorbed proteins activate the intrinsic coagulation, complements and kinin / the kallikrein system.
3. Adhesion of some blood cells such as platelets, granulocytes, or monocytes on the protein layer of the material surface.
4. Fibrin formation as well as the activation of the fibrinolytic system [63, 66].

There are multiple factors that affect the material-blood interaction:

1. Surface and volume characteristics of materials
2. Chemical and physical structure of surface of materials
3. Occurrence form of interaction
4. Blood flow rate
5. Anticoagulant property of material
6. Cell adhesion
7. Symmetric platelet/leucocyte aggregation [67]

Hemocompatibility Experiments

Hemocompatibility assays in the literature include the hemolytic test, platelet adhesion and activation, clotting time test, and anticoagulant assays [68].

Hemolysis Assay

Hemolysis is a phenomenon that occurs in red blood cells as a result of increased osmotic pressure in the cell. During hemolysis, erythrocytes are destroyed and hemoglobin is released from the cell [68, 69]. Hemolysis is divided into *in vivo* and *in vitro* hemolysis; *in vivo* hemolysis is further divided into extravascular hemolysis and intravascular hemolysis [69 - 71]. Extravascular hemolysis is characterized by the destruction of red blood cells in the spleen and other reticuloendothelial organs, as autoimmune hemolytic anemia or in hereditary spherocytosis. Intravascular hemolysis is seen together with another pathology such as a hereditary disorder of the Red Blood Cells (RBC). Erythrocytes can be removed by macrophages in the liver and spleen, or more rarely, can be destroyed in circulation with membrane damage of cells. *In vitro* hemolysis may occur during bloodletting or when blood is being delivered to the laboratory, processed, or stored [72 - 74].

The hemolysis percentage is found by measuring cleaved red blood cells when the material comes into contact with blood. The hemolysis rate is calculated as the count of destroyed red blood cells [68]. According to the ASTMF756-00(2000) standard, materials can be classified into three categories with respect to the hemolytic index. If the hemolysis rate greater than 5%, materials are defined as hemolytic. If materials have a hemolytic rate between 5 and 2%, these materials are considered slightly hemolytic. Materials with a hemolytic rate of less than 2% are non-hemolytic [68].

Platelet Adhesion and Activation Assay

Platelet activation is evaluated according to the extraordinary changes in the morphology of platelets, such as activation proceeds, loss of round shape, pseudopodia form, and spread on the biomaterials. The platelet adhesion test is used for the determination of the activation of the platelets and fibrin clots [75]. Changes in morphology of platelets adherent to the biomaterial are assessed using Scanning Electron Microscopy (SEM) [68]. The morphology of adherent platelets are classified into activation degrees, such as rounded, dendritic, spread-dendritic, spread, and fully spread. In addition to other tests, platelet activation can be determined with a visualized expression of p-selectine activation markers on platelets using the immunofluorescence technique [76].

Clotting Time Assays

The purpose of these tests is to determine any losses in the anticoagulant pathway. Blood coagulation cascade pathways are divided into three classes: intrinsic, extrinsic, and common pathways. The intrinsic and extrinsic pathways play important roles in the metabolic pathways of fibrin clots [77]. An Activated Partial Thromboplastin Time (APPT) is one of the tests performed for determining the hemocompatibility of biomaterials, particularly for detecting the activation time of Factor XII during the biomaterial's contact with blood. A longer APPT shows that biomaterials have anticoagulant activity [78]. Therefore, blood plasma APPT assay is used to measure *in vitro* anticoagulant activity of different biomaterials [68].

A Plasma Recalcification Time (PRT) assay is used to compare the clotting time delays of the platelet's poor plasma after prothrombin activation in the presence of Ca^{+2} caused by the sample. PRT is an important indicator for determining the activation of intrinsic coagulation cascades, and because of this property, is a useful marker for detecting the hemocompatibility of biomaterials [79]. PRT is generally delayed in the absence of fibrinogen, thrombinogen, and other coagulation factors or in the presence of the anticoagulant agent in the medium. A longer PRT shows that the material has a better anticoagulant activation [78].

Lastly, the prothrombin time (PT) test is used to detect the activation of extrinsic and common coagulation. PT reflects the starting time of the extrinsic period, and a longer PT shows increased anticoagulant activity of the biomaterial [80].

Anticoagulant Assay

Clotting time tests are used to determine the anticoagulant properties of biomaterials [81].

Other Assays

Other assays are suitable for testing certain materials used in the cardiovascular system and those that come into contact with blood. These tests include:

- Qualitative and quantitative analysis of immobilized bioactive molecules used for surface modification
- Wettability test by static and/or contact angle tester
- Protein adsorption assay
- Adsorption of fibrinogen and ATIII
- Thrombogenicity of the surface
- Scanning electron microscopy (SEM)
- Atomic force microscopy (AFM)
- X-ray photoelectron spectroscopy (XPS)
- Fourier transform infrared (FTIR) spectroscopy [65].

Standardization of Hemocompatibility Assay

Standard hemocompatibility testing of medical devices was determined with the International Organization for Standardization 10933-4 coded standardization, published in 2002 and updated in 2009 by The American National Standards Institute and the Medical Device Development Association. Blood compatibility tests are grouped under five headings in this standardization. These include thrombosis tests, coagulation tests, platelet activation tests, blood cell changes, and complement activation tests. Tests under these headings are provided in Table **3** [68, 82].

Table 3. Group of blood compatibility tests [68, 82].

Blood-Incompatibility	Tests
Thrombosis	• Percent occlusion • Flow reduction • Pressure drop across device • Antibody binding to thrombus components, thrombus mass • Light microscopy and SEM of adhered platelets, leukocytes, aggregates, erythrocytes, fibrin
Coagulation	• Coagulation PTT (non-activated) • Thrombin generation • Specific coagulation factor assays • FPA • D-dimer • F1+2 • TAT
Platelet activation	• Platelet count/adhesion • Platelet aggregation • Template bleeding time • Platelet function analysis • PF-4 • Thromboxane B2 • Platelet activation markers • Platelet micro particles • Gamma imaging of radiolabeled platelets • 111 In- labelled platelet survival
Blood cell changes	• Leukocyte count with or without differential • Leukocyte activation • Hemolysis • Reticulocyte count

(Table 3) contd.....

Blood-Incompatibility	Tests
Complement activation	• C3a • C 5a • Bb • iC3b • C4d • SC5b-9 • CH50 • C3 convertase • C5 convertase

MECHANICAL EXPERIMENTS

The selection of the biomaterial has important implications for implant design. The construction material for the implant design should provide adequate strength and reduce any adverse responses in the body [83]. Biomaterials must be able to provide sufficient mechanical strength [84]. Otherwise, a mechanical failure of the materials used for implants may cause unwanted effects, such as vascular graft cracking or heart valve failure in body. Biomaterials should have appropriate mechanical properties for avoid such problems [65].

Some important mechanical properties of biomaterials include tensile strength, yield strength, elastic modulus, and fatigue resistance properties [85]. Compressive and tensile tests are used to determine the mechanical strength of a biomaterial [86]. Hardness tests are also used to assess the mechanical properties of certain materials [65]. The uniaxial tensile stress test is the most common test applied to materials and determines many features of the material, such as yield strength, tensile strength, elongation, toughness, and modulus of elasticity. However, the uniaxial tensile test is not solely sufficient for the evaluation of all the properties of biomaterials. Instead of a uniaxial test, a multiaxial stress tensile test should be conducted as it [87].

Mechanical tests of materials include:

- Deformation Testing
- Viscoelasticity Testing
- Failure Testing
- Fracture Testing
- Fatigue Testing
- Wear Testing [87, 88]

Elastic and Plastic Deformation Tests

Elastic deformation occurs when the load applied to the material is removed and the shape of the material is able to return to its previous state. The elasticity module, also known as the Young Module, can be defined as a measurement of elastically changed shape of a material under load. The relationship between stress and strain in elastic deformation is expressed by Hooke's Law [84].

The elasticity module varies between different materials and is a crucial aspect to determining specific features of the selected material. The higher modulus of elasticity of the material means that the higher load carried by materials. It is preferable for a biomaterial to have a modulus of elasticity similar to the elasticity modulus of the target tissues. For example, if a bone implant has higher elasticity modulus than bone, then a process called stress shielding occurs. Because the implant carries the whole load and prevent to carry the load by bones, then in time, the bones may become weak and unable to support the implants [85]. If the material cannot return to its initial shape when the pressure on the material is removed, then it is considered to have incurred plastic deformation. Plastic deformation is permanent [89]. Tensile and compressive tests can be used to detect possible deformation of materials [86].

Viscoelastic Tests

Viscoelastic behavior is a kind of non-elastic behavior that is time dependent [90]. Viscoelastic materials have both solid and liquid characters. When constant stress is applied to these materials, a sudden elastic elongation is observed, following which, elongation continues to increase. During viscoelastic behavior, when the load on the material is removed, sudden elastic behavior appears and then recovery decreases over time [87]. The viscoelastic properties of materials can be investigated with tension experiments [91]. Compressive loading may be used for viscoelastic tests [92].

Failure Tests

It is expected that biomedical materials provide enough resistance without failure [88]. Some factors—such as strain, brittleness, semi-brittleness, or ductility of a material—affects its failure process. Generally, ductile materials yield before breaking under load, as seen in most polymers. In contrast, brittle materials (*e.g.*, ceramics) fracture before they yield. Semi-brittle materials like ionic crystals and some metals show a small amount of plastic or permanent deformation capacity under load before they fracture [87].

Tensile tests may be used to detect a material's failure mode [93]. A compressive tensile test is used to detect failure [94].

Fracture Tests

Fracture mechanics is an important area to be considered in the design of biomedical devices. This is because the fracture of a material may lead to serious consequences for the patient. It should be assumed that there is no failure in the tested material. However, flaws or cracks of the materials may occur inherently or during the production or design processes [87]. Fracture may occur due to sudden or repeated loads or may be time dependent [88].Tensile tests may be used to predict fracture [95]. Alternatively, a compressive test may be used to detect the potential fracture of biomaterials [96].

Fatigue Tests

The fatigue of materials can be defined as decreased strength or damage of the material under repeated stress. Cyclic loads are applied to materials until they break. So cyclic loads reduce mechanical strength. Material properties, type of stress, and environmental conditions may affect the results of fatigue tests [65]. Fatigue was investigated systemically by a German engineer August Wöhler [97] and the following factors may cause fatigue;

• Unsuitable sterilization or manufacturing methods
• Poor materials or careless design
• Initiating sites of material crack
• Insufficient stress analysis [87]

The surface roughness and stress concentrations of the material may be reduced in order to decrease the fatigue [87]. Fatigue has been observed in metals and polymers, but is uncommon in ceramic [88]. Fatigue failure can cause significant problems in the implant. These problems may be summarized as implant loss, stress shielding, and implant failure [85].

Wear Tests

Wear has a major impact on both biological responses and the material itself. After wear of biomaterials, the extracts of the material may induce immune system and inflammatory responses as well as cause local and systemic toxic effects to the cells, tissues, or organs [85]. A high wear resistance and low friction coefficient is preferable for body tissue compatibility. Wear also results in the loosening of implants, changes the geometry of the implant surface, and affects the function and lifetime of the implant [87]. Wear tests are often used to design materials for implants [98].

CHARACTERIZATION TESTS

Adhesion Testing and Surface Testing

The surface properties of the implant are extremely important because the implant surface interacts with the tissue or body fluids as well as microorganisms [97]. In particular, bacterial adhesion may occur in the surface of biomaterials, and device-associated infections may arise in the body. In order to avoid this situation, anti-adhesive surfaces of biomaterials are currently in development, as an anti-adhesive surface would prevent bacterial colonization and biofilm formation on the materials [99].

Electrical Testing

One important consideration when selecting material for devices like cardiac pacemakers or stimulators is the electrical features of materials [89].This is especially crucial for the new generation of smart biomaterials, since electricity can provide beneficial effects like the stimulation of cell growth and enhancement of nerve regeneration [100]. Additionally, materials with high electrical resistance are useful for the isolation of electrical equipment from body fluids. The electrical resistance of such materials differ from each other. Materials are selected according to the location and aim of use [89].

Optical Testing

The optical property is important for aesthetic and functional aspects of biomaterials, especially for those used in the eyes and teeth [89]. For example, light transmittance of a lens affects vision quality, so ophthalmic biomaterials must have clarity and refraction properties [85]. Optical characteristics such as color, translucence, and fluorescence for aesthetic brackets are important factors for reducing visual perception. The tests for optical properties of materials is measured by a spectrophotometer [101].

X-Ray Absorption Testing

X-rays were discovered in 1895 by Wilhelm C. Röntgen. Since the discovery of X-ray imaging it has become one of the most used methods in medical imaging [102]. X-rays used in medicine may examine bones, teeth, lungs, and implants, among other aspects of the body [103]. The selection of the implant material to be used in X-ray absorption must be considered. For example, metal materials strongly absorb X-ray waves and give a good X-ray images. Conversely, polymers cannot absorb X-ray waves well [89].

Ultrasonic Testing

Ultrasound is the second most common imaging method [104]. A diagnostic ultrasound scan is useful for materials that cannot absorb X-rays, such as polymers. Polymer materials in the body may be observed by using ultrasound techniques because the acoustic properties of the polymer is different from the tissues of the body [89].

Diffusion Testing

Diffusion is a transportation type of substance, and the direction of diffusion depends on the concentration gradient [105]. Biological diffusion properties of the implant play a major role in some medical devices like dialyzers [106], oxygenators [107], artificial livers [108], drug delivery systems [109], and tissue scaffolds [110].

Density Testing and Porosity Testing

Even though the volume of an implant may be the same as the target tissue, the mass of the material may be different due to its density [89]. Moreover, the number and size of the pores is a significant feature of the material. For example, the number of pores and pore size of the membrane is significant for hemodialysis [111], heart lung machine [112], and tissue scaffolds [113], since porosity plays a major role in the transport of oxygen, nutrient and waste. It also affects cell migration, vascularization, and mechanical strength in the tissue engineering process. The number and size of the pores is contingent on the material's intended use [114].

Corrosion Testing

Most of the metallic biomaterials are highly corrosive in bodily fluids [115]. Therefore, corrosion resistance of metallic biomaterials is an important part of the selection criteria. This is due to the fact that metal ions are released from the implant after corrosion and can be toxic to living tissues and cause material wear [85]. Due to the high possibility of corrosion, the use of metallic biomaterials is limited [116].

CONCLUDING REMARKS

In vivo and *in vitro* tests are conducted to characterize the biological and mechanical properties of biomaterials. The mechanical compatibility and side effects of the materials may be predicted based on such test results. *In vivo* tests detect possible sensitization, irritation, toxicity, immunogenicity, and pyrogenicity to determine the compatibility between materials and living organisms.

Furthermore, genotoxicity tests show the effects of biomaterials at the DNA level. Carcinogenic potential can be measured using a carcinogenicity test, while teratogenic effects are showed by teratogenicity tests.

Yet, *in vivo* tests have some disadvantages such as their high cost, experimental animal requirements and ethical issues, and longer time required. Thus, *in vitro* methods have been investigated as alternatives to *in vivo* tests. However, *in vitro* tests cannot provide requisite information about more holistic physiological, inflammatory, and immune responses, so they cannot completely replace *in vivo* tests. They do, however, provide preliminary data and can be used as screening tests. More sophisticated and specific *in vitro* tests should be developed in order to provide more alternatives to *in vivo* research.

Some tests such as hemolysis, platelet adhesion and activation, and clotting time tests must be conducted to determine hemocompatibility. Hemolysis tests are used to determine any damage to the blood by biomaterials. Platelet activation, platelet adhesion, and clotting time tests are used to determine clotting potential. These tests are standardized by the American National Standards Institute and the Medical Device Development Association. The ISO 10933 is prepared by the International Organization for Standardization and used as an international guide for selecting test methods correctly for any medical devices that may be in contact with the blood. The ASTM F 756-00 is a standard test method used for evaluating of hemolysis after the direct contact of blood with the material or extract of the material. Regarding, ASTMF2888-13, this assay helps to evaluate a material's ability to induce thrombosis formation, particularly in cardiovascular device materials. In human; decrease of platelets and leukocytes decrease can be evaluated with the help of Active thrombosis. This assay, in accordance with ANSI / AAMI / ISO 10993-4, is part of a test for blood compatibility of materials and devices that come into contact with human blood.

Biomaterials must be able to demonstrate sufficient mechanical properties in relation to their applications. Mechanical problems of materials (*e.g.*, vascular graft cracking and heart valve failure) may cause serious side effects in the body. Some important mechanical properties of biomaterials are tensile and yield strength, elastic modulus, fatigue resistance, failure properties, deformations, and wear. Other specific properties such as optics (for lenses), porosity (for tissue scaffolds), electrical conductivity (pacemaker) are also important features to consider.

There are some standardizations for mechanical tests, but for repeatable results, all procedures should be standardized.

FUTURE RESEARCH

- In biocompatibility tests, to reduce animal use and other disadvantages of *in vivo* tests, alternative *in vitro* tests and standard procedures should be investigated and developed.
- Cell culture models and 3D tissues that are more similar to natural tissues should be developed for *in vitro* toxicity tests.
- Artificial organs (*e.g.*, for the liver or kidney) could provide a potential avenue to determine the effects of materials and their extracts.
- Research should focus on more rapid and automatized test kits for biocompatibility assays.
- The results of *in vivo* and *in vitro* tests of certain materials from all over the world should be submitted to open access database systems.

CONFLICT OF INTEREST

The authors declares no conflict of interest, financial or otherwise.

ACKNOWLEDGEMENTS

Declared none.

REFERENCES

[1]   Özdemir Y. Nurten, biyomateryaller ve biyouyumluluk ankara Üniv.Ecz. Fak Der 1996; 25(2): 57-72.

[2]   Güven, Ş.Y.. Biyouyumluluk ve biyomalzemelerin seçimi. Journal of Engineering Sciences and Design 2014; 2(3): 303-11.

[3]   Schmalz G. Concepts in biocompatibility testing of dental restorative materials. Clin Oral Investig 1997; 1(4): 154-62.
[http://dx.doi.org/10.1007/s007840050027] [PMID: 9555211]

[4]   Zorba YOY. Mehmet, adeziv restoratif materyallerde biyouyumluluk testleri ve kriterleri. Atatürk Üniversitesi Diş Hekimliği Fakültesi Dergisi 2007; 2007(2)

[5]   Lamba NM, Woodhouse KA, Cooper SL. Polyurethanes in biomedical applications. Taylor & Francis 1997.

[6]   Jackson MJ, Ahmed W. Surface engineered surgical tools and medical devices. Springer, US 2007.
[http://dx.doi.org/10.1007/978-0-387-27028-9]

[7]   Salzman E, Merrill E, Kent K. Interaction of blood with artificial surfaces Hemostasis and Thrombosis. 3rd ed., Philadelphia: Lippincott 1994.

[8]   Williams DF. On the mechanisms of biocompatibility. Biomaterials 2008; 29(20): 2941-53.
[http://dx.doi.org/10.1016/j.biomaterials.2008.04.023] [PMID: 18440630]

[9]   Magnusson B, Kligman A. The identification of contract allergens by animal assay. J Occup Environ Med 1970; 12(2): 59.
[http://dx.doi.org/10.1097/00043764-197002000-00023]

[10]   Basketter DA, Gerberick GF, Kimber I, Loveless SE. The local lymph node assay: a viable alternative to currently accepted skin sensitization tests. Food Chem Toxicol 1996; 34(10): 985-97.
[http://dx.doi.org/10.1016/S0278-6915(96)00059-2] [PMID: 9012774]

[11] Basketter DA, Balikie L, Dearman RJ, *et al.* Use of the local lymph node assay for the estimation of relative contact allergenic potency. Contact Dermat 2000; 42(6): 344-8.
[http://dx.doi.org/10.1034/j.1600-0536.2000.042006344.x] [PMID: 10871098]

[12] Kimber I, Dearman RJ, Basketter DA, Ryan CA, Gerberick GF. The local lymph node assay: past, present and future. Contact Dermat 2002; 47(6): 315-28.
[http://dx.doi.org/10.1034/j.1600-0536.2002.470601.x] [PMID: 12581276]

[13] Welss T, Basketter DA, Schröder KR. *In vitro* skin irritation: facts and future. State of the art review of mechanisms and models. Toxicol *In Vitro* 2004; 18(3): 231-43.
[http://dx.doi.org/10.1016/j.tiv.2003.09.009] [PMID: 15046769]

[14] Spielmann H, Hoffmann S, Liebsch M, *et al.* The ECVAM international validation study on *in vitro* tests for acute skin irritation: report on the validity of the EPISKIN and EpiDerm assays and on the Skin Integrity Function Test. Altern Lab Anim 2007; 35(6): 559-601.
[PMID: 18186667]

[15] Williams DF. Biocompatibility and performanceof medical devices. In: Boutrand JP, Ed. Concepts in biocompatibility: new biomaterials, new paradigmsand new testing regimes. London: Woodhead Publishing 2012.

[16] Vinardell MP, Mitjans M. Alternative methods for eye and skin irritation tests: an overview. J Pharm Sci 2008; 97(1): 46-59.
[http://dx.doi.org/10.1002/jps.21088] [PMID: 17701961]

[17] Ratner BD, *et al.* Biomaterials Science: An Introduction to Materials in Medicine. Elsevier Science 2012.

[18] Hartung T, Aaberge I, Berthold S, *et al.* Novel pyrogen tests based on the human fever reaction. The report and recommendations of ECVAM Workshop 43. Altern Lab Anim 2001; 29(2): 99-123.
[PMID: 11262757]

[19] İzgü E. Genel ve Endüstriyel Farmasötik Teknolojileri 1. Ankara: Ankara Üniversitesi Eczacılık Fakültesi Yayınları 1983.

[20] Bedir A, Bilgici B, Yurdakul Z. DNA Hasarı Analizinde μ-FADU ve COMET Yöntemlerinin Karşılaştırılması. Turk Klin Biyokim Derg 2004; 2(3): 97-103.

[21] Yüzbaşıoğlu D, Zengin N, Ünal F. Ünal, Gıda Koruyucuları ve Genotoksisite Testleri. Gıda Dergisi 2014; 39(3)

[22] Şekeroğlu ZA, Şekeroğlu V. Genetik toksisite testleri. TÜBAV Bilim Dergisi 2011; 4(3): 221-9.

[23] Demirel S, Zamani AG. Mikronükleus tekniği ve kullanım alanları. Genel Tıp Dergisi 2002; 12(3): 123-7.

[24] Güldaş E, Keçeci DA. Endodontik tedavidekullanılan kök kanal patlarınınsitotoksik özellikleri – Bölüm I. Türk Diş Hekimliği Dergisi 2011; 81: 72-5.

[25] Gibbons JH, Chandler WU. Conjunctures of Energy and Environment Springer 1981; pp. 103-31.
[http://dx.doi.org/10.1007/978-1-4615-9209-9_7]

[26] Migonney V. Biocompatibility and Norms in Biomaterials John Wiley & Sons, Inc. 2014; pp. 83-100.
[http://dx.doi.org/10.1002/9781119043553.ch4]

[27] Kalter H. Teratology in the twentieth century: congenital malformations in humans and how their environmental causes were established. Elsevier 2003.

[28] Baker J. Principles for the testing of drugs for teratogencity. Report of a WHO Scientific Group 1967.

[29] Cook MJ, Fairweather FA. Methods used in teratogenic testing. Lab Anim 1968; 2(2): 219-28.
[http://dx.doi.org/10.1258/002367768781082834]

[30] Di Silvio L. Cellular response to biomaterials. Elsevier 2008.

[31]   Basu B, Katti DS, Kumar A. Advanced biomaterials: fundamentals, processing, and applications. John Wiley & Sons 2010.

[32]   You ES, *et al*. *In vitro* biocompatibility of surface-modified poly (DL-lactide-co-glycolide) scaffolds with hydrophilic monomers. J Indus Eng Chem Seoul 2007; 13(2): 219.

[33]   Wataha JC, Hanks CT, Craig RG. The effect of cell monolayer density on the cytotoxicity of metal ions which are released from dental alloys. Dent Mater 1993; 9(3): 172-6.
[http://dx.doi.org/10.1016/0109-5641(93)90116-8] [PMID: 8056172]

[34]   Schedle A, Samorapoompichit P, Rausch-Fan XH, *et al*. Response of L-929 fibroblasts, human gingival fibroblasts, and human tissue mast cells to various metal cations. J Dent Res 1995; 74(8): 1513-20.
[http://dx.doi.org/10.1177/00220345950740081301] [PMID: 7560408]

[35]   Chakrabarty S, Roy M, Hazra B, Bhattacharya RK. Induction of apoptosis in human cancer cell lines by diospyrin, a plant-derived bisnaphthoquinonoid, and its synthetic derivatives. Cancer Lett 2002; 188(1-2): 85-93.
[http://dx.doi.org/10.1016/S0304-3835(02)00494-9] [PMID: 12406552]

[36]   Lestari F, Hayes AJ, Green AR, Markovic B. *In vitro* cytotoxicity of selected chemicals commonly produced during fire combustion using human cell lines. Toxicol *In Vitro* 2005; 19(5): 653-63.
[http://dx.doi.org/10.1016/j.tiv.2005.03.002] [PMID: 15893446]

[37]   Tuncer S, Demirci M. Dental materyallerde biyouyumluluk değerlendirmeleri. Atatürk Üniversitesi Diş Hekimliği Fakültesi Dergisi 2011; 2011(2)

[38]   Schmalz G, Arenholt-Bindslev D. Biocompatibility of dental materials. Springer 2009.

[39]   Freshney RI. Culture of specific cell types. Wiley Online Library 2005.
[http://dx.doi.org/10.1002/0471747599.cac023]

[40]   Helgason CD, Miller CL. Basic Cell Culture Protocols. Humana Press 2012.

[41]   Martin AJ. Cytotoxicity testing *in vitro*: Investigation of 5 miniaturized, colorimetric assays. Dublin City University 1992.

[42]   ASTM. Practice for direct contact cell culture evaluation of materials for medical devices 1995.

[43]   Dutta R. Fundamentals of Biochemical Engineering. Springer 2010.

[44]   Karaboz İ, Kayar E, Akar S. Flow sitometri ve kullanım alanları. Elektronik Mikrobiyoloji Dergisi 2008; 6: 1-18.

[45]   Hudson L, Hay F. Isolation and structure of immunoglobulins. Practical Immunology 1980; p. 3.

[46]   Mishell BB, Shiigi SM. Selected methods in cellular immunology. WH Freeman 1980.

[47]   Louis KS, Siegel AC. Cell viability analysis using trypan blue: manual and automated methods. Mammalian Cell Viability. Springer 2011; pp. 7-12.
[http://dx.doi.org/10.1007/978-1-61779-108-6_2]

[48]   Jenkins N. Animal Cell Biotechnology: Methods and Protocols. Humana Press 1999.
[http://dx.doi.org/10.1385/0896035476]

[49]   Mosmann T. Rapid colorimetric assay for cellular growth and survival: application to proliferation and cytotoxicity assays. J Immunol Methods 1983; 65(1-2): 55-63.
[http://dx.doi.org/10.1016/0022-1759(83)90303-4] [PMID: 6606682]

[50]   Alley MC, Scudiero DA, Monks A, *et al*. Feasibility of drug screening with panels of human tumor cell lines using a microculture tetrazolium assay. Cancer Res 1988; 48(3): 589-601.
[PMID: 3335022]

[51]   Freshney RI. Culture of animal cells: A manual of basic technique and specialized applications. Wiley 2011.

[52] Kirkpatrick CJ, Peters K, Hermanns MI, *et al. In vitro* methodologies to evaluate biocompatibility: status quo and perspective. Itbm-Rbm 2005; 26(3): 192-9.
[http://dx.doi.org/10.1016/j.rbmret.2005.04.008]

[53] Cotovio J, Grandidier MH, Portes P, Roguet R, Rubinstenn G. The *in vitro* skin irritation of chemicals: optimisation of the EPISKIN prediction model within the framework of the ECVAM validation process. Altern Lab Anim 2005; 33(4): 329-49.
[PMID: 16185103]

[54] Kandárová H, Liebsch M, Gerner I, *et al.* The EpiDerm test protocol for the upcoming ECVAM validation study on *in vitro* skin irritation tests--an assessment of the performance of the optimised test. Altern Lab Anim 2005; 33(4): 351-67.
[PMID: 16185104]

[55] Kandárová H, Hayden P, Klausner M, Kubilus J, Kearney P, Sheasgreen J. *In vitro* skin irritation testing: Improving the sensitivity of the EpiDerm skin irritation test protocol. Altern Lab Anim 2009; 37(6): 671-89.
[PMID: 20105002]

[56] Morikawa N, Morota K, Morita SI, Kojima H, Nakata S, Konishi H. Prediction of Human Skin Irritancy Using a Cultured Human Skin Model: Comparison of Chemical Application Procedures and Development of a Novel Chemical Application Procedure Using the Vitrolife-Skin™ Model. Alternatives to animal testing and experimentation: AATEX 2002; 9(1): 1-10.

[57] Schaller J, Gerber S, Kämpfer U, Lejon S, Trachsel C. Human Blood Plasma Proteins: Structure and Function. Wiley 2008.
[http://dx.doi.org/10.1002/9780470724378]

[58] Rogers K. Blood: Physiology and Circulation. Britannica Educational Pub. 2010.

[59] Shahid M, Nunhuck A. Physiology. 2008: Mosby.

[60] Chen Z, Zhang R, Kodama M, Nakaya T. Anticoagulant surface prepared by the heparinization of ionic polyurethane film. J Appl Polym Sci 2000; 76(3): 382-90.
[http://dx.doi.org/10.1002/(SICI)1097-4628(20000418)76:3<382::AID-APP13>3.0.CO;2-A]

[61] Vallar L, Rivat C. Regenerated cellulose-based hemodialyzers with immobilized proteins as potential devices for extracorporeal immunoadsorption procedures: an assessment of protein coupling capacity and *in vitro* dialysis performances. Artif Organs 1996; 20(1): 8-16.
[http://dx.doi.org/10.1111/j.1525-1594.1996.tb04412.x] [PMID: 8645134]

[62] Missirlis Y. How to Deal with the Complexity of the Blood—Polymer Interactions, in Biologically Modified Polymeric Biomaterial Surfaces. 1992, Springer. p. 9-12.

[63] Gourlay T, Black RA. Biomaterials and Devices for the Circulatory System. Elsevier Science 2010.
[http://dx.doi.org/10.1533/9780857090553]

[64] Courtney JM, Lamba NM, Sundaram S, Forbes CD. Biomaterials for blood-contacting applications. Biomaterials 1994; 15(10): 737-44.
[http://dx.doi.org/10.1016/0142-9612(94)90026-4] [PMID: 7986936]

[65] Dawids S. Test Procedures for the Blood Compatibility of Biomaterials. Springer Netherlands 2012.

[66] Sundaram S, Courtney JM, Taggart DP, *et al.* Biocompatibility of cardiopulmonary bypass: influence on blood compatibility of device type, mode of blood flow and duration of application. Int J Artif Organs 1994; 17(2): 118-28.
[PMID: 8039940]

[67] Cumming RD. Important factors affecting initial blood-material interactions. Trans Am Soc Artif Intern Organs 1980; 26(1): 304-8.
[PMID: 7245503]

[68] Elahi MF, Guan G, Wang L. HEMOCOMPATIBILITY OF SURFACE MODIFIED SILK FIBROIN MATERIALS: A REVIEW. Rev Adv Mater Sci 2014; 38(2): 148-59.

[69]   Li W, Zhang J, Tse FL. Handbook of LC-MS Bioanalysis: Best Practices, Experimental Protocols, and Regulations. Wiley 2013.
[http://dx.doi.org/10.1002/9781118671276]

[70]   Lippi G, Cervellin G, Favaloro EJ, Plebani M. *In Vitro* and *In vivo* Hemolysis: An Unresolved Dispute in Laboratory Medicine. De Gruyter 2012.
[http://dx.doi.org/10.1515/9783110246148]

[71]   Bennett ST, Lehman CM, Rodgers GM. Laboratory Hemostasis: A Practical Guide for Pathologists. Springer International Publishing 2014.

[72]   Dasgupta A, Sepulveda JL. Accurate Results in the Clinical Laboratory: A Guide to Error Detection and Correction. Elsevier Science 2013.

[73]   McClatchey KD. Clinical Laboratory Medicine. Lippincott. Wiliams & Wilkins 2002.

[74]   Linden J. Blood Safety and Surveillance. CRC Press 2001.
[http://dx.doi.org/10.1201/b13998]

[75]   Okada T, Ikada Y. Modification of silicone surface by graft polymerization of acrylamide with corona discharge. Makromol Chem 1991; 192(8): 1705-13.
[http://dx.doi.org/10.1002/macp.1991.021920804]

[76]   Marois Y, Chakfé N, Guidoin R, *et al.* An albumin-coated polyester arterial graft: *in vivo* assessment of biocompatibility and healing characteristics. Biomaterials 1996; 17(1): 3-14.
[http://dx.doi.org/10.1016/0142-9612(96)80749-6] [PMID: 8962944]

[77]   Kung F-C, Yang M-C. Effect of conjugated linoleic acid immobilization on the hemocompatibility of cellulose acetate membrane. Colloids Surf B Biointerfaces 2006; 47(1): 36-42.
[http://dx.doi.org/10.1016/j.colsurfb.2005.11.019] [PMID: 16386881]

[78]   Liu Y, Yang Y, Wu F. Effects of L-arginine immobilization on the anticoagulant activity and hemolytic property of polyethylene terephthalate films. Appl Surf Sci 2010; 256(12): 3977-81.
[http://dx.doi.org/10.1016/j.apsusc.2010.01.060]

[79]   Sagnella S, Mai-Ngam K. Chitosan based surfactant polymers designed to improve blood compatibility on biomaterials. Colloids Surf B Biointerfaces 2005; 42(2): 147-55.
[http://dx.doi.org/10.1016/j.colsurfb.2004.07.001] [PMID: 15833667]

[80]   Kainthan RK, Gnanamani M, Ganguli M, *et al.* Blood compatibility of novel water soluble hyperbranched polyglycerol-based multivalent cationic polymers and their interaction with DNA. Biomaterials 2006; 27(31): 5377-90.
[http://dx.doi.org/10.1016/j.biomaterials.2006.06.021] [PMID: 16854460]

[81]   Tripodi A, Chantarangkul V, Clerici M, Mannucci PM. Laboratory diagnosis of lupus anticoagulants for patients on oral anticoagulant treatment. Performance of dilute Russell viper venom test and silica clotting time in comparison with Staclot LA. Thromb Haemost 2002; 88(4): 583-6.
[PMID: 12362227]

[82]   Dawids S, *et al.* Blood compatible materials and their testing: Sponsored by the commission of the european communities, as advised by the committee on medical and public health research and the committee on bioengineering evaluation of technology transfer and standardization. Springer 1986.

[83]   Saini M, Singh Y, Arora P, Arora V, Jain K. Implant biomaterials: A comprehensive review. World J Clin Cases 2015; 3(1): 52-7.
[http://dx.doi.org/10.12998/wjcc.v3.i1.52] [PMID: 25610850]

[84]   Bhat SV. Biomaterials. New Delhi, India: Alpha Science International Ltd. 2002; p. 13.
[http://dx.doi.org/10.1007/978-94-010-0328-5]

[85]   Patel NR, Gohil PP. A review on biomaterials: scope, applications & human anatomy significance. Int J Emerg Technol Adv Eng 2012; 2(4): 91-101.

[86]   Patil SG, Sajjan MS, Patil R. The effect of temperature on compressive and tensile strengths of commonly used luting cements: an *in vitro* study. J Int Oral Health 2015; 7(2): 13-9.
[PMID: 25859100]

[87]   Pruitt LA, Chakravartula AM. Mechanics of biomaterials: Fundamental principles for implant design. MRS Bull 2012; 37(07): 698-8.
[http://dx.doi.org/10.1557/mrs.2012.165]

[88]   Hosford WF, Caddell RM. Metal forming: mechanics and metallurgy. Cambridge University Press 2011.
[http://dx.doi.org/10.1017/CBO9780511976940]

[89]   Park J, Lakes RS. Biomaterials: an introduction. Springer Science & Business Media 2007.

[90]   Evaluating the mechanical properties of biomaterials. In: Dubruel P, Vlierberghe SV, Eds. Biomaterials for Bone Regeneration: Novel Techniques and Applications. 1st ed. Woodhead Publishing, 2014: p. 270.

[91]   Boyce BL, Jones RE, Nguyen TD, Grazier JM. Stress-controlled viscoelastic tensile response of bovine cornea. J Biomech 2007; 40(11): 2367-76.
[http://dx.doi.org/10.1016/j.jbiomech.2006.12.001] [PMID: 17240381]

[92]   Linde F. Elastic and viscoelastic properties of trabecular bone by a compression testing approach. Dan Med Bull 1994; 41(2): 119-38.
[PMID: 8039429]

[93]   Aira J, Arriaga F, Íñiguez-González G, Guaita M. Failure modes in halved and tabled tenoned timber scarf joint by tension test. Constr Build Mater 2015; 96: 360-7.
[http://dx.doi.org/10.1016/j.conbuildmat.2015.08.107]

[94]   Harmata AJ, Uppuganti S, Granke M, Guelcher SA, Nyman JS. Compressive fatigue and fracture toughness behavior of injectable, settable bone cements. J Mech Behav Biomed Mater 2015; 51: 345-55.
[http://dx.doi.org/10.1016/j.jmbbm.2015.07.027] [PMID: 26282077]

[95]   Chuluunbat T, Lu C, Kostryzhev A, Tieu K. Investigation of X70 line pipe steel fracture during single edge-notched tensile testing using acoustic emission monitoring 2015; 640: 471-9.
[http://dx.doi.org/10.1016/j.msea.2015.06.030]

[96]   Wawersik W, Fairhurst C. *A study of brittle rock fracture in laboratory compression experiments.* Elsevier 1970.
[http://dx.doi.org/10.1016/0148-9062(70)90007-0]

[97]   Soboyejo W. Mechanical properties of engineered materials. CrC Press 2002; Vol. 152.
[http://dx.doi.org/10.1201/9780203910399]

[98]   Smith SL, Li BL, Buniya A, *et al. In vitro* wear testing of a contemporary design of reverse shoulder prosthesis. J Biomech 2015; 48(12): 3072-9.
[http://dx.doi.org/10.1016/j.jbiomech.2015.07.022] [PMID: 26278181]

[99]   Campoccia D, Montanaro L, Arciola CR. A review of the biomaterials technologies for infection-resistant surfaces. Biomaterials 2013; 34(34): 8533-54.
[http://dx.doi.org/10.1016/j.biomaterials.2013.07.089] [PMID: 23953781]

[100] Balint R, Cassidy NJ, Cartmell SH. Conductive polymers: towards a smart biomaterial for tissue engineering. Acta Biomater 2014; 10(6): 2341-53.
[http://dx.doi.org/10.1016/j.actbio.2014.02.015] [PMID: 24556448]

[101] Lopes Filho H, Maia LE, Araújo MV, Ruellas AC. Influence of optical properties of esthetic brackets (color, translucence, and fluorescence) on visual perception. Am J Orthod Dentofacial Orthop 2012; 141(4): 460-7.
[http://dx.doi.org/10.1016/j.ajodo.2011.10.026] [PMID: 22464528]

[102] Taguchi K, Iwanczyk JS. Vision 20/20: Single photon counting x-ray detectors in medical imaging.

Med Phys 2013; 40(10): 100901.
[http://dx.doi.org/10.1118/1.4820371] [PMID: 24089889]

[103] Chen H, Rogalski MM, Anker JN. Advances in functional X-ray imaging techniques and contrast agents. Phys Chem Chem Phys 2012; 14(39): 13469-86.
[http://dx.doi.org/10.1039/c2cp41858d] [PMID: 22962667]

[104] Wells PN, Liang H-D. Medical ultrasound: imaging of soft tissue strain and elasticity. J R Soc Interface 2011; 8(64): 1521-49.
[http://dx.doi.org/10.1098/rsif.2011.0054] [PMID: 21680780]

[105] Wijmans J, Baker R. The solution-diffusion model: a review. J Membr Sci 1995; 107(1): 1-21.
[http://dx.doi.org/10.1016/0376-7388(95)00102-I]

[106] Davenport A. How can dialyzer designs improve solute clearances for hemodialysis patients? Hemodial Int 2014; 18(S1) (Suppl. 1): S43-7.
[http://dx.doi.org/10.1111/hdi.12223] [PMID: 25330831]

[107] Robak O, Lakatos PK, Bojic A, *et al.* Influence of different oxygenator types on changing frequency, infection incidence, and mortality in ARDS patients on veno-venous ECMO. Int J Artif Organs 2014; 37(11): 839-46.
[http://dx.doi.org/10.5301/ijao.5000360] [PMID: 25362902]

[108] Hay PD, Veitch AR, Smith MD, Cousins RB, Gaylor JD. Oxygen transfer in a diffusion-limited hollow fiber bioartificial liver. Artif Organs 2000; 24(4): 278-88.
[http://dx.doi.org/10.1046/j.1525-1594.2000.06499.x] [PMID: 10816201]

[109] Siepmann J, Siepmann F. Modeling of diffusion controlled drug delivery. J Control Release 2012; 161(2): 351-62.
[http://dx.doi.org/10.1016/j.jconrel.2011.10.006] [PMID: 22019555]

[110] Cheema U, Rong Z, Kirresh O, Macrobert AJ, Vadgama P, Brown RA. Oxygen diffusion through collagen scaffolds at defined densities: implications for cell survival in tissue models. J Tissue Eng Regen Med 2012; 6(1): 77-84.
[http://dx.doi.org/10.1002/term.402] [PMID: 21312340]

[111] Hedayat A, Shoker A. Polyflux® 210H hemodialysis membrane targets to improve filtration. Saudi J Kidney Dis Transpl 2014; 25(1): 156-60.
[http://dx.doi.org/10.4103/1319-2442.124551] [PMID: 24434402]

[112] Kyrolainen M, Hkanson H, Ekroth R, Mattiasson B. Biosensor monitoring of blood lactate during open-heart surgery. Analytical Biotechnology 2012; 279: 149-53.

[113] Rnjak-Kovacina J, Wise SG, Li Z, *et al.* Tailoring the porosity and pore size of electrospun synthetic human elastin scaffolds for dermal tissue engineering. Biomaterials 2011; 32(28): 6729-36.
[http://dx.doi.org/10.1016/j.biomaterials.2011.05.065] [PMID: 21683438]

[114] Mediaswanti K, Wen C, Ivanova EP. A review on bioactive porous metallic biomaterials. J Biomim Biomater Tissue Eng 2013; 18(104): 2.

[115] Black JH. The physical state of primordial intergalactic clouds. Mon Not R Astron Soc 1981; 197(3): 553-63.
[http://dx.doi.org/10.1093/mnras/197.3.553]

[116] Staiger MP, Pietak AM, Huadmai J, Dias G. Magnesium and its alloys as orthopedic biomaterials: a review. Biomaterials 2006; 27(9): 1728-34.
[http://dx.doi.org/10.1016/j.biomaterials.2005.10.003] [PMID: 16246414]

CHAPTER 8

Immune Aspects of Scaffold Design

Nasrin Mokhtari[1], **Hamidreza Mokhtari**[2] and **Mehdi Razavi**[3,*]

[1] Department of Dentistry, Khorasgan University of Dentistry Sciences, Isfahan 81551-39998, Iran

[2] Department of Material Engineering, Isfahan University of Technology, Isfahan 84156-83111, Iran

[3] Department of Radiology, School of Medicine, Stanford University, Palo Alto, California 94304, USA

Abstract: Long-term survival of scaffolds depends on having no detrimental immune response. Designing biomaterials that are able to modulate host responses and thus support the healing process is essential for tissue remodeling. In depth understanding of immune response to the biomaterials and their transplanted cells is important since the interaction between host response and transplanted cells demonstrates the biocompatibility of the implanted scaffold. In this chapter, we mainly aim to focus on innate and adaptive immune response and wound healings processes. In detail we discuss about variables that effect on the immune responses and the current strategies for modulating.

Keywords: Immune responses, Scaffold, Tissue engineering.

INTRODUCTION

One of the most significant current discussion in tissue engineering is modulating the host response. As we know, combination of soluble factors and scaffold and cells are components of tissue engineering .some of these agents could stimulate the immune response, as a foreign object. Eventually, modulating immune reactions can help to improve implant long-term survival and enhance their function [1]. Accordingly, deep understanding on the wound healing and immune reactions toward implants is necessary for improving the immunomodulatory potentials of biomaterials [2]. The immune system could be affected by effective materials, they could encourage healing and scaffold integration although, sustaining its continuation leading to chronic inflammation and foreign body reactions and eluding specific implant function [2, 3]. Furthermore, numerous

* **Corresponding author Mehdi Razavi:** Department of Radiology, School of Medicine, Stanford University, Palo Alto, California 94304, USA; Tel: +16504847293; E-mails: merazavi@stanford.edu; mrazavi2659@gmail.com

studies have attempted to highlight importance of testing the biomaterials on specific and non-specific immune reactions as a factor of biocompatibility assessment [2, 4, 5]. The host response against an implant (without transplanted cells) begins with an acute inflammation and Direct to a chronic inflammation in some cases and granulation tissue development, a foreign body reaction and fibrous capsule development [6]. Previous studies have found that, this host response have impact on repair or regeneration of the wound that caused by surgical procedures for biomaterial implantation [7]. Defense against foreign bodies is intervened by the immediate reactions of non-specific immunity and the subsequent responses of acquired immunity [8]. Briefly, the non-specific immunity(innate or in-born immunity) defends host from pathogens by anatomical host barriers(skin, other epithelial surfaces) and cells (neutrophils, macrophages, dendritic cells, *etc.*) and plasma proteins(the complement proteins, *etc.*),while, adaptive immunity (acquired immunity) works by humoral and cellular immunity humoral immune system includes B lymphocyte and antibodies, and cellular immune system comprises T lymphocyte and cytokines [9].

IMMUNE MECHANISMS

Initially, the implant surface is covered by proteins witch exit from the vessels or present in tissue fluids [2]. The activation of clotting cascade, complement system, and immune cells is controlled by these proteins that absorbed on the implant surface. A temporary provisional matrix around the biomaterials is created by the interactions of these systems and their products (such as fibrin) [2, 10, 11]. Moreover, studies have found that some glycoproteins such as fibronectin and vitronectin could absorbed to implant surfaces [2, 12]. While fibrinogen and complement mostly employed to the activating of inflammatory cells, fibronectin and vitronectin are important factors in regulating the inflammatory reactions against implants [2]. Firstly, immune cells adhere to the implant surface by adhesion receptors witch attaches to the absorbed proteins, and these cells release chemokines that attract other phagocytic cells [7]. And in the case of large implants, could occur a "frustrated phagocytosis" that phagocytes release the toxic agents in environment [13]. The Initial stage of wound healing is acute inflammation whereas neutrophils and then monocytes, transmigrate across the endothelium, and fibrin clot and extracellular matrix are then formed in the inflammatory site. The inflammatory mediators stimulate synthesis of some cell surface proteins caused by leukocytes interplay with the endothelium and other inflammatory cells and also extracellular matrix proteins [14]. Neutrophils can remove some foreign materials and pathogens [14 - 16]. Polymorph nuclear leukocytes (PMNs) eliminate the foreign materials by phagocytosis and release of reactive oxygen species (ROS) and inflammatory cytokines [17]. Macrophages are recruited to the implant site following the neutrophils infiltration process [18]. Although for neutrophils infiltration, surgical wounding is enough, but implanted biomaterials is necessary for macrophages recruitment [19]. Then, after monocytes are recruited to locus of damage, they change to macrophages [15]. The amount of macrophages usually increases in the first week, however, they remain in the locus of damage for months [15, 16]. They as well as neutrophils release ROS and cytokines could participate in secondary damage. Although, they also help to regeneration due to releasing growth factors and they can also, engulf and digest pathogens [7, 20, 21]. Durability of an inflammatory stimulus causes chronic inflammation that is indicated by the exit of granulocytes and some macrophages from the locus of damage, with the proliferation of blood vessels and connective tissue [14], and recruitment of lymphocytes and plasma cells which are principle elements of acquired immunity. According to residual macrophages phenotype, they produce cytokines [7, 22]. Macrophage polarization is related to micro-environmental factors. The Th1 cytokines (Interferon gamma) improve The (M1) phenotype activation (Classically activated macrophages), in contrast to (M2) macrophages activation (Alternatively activated macrophages) that relates to Th2 response [7, 23]. There are some differences between M1 and M2 macrophages such as type of releasing cytokines and surface markers and their metabolism. M1 macrophages have inflammatory functions and phagocytosis cell debris and pathogens, but M2 macrophages have anti-inflammatory functions and their roles in tissue repair and remodeling is significant. Typically the cell surface markers of M1 phenotype is CD80, CD86, but M2 phenotype has different markers that based on their subsets.M1 macrophages produce pro-inflammatory cytokines (such as tumor necrosis fsctors,interlukin-12), in contrast M2 macrophages release anti-inflammatory cytokines(such as interlukin-10,transforming growth factor) [24]. Previous studies have found that characteristics of microenvironment would influence on macrophages polarization. The stiffness and rigidity of substrate could effects on macrophage phenotype and its function. Several evidences suggest that increasing tissue rigidity can increase phagocytosis and elongation of these cells [25, 26]. Furthermore, macrophage polarization is dependent on its morphology. Also, Micro and nano topography have large impact on polarization *via* macrophage morphology. McWhorter *et al* examine this impact by micro patterning of substrate, and demonstrate that rounded shaped cells have M1 characteristics, and elongated shaped cells have M2 characteristics [27]. Sussman *et al.* demonstrate that 34 µm pores in compared with 160 µm pores, leads polarization towards M1 cells [28]. Modulating mechanical forces influence on macrophages polarization as, V.Ballotta *et al* demonstrate that 7% cyclical load leads to increase in anti-inflammatory phenotype presence [29]. Altering adsorbed proteins influenced by surface chemistry modification affects the macrophages. Rostam HM *et al.* use two different chemical composition to show this impact. Untreated hydrophobic polystyrene shifts macrophages into M2 activation and hydrophilic O_2 plasma-etched polystyrene shits them into M1 activation [30]. During the healing process, the granulation tissue is started to form. This connective tissue has diverse cells such as macrophages for immune approaches and fibroblasts that produce the extracellular matrix, and endothelial cells for angiogenesis [14]. The final stage of the *in vivo* biomaterial host response, is comprised of foreign body giant cells interacted with the biomaterial surface, surrounded by granulation tissue and fibrous encapsulation of the implant [14]. T lymphocytes response is one of the critical factors in adaptive immune response. T lymphocytes have been known to adhere to synthetic biomaterials *in vitro* [13]. Not only, they aren't attached to the implant but also, they are attached to macrophages. The interactions between Tell and macrophages leads to increase macrophage adhesion and the foreign body reaction and formation of multinucleated giant cells [2, 31]. It is significant that synthetic biomaterials are not considered as an antigen. Also functional groups on the synthetic biomaterials surfaces may acting as mitogens during lymphocyte activation [32]. Type 1 helper T cells release diverse cytokines such as interlucin-2(IL-2), interferon (IFN), and tumor necrosis factor (TNF) that can activate the macrophage, and cell-mediated immunity [33, 34]. In allogeneic and xenogeneic implants rejection, functions of these cells have been showed [35 - 37]. Th2 cells release IL-4, IL-5, IL-6, and IL-10 and macrophages activation is not demonsterated. Th2 cells participate in humoral immunity. Function of these cells is contributed to the transplant acceptance [38, 39]. The SIS-ECM is the ECM scaffold which is able to determine the Th1/Th2 response [40, 41]. SIS-ECM is a type of biomaterial which including porcine small intestinal submucosa [42]. Dendritic cells (DCs) play a great role in innate and adaptive immunity [2]. Although, DCs activate T cells as antigen presenting cells, they have immunoregulatory potentials and participate in central and peripheral tolerance mechanisms [43, 44]. Many agents can influence on inducing these two different roles of DCs [44]. For example, immature DCs express no co-stimulatory molecules and semi-mature DCs are not able to express pro-inflammatory cytokines that are necessary for T-cell fully activation [45 - 48]. Therefore function of these cells lead to tolerance but function of mature DCs promote immunity [43, 49, 50]. IL-10 and transforming growth factor-b (TGF- b) and low amount of IL-6 and TNF-a, also IL-16, colony-stimulating factor-3 and scatter factor induce tolerogenic functions of DCs [44 - 46]. Due to the scaffolding applications, increasing of DCs with tolerogenic phenotypes can be helpful for modulation of host response [2].

CELL THERAPY AND IMMUNE RESPONSE

Another essential issue is about cell transplantation. There are many reasons for host responses to cell transplantation rejection. Alpha-Gal oligosaccharides are cell surface markers that are expressed in majority species except human and old world monkey, could lead to xenotransplantation hyper acute rejection [24]. Humans and Old World monkeys produce huge concentration of anti-Gal antibodies, consist of: IgG, IgM, and IgA [51 - 53]. Xenotransplants of Gal knockout hearts [54, 55] and kidneys [56] have been rejected over periods of 6 months and 1 month, respectively, because of the immune response including the formation of anti-non-Gal Ab specific to porcine antigens. Even porcine glutaraldehyde-fixed heart valve bioprostheses due to the existence of alpha-Gal oligosaccharides have not complete biocompatibility and demonstrate anti-Gal IgM [24]. This immune mechanism towards these biological prosthesis include calcific and degenerative changes and collagen destruction [57]. Treatment the bioprostheses with galactosidase has been planned to decrease detrimental impacts of immune system [58, 59]. The enzymatic therapy could efficiently eliminate these oligosaccharides from porcine cartilage and anterior cruciate ligament (ACL) tissue; however the Gal epitope is not replaced through natural turnover, since the cells within the tissue graft are not viable [60]. Another reason is remnant DNA which within scaffolding biomaterials after the decellularization has been showed as the reason of "immune responses" since the of porcine-derived acellular scaffolds are implanted for orthopaedic usages [61]. Due to they are usually in small size, they can have not large impacts in adverse tissue remodeling response [62]. The decellularization technique is able to inhibit the detrimental impacts in host tissue [63], though, some additional techniques are desirable for removal of cell remnants [24].

TECHNIQUES AND EFFICIENT VARIABLES IN TISSUE ENGINEERING

The period and extent of immune reactions is related to the amount of injury, the chemical cues of biomaterial, surface free energy, surface charge, porosity, roughness, and surface topography [64]. Surface chemistry effects on attached proteins and consequently attachment and activation of different immune cells are related to these proteins [7]. Commonly researches are shown that the hydrophobic implants lead to increase the monocyte adhesion compared to hydrophilic implants induce a local immune reaction and *in vitro* studies demonstrate that this hydrophilic condition minimize the monocyte/macrophage adhesion and foreign body reaction [65, 66]. One of the strategies that improve the mechanical properties of biological materials is chemical crosslinking treatment; however, it can influence on the host response [7]. For instance, carbodiimide (CDI) cross-linking of scaffolds leading to increase M1 macrophages, while a cellular extra cellular matrix scaffolds which were not modified induced an M2 phenotype [67]. As mentioned, Micro and nano topography of implants have impact on host response [7]. Micro- porosity of an implant is fundamental for intended reconstruction, while micron-scale architectures could impact on host response [7]. The micro architecture of the structure tend to decrease the cell fusion compared to the flat surfaces [68] and induce a type of macrophage that is different from classically and alternatively activated macrophages, while nano-scale did not have such impact [69]. Enhancing the hydrophilicity of the biomaterials has been utilized to reduce DCs maturation [70]. Coating the implant surface have been used to protect it from protein adsorption and the host response and lead implant to be invisible. Another common method for improving immunomodulatory properties of biomaterial is coupling of anti-inflammatory drugs to biomaterials. Glucocorticoids is most common anti-inflammatory drug that has large immunosuppressive impacts. These effects are caused by inhibition of a type of transcription factor that influences in translation of many mediators and some immune proteins. The systemic anti-inflammatory drug delivery can modulate the host response but can have some adverse impacts on tissue regeneration [7]. We can eliminate these adverse effects by local drug delivery that doesn't influence on whole of immune system [7]. Also the delivery of mesenchymal stem cells has been used to increase tissue regenerative potentials [71], often through the secretion of trophic factors [72]. These scaffold implantation or organ xenotransplantation rejection problems could also be solved by the advanced scaffold fabrication techniques [73 - 84]. Tae-Ha Song, *et al.* have found that a 3D printing technique could increase the efficiency of immunosuppressive drugs local-delivery in the scaffolds, resulting in successful tissue regeneration by scaffold implantation with much fewer side effects [85].

CONCLUSION

One of the detrimental factors that plays an important role in tissue remodeling is immune response. The innate and adaptive immune responses can lead to fibrosis or rejection of the implants. Growing knowledge on these processes is essential for developing materials that affect the host responses. Current strategies are focused on modification of biomaterial chemical composition, porosity, roughness and some other engineering techniques to assess the immune responses of the scaffolds.

CONFLICT OF INTEREST

The authors declare no conflict of interest, financial or otherwise.

ACKNOWLEDGEMENTS

Declared none.

REFERENCES

[1] Sefton MV, Babensee JE, Woodhouse KA. Innate and adaptive immune responses in tissue engineering. Semin Immunol 2008; 20(2): 83-5.
[http://dx.doi.org/10.1016/j.smim.2007.12.008] [PMID: 18221888]

[2] Franz S, Rammelt S. Immune responses to implants e A review of the implications for the design of immunomodulatory biomaterials. Biomaterials 2011; 32: 6692-709.

[3] Williams DF. On the mechanisms of biocompatibility. Biomaterials 2008; 29: 2941-53.
[http://dx.doi.org/10.1016/j.biomaterials.2008.04.023]

[4] Smith MJ, White KL Jr, Smith DC, Bowlin GL. *In vitro* evaluations of innate and acquired immune responses to electrospunpolydioxanone-elastin blends. Biomaterials 2009; 30: 149-59.

[5] Smith MJ, Smith DC, Bowlin GL, White KL. Modulation of murine innate and acquired immune responses following *in vitro* exposure to electrospun blends of collagen and polydioxanone. J Biomed Mater Res A 2010; 93: 793-806.

[6] Anderson JM. Mechanisms of inflammation and infection with implanted devices. Cardiovasc Pathol 1993; 2: 33S-41S.
[http://dx.doi.org/10.1016/1054-8807(93)90045-4]

[7] Boehler R M, Graham J G. Tissue engineering tools for modulation of the immune response. Biotechniques 2011 October; 51(4): 239-passim.

[8] Paulukat J. Regulation of IL-18 binding protein by IFN-gamma. 2003.

[9] Abul KA, Andrew HL, Shiv P. Cellular and Molecular Immunology. 1600 John F. Kennedy Blvd. Ste 1800 Philadelphia : Jeff Patterson ; 2015 . chapter1,page 2 . Eight Edition.

[10] Wilson CJ, Clegg RE, Leavesley DI, Pearcy MJ. Mediation of biomaterialecell interactions by adsorbed proteins: a review. Tissue Eng 2005; 11: 1-18.

[11] Gorbet MB, Sefton MV. Biomaterial-associated thrombosis: roles of coagulationfactors, complement, platelets and leukocytes. Biomaterials 2004; 25: 5681-703.
[http://dx.doi.org/10.1016/B978-008045154-1.50025-3]

[12] McFarland CD, Thomas CH, DeFilippis C, Steele JG, Healy KE. Protein adsorption and cell attachment to patterned surfaces. J Biomed Mater Res 2000; 49: 200-10.

[13] Anderson JM, Rodriguez A, Chang DT. Foreign body reaction to biomaterials. Semin Immunol 2008; 20(2): 86-100.
[http://dx.doi.org/10.1016/j.smim.2007.11.004] [PMID: 18162407]

[14] Mikos AG, McIntire LV, Anderson JM, Babensee JE. Host response to tissue engineered devices. Adv Drug Deliv Rev 1998; 33(1-2): 111-39.
[http://dx.doi.org/10.1016/S0169-409X(98)00023-4] [PMID: 10837656]

[15] Donnelly DJ, Popovich PG. Inflammation and its role in neuroprotection, axonal regeneration and functional recovery after spinal cord injury. Exp Neurol 2008; 209(2): 378-88.
[http://dx.doi.org/10.1016/j.expneurol.2007.06.009] [PMID: 17662717]

[16] Beck KD, Nguyen HX, Galvan MD, Salazar DL, Woodruff TM, Anderson AJ. Quantitative analysis of cellular inflammation after traumatic spinal cord injury: evidence for a multiphasic inflammatory response in the acute to chronic environment. Brain 2010; 133(Pt 2): 433-47.
[http://dx.doi.org/10.1093/brain/awp322] [PMID: 20085927]

[17] Pineau I, Lacroix S. Proinflammatory cytokine synthesis in the injured mouse spinal cord: multiphasic expression pattern and identification of the cell types involved. J Comp Neurol 2007; 500(2): 267-85.
[http://dx.doi.org/10.1002/cne.21149] [PMID: 17111361]

[18] Jones KS. Effects of biomaterial-induced inflammation on fibrosis and rejection. Semin Immunol 2008; 20(2): 130-6.

[http://dx.doi.org/10.1016/j.smim.2007.11.005] [PMID: 18191409]

[19]   Robitaille R, Dusseault J, Henley N, Desbiens K, Labrecque N, Hallé JP. Inflammatory response to peritoneal implantation of alginate-poly-L-lysine microcapsules. Biomaterials 2005; 26(19): 4119-27.
[http://dx.doi.org/10.1016/j.biomaterials.2004.10.028] [PMID: 15664639]

[20]   Duffield JS. The inflammatory macrophage: a story of Jekyll and Hyde. Clin Sci 2003; 104(1): 27-38.
[http://dx.doi.org/10.1042/cs1040027] [PMID: 12519085]

[21]   Xu W, Roos A, Schlagwein N, Woltman AM, Daha MR, van Kooten C. IL-10-producing macrophages preferentially clear early apoptotic cells. Blood 2006; 107(12): 4930-7.
[http://dx.doi.org/10.1182/blood-2005-10-4144] [PMID: 16497970]

[22]   Anderson JM. Inflammatory and immune responses to tissue engineered devices Tissue engineering and artificial organs Taylor and Francis, Boca Raton 2006.
[http://dx.doi.org/10.1201/9781420003871.ch36]

[23]   Martinez FO, Sica A, Mantovani A, Locati M. Macrophage activation and polarization. Front Biosci 2008; 13: 453-61.
[http://dx.doi.org/10.2741/2692] [PMID: 17981560]

[24]   Badylak SF, Gilbert TW. Immune response to biologic scaffold materials. Semin Immunol 2008; 20(2): 109-16.
[http://dx.doi.org/10.1016/j.smim.2007.11.003] [PMID: 18083531]

[25]   Patel NR, Bole M, Chen C, *et al.* Cell elasticity determines macrophage function. PLoS One 2012; 7(9): e41024.
[http://dx.doi.org/10.1371/journal.pone.0041024] [PMID: 23028423]

[26]   Gruber E, Sinha S, Ehrlich E, Leifer C. Extracellular Substrate Stiffness Alters Macrophage Morphology and Function. The FASEB Journal 2015; 29(1 Supplement): 571.

[27]   McWhorter FY, Wang T, Nguyen P, Chung T, Liu WF. Modulation of macrophage phenotype by cell shape. Proc Natl Acad Sci USA 2013; 110(43): 17253-8.
[http://dx.doi.org/10.1073/pnas.1308887110] [PMID: 24101477]

[28]   Sussman EM, Halpin MC, Muster J, Moon RT, Ratner BD. Porous implants modulate healing and induce shifts in local macrophage polarization in the foreign body reaction. Ann Biomed Eng 2014; 42(7): 1508-16.
[http://dx.doi.org/10.1007/s10439-013-0933-0] [PMID: 24248559]

[29]   Ballotta V, Driessen-Mol A, Bouten CV, Baaijens FP. Strain-dependent modulation of macrophage polarization within scaffolds. Biomaterials 2014; 35(18): 4919-28.
[http://dx.doi.org/10.1016/j.biomaterials.2014.03.002] [PMID: 24661551]

[30]   Rostam HM, Singh S, Salazar F, *et al.* The impact of surface chemistry modification on macrophage polarisation. Immunobiology 2016; 221(11): 1237-46.
[http://dx.doi.org/10.1016/j.imbio.2016.06.010] [PMID: 27349596]

[31]   Brodbeck WG, Macewan M, Colton E, Meyerson H, Anderson JM. Lymphocytes and the foreign body response: lymphocyte enhancement of macrophage adhesion and fusion. J Biomed Mater Res A 2005; 74: 222-9.

[32]   Rodriguez A, Anderson JM. Evaluation of clinical biomaterial surface effects on T lymphocyte activation. J Biomed Mater Res A 2010; 92: 214-0.

[33]   Abbas AK, Murphy KM, Sher A. Functional diversity of helper T lymphocytes. Nature 1996; 383(6603): 787-93.
[http://dx.doi.org/10.1038/383787a0] [PMID: 8893001]

[34]   Matsumiya G, Shirakura R, Miyagawa S, Izutani H, Nakata S, Matsuda H. Assessment of T-cell subsets involved in antibody production and cell-mediated cytotoxicity in rat-to-mouse cardiac xenotransplantation. Transplant Proc 1994; 26(3): 1214-6.

[PMID: 8029892]

[35] Strom TB, Roy-Chaudhury P, Manfro R, *et al.* The Th1/Th2 paradigm and the allograft response. Curr Opin Immunol 1996; 8(5): 688-93.
[http://dx.doi.org/10.1016/S0952-7915(96)80087-2] [PMID: 8902395]

[36] Zhai Y, Ghobrial RM, Busuttil RW, Kupiec-Weglinski JW. Th1 and Th2 cytokines in organ transplantation: paradigm lost? Crit Rev Immunol 1999; 19(2): 155-72.
[PMID: 10352902]

[37] Chen N, Gao Q, Field EH. Prevention of Th1 response is critical for tolerance. Transplantation 1996; 61(7): 1076-83.
[http://dx.doi.org/10.1097/00007890-199604150-00016] [PMID: 8623189]

[38] Bach FH, Ferran C, Hechenleitner P, *et al.* Accommodation of vascularized xenografts: expression of "protective genes" by donor endothelial cells in a host Th2 cytokine environment. Nat Med 1997; 3(2): 196-204.
[http://dx.doi.org/10.1038/nm0297-196] [PMID: 9018239]

[39] Piccotti JR, Chan SY, VanBuskirk AM, Eichwald EJ, Bishop DK. Are Th2 helper T lymphocytes beneficial, deleterious, or irrelevant in promoting allograft survival? Transplantation 1997; 63(5): 619-24.
[http://dx.doi.org/10.1097/00007890-199703150-00001] [PMID: 9075827]

[40] Allman AJ, McPherson TB, Badylak SF, *et al.* Xenogeneic extracellular matrix grafts elicit a TH2-restricted immune response. Transplantation 2001; 71(11): 1631-40.
[http://dx.doi.org/10.1097/00007890-200106150-00024] [PMID: 11435976]

[41] Allman AJ, McPherson TB, Merrill LC, Badylak SF, Metzger DW. The Th2-restricted immune response to xenogeneic small intestinal submucosa does not influence systemic protective immunity to viral and bacterial pathogens. Tissue Eng 2002; 8(1): 53-62.
[http://dx.doi.org/10.1089/107632702753503054] [PMID: 11886654]

[42] McPherson TB, Liang H, Record RD, Badylak SF. Galalpha(1,3)Gal epitope in porcine small intestinal submucosa. Tissue Eng 2000; 6(3): 233-9.
[http://dx.doi.org/10.1089/107632700050044416] [PMID: 10941218]

[43] Lutz MB, Schuler G. Immature, semi-mature and fully mature dendritic cells:which signals induce tolerance or immunity?. Trends Immunol 2002; 23: 445-9.

[44] Rutella S, Danese S, Leone G. Tolerogenic dendritic cells: cytokine modulation comes of age. Blood 2006; 108: 1435-40.
[http://dx.doi.org/10.1182/blood-2006-03-006403]

[45] Hawiger D, Inaba K, Dorsett Y, Guo M, Mahnke K, Rivera M. Dendritic cells ind peripheral T cell unresponsiveness under steady state conditions *in vivo*. J Exp Med 2001; 194: 769-9.

[46] Steinman RM, Hawiger D, Liu K, *et al.* Dendritic cell function *in vivo* during the steady state: a role in peripheral tolerance. Ann N Y Acad Sci 2003; 987: 15-25.

[47] Jonuleit H, Schmitt E, Schuler G, Knop J, Enk AH. Induction of interleukin 10-producing, nonproliferatingCD4(þ) T cells with regulatory properties by repetitive stimulation with allogeneic immature human dendritic cells. J Exp Med 2000; 192: 1213-22.

[48] Vigouroux S, Yvon E, Biagi E, Brenner MK. Antigen-induced regulatory T cells. Blood 2004; 104: 26-33.
[http://dx.doi.org/10.1182/blood-2004-01-0182]

[49] Geissmann F, Revy P, Regnault A, *et al.* TGFbeta 1 prevents the noncognate maturation of human dendritic Langerhans cells. J Immunol 1999; 162: 4567-75.

[50] Frick JS, Grunebach F, Autenrieth IB. Immunomodulation by semi-mature dendritic cells: a novel role of toll-like receptors and interleukin-6. Int J Med Microbiol 2010; 300: 19-24.

[http://dx.doi.org/10.1016/j.ijmm.2009.08.010]

[51]   Galili U, Macher BA, Buehler J, Shohet SB. Human natural anti-alpha-galactosyl IgG. II. The specific recognition of alpha (1----3)-linked galactose residues. J Exp Med 1985; 162(2): 573-82.
[http://dx.doi.org/10.1084/jem.162.2.573] [PMID: 2410529]

[52]   Gabrielli A, Candela M, Ricciatti AM, Caniglia ML, Wieslander J. Antibodies to mouse laminin in patients with systemic sclerosis (scleroderma) recognize galactosyl (alpha 1-3)-galactose epitopes. Clin Exp Immunol 1991; 86(3): 367-73.
[http://dx.doi.org/10.1111/j.1365-2249.1991.tb02939.x] [PMID: 1721011]

[53]   Koren E, Neethling FA, Ye Y, *et al.* Heterogeneity of preformed human antipig xenogeneic antibodies. Transplant Proc 1992; 24(2): 598-601.
[PMID: 1566446]

[54]   Kuwaki K, Tseng YL, Dor FJ, *et al.* Heart transplantation in baboons using alpha1,3-galactosyltransferase gene-knockout pigs as donors: initial experience. Nat Med 2005; 11(1): 29-31.
[http://dx.doi.org/10.1038/nm1171] [PMID: 15619628]

[55]   Tseng YL, Kuwaki K, Dor FJ, *et al.* alpha1,3-Galactosyltransferase gene-knockout pig heart transplantation in baboons with survival approaching 6 months. Transplantation 2005; 80(10): 1493-500.
[http://dx.doi.org/10.1097/01.tp.0000181397.41143.fa] [PMID: 16340796]

[56]   Chen G, Qian H, Starzl T, *et al.* Acute rejection is associated with antibodies to non-Gal antigens in baboons using Gal-knockout pig kidneys. Nat Med 2005; 11(12): 1295-8.
[http://dx.doi.org/10.1038/nm1330] [PMID: 16311604]

[57]   Konakci KZ, Bohle B, Blumer R, *et al.* Alpha-Gal on bioprostheses: xenograft immune response in cardiac surgery. Eur J Clin Invest 2005; 35(1): 17-23.
[http://dx.doi.org/10.1111/j.1365-2362.2005.01441.x] [PMID: 15638815]

[58]   Stone KR, Abdel-Motal UM, Walgenbach AW, Turek TJ, Galili U. Replacement of human anterior cruciate ligaments with pig ligaments: a model for anti-non-gal antibody response in long-term xenotransplantation. Transplantation 2007; 83(2): 211-9.
[http://dx.doi.org/10.1097/01.tp.0000250598.29377.13] [PMID: 17264818]

[59]   Stone KR, Walgenbach AW, Turek TJ, Somers DL, Wicomb W, Galili U. Anterior cruciate ligament reconstruction with a porcine xenograft: a serologic, histologic, and biomechanical study in primates. Arthroscopy 2007; 23(4): 411-9.
[http://dx.doi.org/10.1016/j.arthro.2006.12.024] [PMID: 17418335]

[60]   LaVecchio JA, Dunne AD, Edge AS. Enzymatic removal of alpha-galactosyl epitopes from porcine endothelial cells diminishes the cytotoxic effect of natural antibodies. Transplantation 1995; 60(8): 841-7.
[http://dx.doi.org/10.1097/00007890-199510270-00014] [PMID: 7482745]

[61]   Zheng MH, Chen J, Kirilak Y, Willers C, Xu J, Wood D. Porcine small intestine submucosa (SIS) is not an acellular collagenous matrix and contains porcine DNA: possible implications in human implantation. J Biomed Mater Res B Appl Biomater 2005; 73(1): 61-7.
[http://dx.doi.org/10.1002/jbm.b.30170] [PMID: 15736287]

[62]   Gilbert TW, Freund JM, Badylak SF. Quantification of DNA in biologic scaffold materials. J Surg Res 2009; 152(1): 135-9.
[http://dx.doi.org/10.1016/j.jss.2008.02.013] [PMID: 18619621]

[63]   Gilbert TW, Sellaro TL, Badylak SF. Decellularization of tissues and organs. Biomaterials 2006; 27(19): 3675-83.
[PMID: 16519932]

[64]   Anderson JM. Inflammatory response to implants, Trans. Am. Soc. Intern Organs 1988; 24: 101-7.

[65]   Hezi-Yamit A, Sullivan C, Wong J, *et al.* Impact of polymer hydrophilicity on biocompatibility:

implication for DES polymer design. J Biomed Mater Res A 2009; 90(1): 133-41.
[http://dx.doi.org/10.1002/jbm.a.32057] [PMID: 18491390]

[66]   Jones JA, Chang DT, Meyerson H, *et al.* Proteomic analysis and quantification of cytokines and chemokines from biomaterial surface-adherent macrophages and foreign body giant cells. J Biomed Mater Res A 2007; 83(3): 585-96.
[http://dx.doi.org/10.1002/jbm.a.31221] [PMID: 17503526]

[67]   Brown BN, Valentin JE, Stewart-Akers AM, McCabe GP, Badylak SF. Macrophage phenotype and remodeling outcomes in response to biologic scaffolds with and without a cellular component. Biomaterials 2009; 30(8): 1482-91.
[http://dx.doi.org/10.1016/j.biomaterials.2008.11.040] [PMID: 19121538]

[68]   Chen S, Jones JA, Xu Y, Low HY, Anderson JM, Leong KW. Characterization of topographical effects on macrophage behavior in a foreign body response model. Biomaterials 2010; 31(13): 3479-91.
[http://dx.doi.org/10.1016/j.biomaterials.2010.01.074] [PMID: 20138663]

[69]   Paul NE, Skazik C, Harwardt M, *et al.* Zwadlo-KlarwasserG.Topographical control of human macrophages by a regularly microstructuredpolyvinylidene fluoride surface. Biomaterials 2008; 29: 4056-64.
[http://dx.doi.org/10.1016/j.biomaterials.2008.07.010] [PMID: 18667233]

[70]   Kou PM, Babensee JE. Macrophage and dendritic cell phenotypic diversity in the context of biomaterials. J Biomed Mater Res A 2011; 96(1): 239-60.
[http://dx.doi.org/10.1002/jbm.a.32971] [PMID: 21105173]

[71]   Berman DM, Willman MA, Han D, *et al.* Mesenchymal stem cells enhance allogeneic islet engraftment in nonhuman primates. Diabetes 2010; 59: 2558-68.
[http://dx.doi.org/10.2337/db10-0136]

[72]   Bartholomew A, Polchert D, Szilagyi E, Douglas GW, Kenyon N. Mesenchymal stem cells in the induction of transplantation tolerance. Transplantation 2009; 87(9) (Suppl.): S55-7.
[http://dx.doi.org/10.1097/TP.0b013e3181a287e6] [PMID: 19424008]

[73]   Yazdimamaghani M, Razavi M, Vashaee D, Moharamzadeh K, Boccaccini AR, Tayebi L. Porous magnesium-based scaffolds for tissue engineering. Mater Sci Eng C 2017; 71: 1253-66.
[http://dx.doi.org/10.1016/j.msec.2016.11.027] [PMID: 27987682]

[74]   Jazayeri H, Tahriri M, Razavi M, *et al.* A current overview of materials and strategies for potential use in maxillofacial tissue regeneration. Mater Sci Eng C
[http://dx.doi.org/10.1016/j.msec.2016.08.055]

[75]   Yazdimamaghani M, Razavi M, Vashaee D, *et al. In vitro* analysis of Mg scaffolds coated with polymer/hydrogel/ceramic composite layers, Surface and Coatings Technology (Low-temperature deposition of bioceramic coatings) 301. 2016; 126-32.
[http://dx.doi.org/10.1016/j.surfcoat.2016.01.017]

[76]   Heidari F, Razavi M, E Bahrololoom M, *et al.* Mechanical properties of natural chitosan/hydroxyapatite/magnetite nanocomposites for tissue engineering applications. Mater Sci Eng C 2016; 65: 338-44.
[http://dx.doi.org/10.1016/j.msec.2016.04.039] [PMID: 27157760]

[77]   Fahmy MD, Jazayeri HE, Razavi M, Masri R, Tayebi L. Three-dimensional bioprinting materials with potential application in preprosthetic surgery. J Prosthodont 2016; 25(4): 310-8.
[http://dx.doi.org/10.1111/jopr.12431] [PMID: 26855004]

[78]   Khodaei M, Meratian M, Savabi O, Razavi M. The effect of pore structure on the mechanical properties of titanium scaffolds. Mater Lett 2016; 171: 308-11.
[http://dx.doi.org/10.1016/j.matlet.2016.02.101]

[79]   Jazayeri HE, Fahmy MD, Razavi M, *et al.* Dental applications of natural-origin polymers in hard and

soft tissue engineering. J Prosthodont 2016; 25(6): 510-7.
[http://dx.doi.org/10.1111/jopr.12465] [PMID: 27003096]

[80] Yazdimamaghani M, Razavi M, Mozafari M, Vashaee D, Kotturi H, Tayebi L. Biomineralization and biocompatibility studies of bone conductive scaffolds containing poly(3,4-ethylenedioxythiophene):poly(4-styrene sulfonate) (PEDOT:PSS). J Mater Sci Mater Med 2015; 26(12): 274-84.
[http://dx.doi.org/10.1007/s10856-015-5599-8] [PMID: 26543020]

[81] Yazdimamaghani M, Razavi M, Vashaee D, Pothineni VR, Rajadas J, Tayebi L. Significant degradability enhancement in multilayer coating of polycaprolactone-bioactive glass/gelatin-bioactive glass on magnesium scaffold for tissue engineering applications. Appl Surf Sci 2015; 338: 137-45.
[http://dx.doi.org/10.1016/j.apsusc.2015.02.120]

[82] Yazdimamaghani M, Razavi M, Vashaee D, Tayebi L. Surface modification of biodegradable porous Mg bone scaffold using polycaprolactone/bioactive glass composite. Mater Sci Eng C 2015; 49: 436-44.
[http://dx.doi.org/10.1016/j.msec.2015.01.041] [PMID: 25686970]

[83] Yazdimamaghani M, Razavi M, Vashaee D, Tayebi L. Development and degradation behavior of magnesium scaffolds coated with polycaprolactone for bone tissue engineering. Mater Lett 2014; 132: 106-10.
[http://dx.doi.org/10.1016/j.matlet.2014.06.036]

[84] Yazdimamaghani M, Razavi M, Vashaee D, Tayebi L. Microstructural and mechanical study of PCL coated Mg scaffolds. Surf Eng 2014; 30: 920-6.
[http://dx.doi.org/10.1179/1743294414Y.0000000307]

[85] Song T-H, Jang J, Choi Y-J, Shim J-H, Cho D-W. 3D-printed drug/cell carrier enabling effective release of cyclosporin A for xenogeneic cell-based therapy. Cell Transplant 2015; 24(12): 2513-25.
[http://dx.doi.org/10.3727/096368915X686779] [PMID: 25608278]

CHAPTER 9

Future Perspectives of Porous Scaffolds

Farnaz Naghizadeh*

Biomedical Engineering Faculty, Amirkabir University of Technology (Tehran Polytechnic), Tehran, Iran

Abstract: In the present chapter, the future perspective and the current challenges of porous scaffolds design will be described. In addition, the state of the art in this field and what we can expect from future generations of porous scaffolds will be discussed. The difficulties in bridging the gap between research and clinical practice have also been outlined.

Keywords: Challenges, Porous scaffolds, Regenerative medicine and future perspectives, Tissue engineering.

INTRODUCTION

The aim of tissue engineering is to mimic what takes place in natural tissues [1]. In previous chapters, a variety of materials that were used for scaffolds fabrication have been described; however, shortage of good quality and efficacy is still the main issue in fabricated scaffolds. Generally, a desired kind of scaffold has proper mechanical strength, flexibility, degradation rate, cell binding, cellular uptake and biocompatibility that can maintain, induce and repair biological functions where growth factors, cells and ECM are required [2, 3].

The solution of appropriate materials in hybrid form is essential to prepare appropriate scaffolds for use in different sites of the body. Combining the advantage of materials alongside tailored structure for specific application is the main challenge for scaffold fabrication among researchers. Depending on defected site, specific properties are needed to facilitate matching of scaffold to surrounded tissue. Consequently, depending on the scaffold application, different challenges and limitations are arisen.

Properties of prepared scaffold strongly depend on applied basics for the design of scaffold. Through incorporating experiments and computer modeling (simulation-

* **Corresponding author Farnaz Naghizadeh:** Biomedical Engineering Faculty, Amirkabir University of Technology (Tehran Polytechnic), Tehran, Iran; Tel: +989126983254; Fax: +9821-22214511; E-mails: f.naghizadeh@aut.ac.ir; f.naghizadeh@gmail.com

based) acts, more effective method to develop scaffolds will be enabled. However, plenty of essential researches are still required prior to comprehensive understanding of all the biological specifications for a precise scaffold design [4].

SCAFFOLDING BIOMATERIALS AND TECHNOLOGY

Polymer-based Biomaterials

One of the most attractive categories of composite scaffolds in tissue engineering is combination of biodegradable polymers and inorganic bioactive materials because of their bioactive property, modifiable biodegradation rate and shapability [5, 6]. However, their vital role may be enhanced by combining with stem cell seeding as described in previous studies [7]. Uneven degradation rate of most polymers and their faster degradation rate in comparison with most of the ceramic materials in polymer/ceramic composites cause problems like osteolysis. Thus, matching degradation rate of polymers and ceramics is essential for an equal resorption process in the scaffolds.

The major challenge during fabrication of polymer/bioceramic composite scaffolds is balancing the appropriate amount of porosity and mechanical properties to ensure that the scaffold not only withstands physiological loads, but also allow for new tissue growth. As these properties exhibit an inverse relationship, it is often not feasible to have desirable properties in both respects, and in many cases, one property must be selected over another. Future challenges include how to improve the mechanical properties of the scaffolds without sacrificing the porosity or degradation rate [6].

New investigation on the interaction between stem cells and polymer/inorganic composite interfaces has become a hot topic among researchers. Seeding stem cells on the composite scaffolds allows the scaffolds to mimic complex native biological functions that may lead to tissue regeneration. Moreover, lack of information regarding the long-term effects of bioceramic scaffolds in the body is another interesting area of current research. For instance, implanted HA scaffold in human body could degrade only about 10% after 4 years. Consequently, release of the HA crystals in implanted area may lead to inflammation. Thus, further investigation on the interaction between seeded stem cells and the biopolymer/ inorganic composites associated with long term *in vitro* and *in vivo* assays is unavoidable to facilitate fabrication of the appropriate scaffold with potential use in clinic [8].

The mechanical integrity of man-made composite scaffolds is still at least one order of magnitude lower than that of cancellous or cortical bone. Achieving the mechanical properties of bone might also allow replacement of bigger parts of damaged bone tissue than what is possible today. Thus, despite the increase of interfacial bonding and overall mechanical properties of composites achieved by introduction of nano size particles as surfactants, their impact on degradation kinetics and cytotoxicity of the composite are mostly unknown and remain unexplored. Moreover, another related challenge that requires further investigation is the long-term *in vitro* and *in vivo* characterization of the porous 3D scaffold composites specifically regarding the long-term effect of the incorporation of inorganic bioactive phases on the degradation and ion release kinetics and the local impact of growth factors on the cell and tissue systems in these highly porous systems. In conclusion, despite the recent progress in tissue engineering, an appropriate design and fabrication method to ensure preparation of reproducible bioactive and biodegradable constructs with tailored structure remains a challenge. Moreover, the fabricated 3D constructs need to be stable for expected time even under load-bearing surroundings [7].

Amorphous Calcium Phosphate (ACP) is another important polymer based biomaterial that has been used as filler in dental monomers in different composite forms due to its outstanding biocompatibility. It could help in the formation of biological hydroxyapatite in bioactive polymeric composites. Previously, different tactics have been used to improve the properties of the ACP by hybridizing with altered elements like silica and zirconia, which led to generation of composites with improved mechanical and remineralizing properties. In the last few years, additional adjustments in resin formulations were carried out through diverse studies to solve the crucial problem of polymerization shrinkage (*PS*) of the ACP composites. Current researches have focused on applying ACP as sealants and/or base/liner. Subsequently, ongoing studies concentrate on reformulation of resins/ACP composites to prevent demineralization in orthodontically treated teeth and to increase remineralization of white spots [9].

Hydrogels

Hydrogels are ideal candidate materials in the field of tissue engineering as none of the natural hydrogels have sufficient stiffness to function immediately *in vivo*. Mixing natural polymers with synthetic polymers was an applied tactic to reach better stiffness. However, in order to produce sufficiently stiff synthetic scaffold, the problem is that almost all cross-linking agents are cytotoxic at the required levels. Thus, further investigation was suggested to prepare toxic free hydrogels [10, 11].

Metallic Scaffolds

Similar to other scaffolds, metallic scaffolds have their own challenges. For instance, porous metallic scaffolds are used to replace the damaged bone and they meet the mechanical necessities of bone, but fail to offer the required integration between implant and tissue along with the issue of metal ion leaching. Biochemically-modified porous metallic scaffolds were reported to be more suitable for load-bearing applications compared to biodegradable scaffolds. The biochemically modified Ti scaffolds by the use of growth factors and osteoprogenitor cells were reported as a potential bone-healing construct. However, a key requirement of the use of this scaffold in a clinical environment is an outstanding long-term result, which has not as yet been obtained. Moreover, the (Mg) scaffolds were one of the interesting metallic scaffolds in the last few years and in spite of the recent report for *in vivo* biocompatibility of magnesium, further *in vitro* and *in vivo* assays are strongly required for upcoming researches to evaluate this construct properly. Current researches in the metallic scaffolds field focus on improving the rapid prototyping technique (RP) for fabrication of particular low costs structures, which give long-term mechanical consistency in the metal-bone interface. Furthermore, the efficient combinations of osteoinductive materials and growth factors with the metallic scaffolds, along with using cell-based tissue regeneration approach, will probably help to repair damaged bone tissues in the future studies. Consequently, the remaining challenges for metallic scaffolds include metal ion release, limited bioactivity and biodegradation that are under extensive researches. However, a perfectly controlled metallic scaffold still remains to be developed [12].

Gradient Fabrication of Scaffolds

In tissue engineering approaches, certain tissues of the body such as osteochondral (OC) tissue with interface between the soft and hard tissue (cartilage and bone) require complex design and technique for the replacing scaffold. The multilayer or stratified scaffolds were designed to fulfill present day requirements for scaffolds aimed at OC defect repair through different researches. However, fabrication of scaffolds with graded composition or structure to create integrated interface between the two tissues remains a key challenge that requires further study. Designing proper gradient scaffold can eliminate the delamination problem in the currently available multilayer scaffolds [13, 14].

STEM CELL-BASED TISSUE ENGINEERING

Stem Cells

Stem cell incorporation into scaffolds is a promising trend for fabrication of future composite biomaterials due to their great adaptability to the biological environment [15, 16]. Differentiation of stem cells led to local cell function adaptation on the stem cell-seeded scaffolds and as a result, mimicking the complicated local biological functions became possible on the surface of scaffolds. This new finding may facilitate growth of new tissues and organs in both *in vitro* and *in vivo* assays [7, 17].

Subsequently, the interface of stem cells and scaffolds are at the moment the center of attention, including growth factor incorporation and cell adhesion [7]. Among different cell lines, embryonic and adult stem cells represent an ideal cell source for tissue engineering according to previous reports. However, biomaterials and their characteristics can potentially influence, for example, stem cell proliferation and differentiation in both positive and negative ways. Thus, stem cell-based therapies using biomaterial scaffolds require a strict and complete assessment of parameters such as material topography, cell adhesion, morphology, viability, proliferation, cytotoxicity and apoptosis. All these parameters have to be analyzed and matched into a basic assessment to further knowledge in this field [18].

Dental

The dental stem cell–based therapy introduced novel concepts in regenerative dentistry for the treatment of tooth loss, cavities, periodontitis and the craniofacial regions. Moreover, application of dental stem cells has recently been initiated in clinic with certain essential challenges regarding cell migration or dying in the recipient site, obtaining the adequate number of stem cells, short-term viability of cells and insufficient differentiation capability of cells for tissue regeneration. Thus, the process of mimicking correct tooth morphogenesis is in early stages by current tactics and several obstacles are still to be overcome such as immune rejection and ethical issues on the use of human embryos, unsuitable embryonic environment that limit the differentiation capability of bone marrow cells into tooth germ cells and inappropriate substitute for the embryonic oral epithelium, which has a unique set of signals for odontogenesis. In spite of solving all these problems, the meaning of the appropriate scaffold and the induction of adequate neovascularization are the remained questions to be answered. Thus, additional researches in this area are inevitable in order to overcome all these obstacles [19].

Neural System

In spite of the altered progress in nerve regeneration, the clinical outcomes were unsatisfactory and there is a long way to reach effective peripheral nervous system (PNS) regeneration. To overcome the inherent regenerative intricacy of human nerves, the precise design of both scaffolds and animal experiments is strongly required. As a new approach, the exogenous bioactive agents were added to the PNS regeneration devices, however due to the complexity of such constructs, their clinical application is quite challenging and not reachable in near future. Subsequently, precise design of scaffold porosity with optimized surface area and contact guidance may decrease the remaining gap between man-made conduits and efficient auto grafts [20].

Moreover, the mechanisms of neurogenesis and brain development have been investigated in general. Thus, crucial questions endure regarding the generation of neuronal diversity and how this can be duplicated *in vitro*. The researchers reported the NSC potency is directly related to the spatial and temporal location of NSCs *in vivo* or to the methods of their derivation and subsequent handling *in vitro*. According to *in vivo* findings, the exact order of neurogenesis, neuronal fate determination, and final locating are critical factors for proper formation of efficient connections. Consequently, the direct differentiation of specific types of neurons and to place them in the suitable location for their functional integration is the remaining big challenge. Furthermore, basic mechanisms of cell fate choices to the details of circuit formation are questions that must be answered precisely. Many of these upcoming understandings may simplify the way to clinical use of transplanted cells in neural system [21].

Cardiovascular System

Cell-based therapy has recently demonstrated promising results about inhibition of the heart failure progress. In this regard, the MSCs are under extensive researches with an optimistic potential in terms of cardiovascular tissue repair [22]. Moreover, bone marrow-derived progenitor cells and other progenitor cells can differentiate into vascular cell types and restore blood flow. More recently, resident cardiac stem cells have been shown to differentiate into multiple cell types present in the heart including cardiac muscle cells. Despite all progress, the number of differentiated and functionally integrated myocytes derived from transplanted stem cells is too small to explain the observed improvements in cardiac function in most studies [23].

Conclusively, achieving the longer-term goal of true cardiac regeneration will probably require more than simply injecting the right type of cells in the right place. Thus, key knowledge is required to understand cardiomyocyte development and turnover both in normal and after injury development. Moreover, investigation on cells regeneration potential of bone-marrow-derived progenitor cell, choosing the best progenitor cells for therapy, ethical barriers, extreme risk for teratoma formation in using of embryonic stem (ES) cells, optimal isolation and culture procedures of cancer stem cells (CSCs), understanding the mechanisms by which each of the stem-cell or progenitor-cell types can affect myocardial performance, determining the optimal route for delivery of cells, obtaining an adequately large cell graft with suitable structural and functional characteristics, long-term survival of transplanted cells, long-term electromechanical strength and proper electromechanical integration with host tissue are essential remaining challenges that need further investigation to address obstacles in cardiac regeneration [23].

Liver and Kidney

Liver is a complex and central organ in the body with a high-density blood vessel network. Thus, fabrication of a functional liver scaffold as a substitute is one of the most difficult approaches that have not been achieved via available methods and knowledge. Available strategies for liver tissue engineering are followed worldwide, including live donor organ transplantation, partial liver grafts, hepatocyte transplantation, extracorporeal devices and stem cell therapy [24]. Recently, decellularized liver tissue was reported as a potential scaffold for creating a practical liver tissue using tissue engineering technology [25]. However, cell-based therapies demonstrated great prospective for treatment of liver failure *via* adult, embryonic and induced pluripotent stem cells that have been successfully differentiated into functional hepatocytes. Recently, induced pluripotent stem cells (iPSCs) have been suggested to be an excellent cell source for liver tissue engineering and have been differentiated to hepatocytes by several groups [25]. However, concerns over the use of viral vectors, changes in cell cycle regulators and teratoma formation are still limiting the application of iPS cells for liver regenerative therapy [24]. Thus, using genetically identical (isogenic) cells is a potentially important point in developing future autologous therapies [26].

Consequently, the availability of suitable cell types, achieving completely efficient protocol for the differentiation of stem cells into functionally mature hepatocytes and deep understanding of the cellular signaling during the differentiation of stem cells into functional hepatocytes and maintenance of mature hepatocyte function are essential challenges in liver tissue regeneration that need to be investigated in depth in future researches [24].

Moreover, kidney is another organ with complex tissues in the human body. Kidney regeneration approaches were categorized as cell-on-scaffold seeding technology (CSST), developmental biology, stem cell, 3D printing and kidney-o--a-chip technologies. Stem cells may represent a valuable source of cells for the reconstitution of the kidney tissue. However, cells succeed only when they are located in their natural niche, the native ECM, for which they have been specifically designed.

Several synthetic or natural scaffolds are used for kidney regeneration. However, due to specific characteristics of natural ECM scaffolds, they are considered as preferred platforms for CSST. The ECM plays an essential role in keeping the organism alive *via* providing mechanical and structural support to cells and tissues along with controlling cellular physiology and fate. Despite progress in the development of transplantable kidney organoids using acellular ECM scaffolds, several key challenges need to be overcome. An in-depth understanding of the human kidney development process, the self-repair mechanisms of the kidney, *in vivo* test on large animal models, calculation of needed oxygen, nutrients and energy to complete the kidney regeneration, modifying the strategies to recellularize ECM scaffolds, proper cell choice without risk of tumorigenesis and obtaining efficient bioreactors and mathematical models are some of the important challenges. Consequently, researchers require in-depth knowledge to overcome the above mentioned challenges that exist in kidney tissue engineering field [27].

Skin Tissue

At the present time, there are no models of a synthetic skin that are able to completely duplicate the natural intact skin properties. Along with natural polymers, several synthetic degradable gels to deliver cells and/or molecules *in situ* were developed as smart matrixes.

In cell therapy researches for skin, the autologous cells have represented the potential advantages for burns and trauma repairs with the capability to easily scale up for clinic. Generally, tissue or organ repair is accompanied by fibrotic reactions that led to scar formation. However, embryonic or fetal skin and the ear of the MRL/MpJ mouse were reported as successful examples for complete regeneration along with elimination of fibrosis and scarring in host tissue. In addition, non-viral gene delivery and stem cell technologies may also contribute to novel approaches that would generate a skin replacement. Identification of the factors and cytokines expressed during regeneration and including them to create a smart matrix for skin regeneration, understanding and exploiting the mechanisms of embryonic development, stem cell biology and biomaterial engineering are considered as key points to achieve next generation skin substitutes.

Despite of all progress in skin tissue engineering, current techniques cannot restore all functions of natural skin by means of existing skin substitutes. Thus, complete regeneration of functional skin and a scar-free integration with the surrounding host tissue requires advanced future investigations [28].

Musculoskeletal System

MSC transplantation is one of the new approaches for the treatment of osteoporosis. Obtaining high amount of MSCs with engraftment capability and potential differentiation ability are two key points that should be considered carefully to promise successful engraftment. Certainly, the focus of researchers on advanced biomaterials and bioreactor design will facilitate the bone regeneration capability and osseointegration in the cell-seeded scaffolds through increasing the osteogenic commitment of MSCs in *ex vivo* cultivation conditions.

Conclusively, the existed challenges in bone regeneration through cell implantation include heightened amount of cell engraftment in implanted bone location, enhanced ability of cells to reconstruct osteoid tissue and increased understanding of basic mechanisms regarding the survival proliferation and differentiation capability of the MSCs. Thus, further researches will ease limitless generation of the capable MSCs for bone treatment in clinic [29]. In the following section, bone scaffolds and the related challenges will be described in detail.

Bone Scaffolds

Bone scaffolds are one of the most successful samples among all scaffolds today. In bone tissue engineering, the main concern after biocompatibility is mimicking the natural mechanical properties of bone tissue. The mechanical support and interior space are considered as two key factors for cell adhesion, proliferation and differentiation, along with tissue formation. Moreover, pore sizes and porosity have inverse effect on mechanical properties. Thus, an optimized structure should be designed for appropriate mechanical properties and bone tissue ingrowth concurrently. Optimized hybrids from bone-mineral like materials and ECM-derived biomolecules have been considered as proper scaffold materials in recent years.

However, surface functionalization has an important role in fabrication of future biomimetic scaffolds by creating tailored surface chemistry and structure leading to effective bone tissue regeneration. A promising approach of surface functionalization is related to the movement restriction of proteins and growth factors on the surface of scaffold, which apply as a post processing method.

Parallel infection control of the wound and bone regenerating after surgery is another essential point in bone tissue engineering that requires further study. To avoid infection, the addition of drugs into scaffolds has been proposed (*i.e.* antibiotics) as a tactic to reduce the probability of infection.

To control the degradation rate of materials, understanding their degradation mechanisms is essential. The degradation rate can be improved by proper design of structures, chemical constituents and coatings depending on specific applications [2].

Sufficient vascular infiltration and bone ingrowth are desirable properties in the prepared scaffolds. Thus, lack of proper vascularity is still a foremost challenge in scaffolds preparation and the strategies for obtaining modified vascularization are considered as one of the widespread research areas in tissue engineering field. One method to increase vascularization might to be engineer microvasculature by cells in the scaffolds before implantation process [1].

Current researchers have suggested different tactics to prevent fibrous tissue formation along with enhanced vascularization in implanted scaffolds. For instance, addition of growth factors and modified cells (with higher release levels of angiogenic vascular endothelial growth factor) *via* the scaffold or coating the scaffold with anti-inflammatory molecules were helpful tactics at the present time.

Achieving homogenous blend of materials in hybrid composite scaffolds is essential to improve the mechanical properties and obtain better quality scaffolds. For example, polymeric-metal composites could achieve homogenous blends with remarkable mechanical properties using cryomilling technology as reported previously [30]. Although many studies about different blends of hybrids have been reported, there is not enough information about homogenous blends and its effect on scaffold properties.

Recently, using bioreactors along with scaffolds, stem cells and growth factors were recommended to confirm cellular distribution and enhanced bone formation [30]. To increase the bone-healing rate, addition of biomolecules like growth factors has been suggested in recent years. Although several researches have accomplished biomolecule incorporation during scaffold preparation, this is still a challenging area of research due to sensitivity of biomolecules to high temperatures and risky chemical environments.

The incorporation of osteoinductive proteins along with an osteoconductive carrier medium has been recommended to aid proper delivery or appropriate material for bone scaffold formation. For example, the BMP as an extremely active osteoinductive growth factor can initiate prompt regeneration of bone. Despite progress in bone regeneration, the repair is limited to small bone defects because of poor vascularization. Moreover, lack of adequate mechanical stability in most of the prepared scaffolds and the presence of non-biodegradable materials in some of them that may lead to infection in long-term are two remaining challenges [30]. Thus, to achieve regeneration of bigger bone defects, the mechanical integrity similar to real bone is an inevitable factor for the fabricated scaffolds, which is not easily reachable currently.

Choosing proper animal models to assess new bone tissue engineering approaches is another serious challenge in pre-clinical researches. Despite several *in vivo* studies accomplished on small animals like mice, the results are not adequately reliable due to big differences in graft size and healing process. Thus, using large animal models due to similarity with humans has been suggested as preferable choice in preclinical studies [31].

Therefore, novel borderlines of research should focus on improved bone tissue regeneration *via* mimicking the natural process of bone healing. For example, combining angiogenesis and osteogenesis properties along with progenitor cell recruitment and differentiation has been suggested [32].

Moreover, delivery of the biomolecules gradually and continually has significant role in controlling the natural bone remodeling process through an unknown mechanism.

Homogeneous distribution of porosity throughout most man-made scaffolds is not desirable due to dissimilarity to natural bone. Natural bone possesses higher porosity in the core with a durable and dense outer shell. Thus, fabrication of similar constructs with mechanical integrity and interconnectivity requires complex design and fabrication process. To obtain desirable bone scaffolds, appropriate selection of biomaterials, proper geometry, pore size and size distribution and controlled release of biomolecules are the main required factors [33].

As a final point, despite several reports for short term success of scaffolds for bone regeneration, long term success is main requirement to guarantee the potential usage of bone scaffolds [34]. Reaching this goal and optimized properties for bone scaffolds is not easily reachable without applying interdisciplinary approaches in future scaffold development [32].

Evaluation Techniques

In Vitro and In Vivo Experiments

In vitro and *in vivo* experiments are necessary to access and identify the cellular and molecular events in the physiological processes (angiogenesis, osteogenesis *etc.*) occurring in the tissues exposed to biomaterials [35]. *In vitro* studies are reproducible test conditions that can address the challenges of *in vivo* complexity and anticipate what will be happen *in vivo* for the *in vitro*-grown scaffolds. Briefly, bioreactors, scaffolds, and mechanical conditioning are three *in vitro* culture parameters, and by manipulation of these parameters, it is possible to change the growth rate, integration and functionality of the engineered tissues. Recently, these parameters are discovered in combination with novel growth factors, biomaterials, gene therapies and other emerging technologies [36].

In vivo studies reveal the safety and efficacy of a tissue engineered construct in rigorous animal models. Further understanding of evolving *in vivo* healing process for different tissues lead to fabrication of proper construct *in vitro*. However, most of the prepared constructs do not have *in vivo* reports yet. In addition, the controversial result for *in vitro* and *in vivo* studies is another obstacle that emphasizes the importance of additional precise researches [37].

Several growth factors could accelerate the normal process of wound healing *in vivo*, which is in line with the findings *in vitro*. However, the mechanisms by which grows factors initiate and propagate the processes are still unrevealed points. Thus, experimental strategies continue to focus on *in vitro* and *in vivo* properties of growth factors.

Conclusively, the challenge for the future is to develop tissue substitutes that restore the normal biochemical functions of living tissues in addition to their structural features. Thus, additional development of proper *in vitro* and *in vivo* models is required to further realize the intricacy of cell-scaffold interactions and the process of induced regeneration. Moreover, design of scaffold should be based on a detailed understanding of the molecular and cellular basis of tissue regulation that is possible through the new upcoming *in vitro* and *in vivo* methodologies [38].

Immune Aspects of Scaffold Design

The immune system response is a key factor that has direct influence on regeneration process of the tissues. To overcome rejection of scaffolds by immune reaction, several strategies have been applied such as particular material design, anti-inflammatory cytokine delivery and immune cell recruitment/transplantation to control the local immune response in order to promote regeneration. Generally, the process of transplanting cells, implanting biomaterial scaffolds, or delivering inductive factors can stimulate the immune reaction. Some technologies have the potential to turn the immune response into an asset for regeneration, leading to the differentiation of cells toward a more regenerative and less inflammatory phenotype. For example, recruitment or delivery of immune cells can be employed as a means to prevent rejection of transplanted cells by host tissue.

So the current technologies have broad implications for numerous applications of biomaterials in medicine, and also in emerging area of cell-based therapies [39]. The potential of biomaterials to modulate immune cell function encouraging the design of biomaterials capable of eliciting appropriate immune responses at implantation sites was confirmed previously. Thus, such biomaterials should be designed with altered material and surface properties to target cell behavior in a scientific way.

Some solutions were suggested such as immunomodulation by surface modifications of biomaterials, immunomodulation by incorporation of bioactive molecules, provision of integrin adhesion sites, coupling of anti-inflammatory drugs to biomaterials, delivery of growth factors, designing "immunomodulating" biomaterials based on artificial ECM, using hydrogels and the artificial ECM coatings for synthetic implants and immunomodulating effects of the ECM coatings. Of all the mentioned tactics, functionalization of biomaterials with artificial ECM coatings appears to be particularly promising method [40].

Additional Topics in Scaffolding Technology

The three other important points regarding scaffolds are nano powders combination in scaffolds, scaffolds for delivery systems and the recent fabrication techniques that will be briefly described in the following sections.

Nano Powders

Nano powders are one of materials that have been widely used in scaffolds fabrication to manipulate and improve scaffolds properties in recent years; however, corporation of nanoparticles in hybrid scaffolds like inorganic / polymer scaffolds is one of the unknown concerns that require more consideration in future researches. There is as yet no decisive evidence of a recognized human toxic response caused by nanoparticles. On the other hand, effects on animals are simply not comparable with a human case. In addition, there are some adverse reports about the toxicity of nano powders. Therefore, lack of standardization in characterization of nano powders and their testing methods with biological systems require specific investigation. The corporation of nanoparticles led to hold biological components on the surface and heighten cellular adhesion and proliferation, which also requires extensive research. Most nano powders that are used in tissue engineering are bio-ceramic, which is an important subset for tissue regeneration and drug release; however, there is shortage of information about their long-term influences on the body. In a previous report, inflammation in implanted area was reported for Hydroxyapatite (HA). Therefore extra *in vitro* and *in vivo* studies and further studies in biological system are unavoidable to achieve clinical application of scaffolds [8].

Delivery Systems

Using scaffolds as delivery systems has attracted the attention of researchers in the last few years. Generally, they have recently been used to deliver peptides, growth factors, cytokines and therapeutic genes. Pore size and existed micropores in scaffolds are essential factors to control the delivery efficiency and determine the rate of delivery. The optimized micropores in scaffolds can deliver the biomolecules in a time-dependent manner, which is vital for the development of future scaffolds. Moreover, the cells behavior can be controlled by means of precise mechanical properties in scaffolds and by biological and biochemical signals from the extracellular matrix [1].

Scaffold Fabrication Techniques

Recently, some modified and additive (combined) techniques (AM) have been introduced to eliminate the shortcomings and limitations of the existing conventional techniques for fabrication of scaffolds [41].

The regular scaffolds fabrication techniques in combination with the AM techniques have recently been used to achieve balanced composite structures. This approach has helped to duplicate complex tissue structures and to improve the vascularization or other biological processes in scaffolds [4]. Several remarkable improvements were reported for the scaffolds fabricated by AM techniques such as preparation of tailored structures, enhanced control over the macroscopic and microscopic shape of the scaffolds and the optimization of properties applicable in bone tissue engineering on a micro and nanometre scale such as osteoconductivity, osteoinductivity *etc.* It is predicted that AM techniques may help to initiate new paths not only in regenerative medicine but also in Personalized Medicine [42].

Despite progress in several areas, controlling structure of scaffolds along with their surface chemistry has not yet been achieved by conventional techniques. However, further researches are required to fabricate scaffold with detailed and graded structures [43]. As a result, the convergence of electrospinning with rapid prototyping technologies could be a promising approach to merge the strengths of both methodologies and minimize their weaknesses [4]. In brief, the ideal strategy should aim at a 'cell-friendly' production process that should ideally take place in a sterile environment [11].

Recommendations for Future Works

There are some overall suggestions for future work on the scaffolds design especially for bone tissue engineering scaffolds. Although some of these suggestions are the subject of ongoing researches, either at the present time or within the last few years, further study is required in order to expand the scaffolds applications. They are summarized as below:

1. Improve the quality and efficacy of available scaffolds.
2. Investigation on toxicity effect of nano powder additives.
3. Further vascularity in scaffolds.

4. Match mechanical property with surrounded tissue.
5. Optimization of mechanical and biological properties.
6. Utilization of bioreactors more extensively.
7. Investigation on nanopowders' effect on cell adhesion.
8. Novel hybrid materials with proper structure for specific applications.
9. Combining experiments and simulation techniques for improved design of scaffolds.
10. Expansion of Additive Manufacturing techniques and improving current scaffold fabrication techniques.
11. Scaffold's surface functionalization and modification.
12. Investigation on obtaining homogenous blend of materials and integrity in scaffolds.
13. Development of scaffolds for repair of large defects.
14. Investigation on long term effects of biomaterials in the body.
15. Adding "stimuli responsive property" in scaffolds for new tissue growth.
16. Investigation on biomechanical, biological and biochemical signals and their effects on cell behaviour.
17. Stem cell and biomolecule incorporation and investigation on their effects.
18. Further *in vitro* and *in vivo* tests especially on large animals.
19. Controlled degradation rate of scaffolds to match the regeneration rate of natural tissue.
20. Matching polymers and ceramics degradation rates in composite scaffolds to avoid residual material issue.
21. Tailored porous structure that mimics natural tissue structure.
22. Further investigation on scaffold/cell interaction in artificial 3D environment.
23. Obtaining long-term success of scaffolds in bone regeneration.
24. Cost effective Tissue Engineering strategies.

CONCLUDING REMARKS

In conclusion, designing biomimetic scaffolds for different organs is a very complicated process and the interaction of several factors leads to increased intricacy. Despite the availability of some clinically engineered biomimetic products, there is still a long way to go to reach the ideal scaffold(s) for tissue engineering *via* new materials, improved techniques and precisely balanced factors [2]. Nevertheless, considerable progress has been made throughout last decade and further *in vitro* and *in vivo* studies are strongly needed to reach the ideal constructs. Finally, we predict that the future discussion will turn towards the identification of the most cost-effective tissue engineering strategies.

CONFLICT OF INTEREST

The author declares no conflict of interest, financial or otherwise.

ACKNOWLEDGEMENTS

The author would like to thank Iran's National Elites Foundation (INEF) for financial support and the Department of Biomedical Engineering, Amirkabir University of Technology (Tehran Polytechnic) for their facilities.

REFERENCES

[1]   O'brien FJ. Biomaterials & scaffolds for tissue engineering. Mater Today 2011; 14(3): 88-95.
[http://dx.doi.org/10.1016/S1369-7021(11)70058-X]

[2]   Billström GH, Blom AW, Larsson S, Beswick AD. Application of scaffolds for bone regeneration strategies: current trends and future directions. Injury 2013; 44 (Suppl. 1): S28-33.
[http://dx.doi.org/10.1016/S0020-1383(13)70007-X] [PMID: 23351866]

[3]   Oshida Y. Bioscience and bioengineering of titanium materials. Elsevier 2010.

[4]   Giannitelli SM, Accoto D, Trombetta M, Rainer A. Current trends in the design of scaffolds for computer-aided tissue engineering. Acta Biomater 2014; 10(2): 580-94.
[http://dx.doi.org/10.1016/j.actbio.2013.10.024] [PMID: 24184176]

[5]   Yunos DM, Bretcanu O, Boccaccini AR. Polymer-bioceramic composites for tissue engineering scaffolds. J Mater Sci 2008; 43(13): 4433-42.
[http://dx.doi.org/10.1007/s10853-008-2552-y]

[6]   Naghizadeh F, Sultana N, Abdul Kadir MR, Muzaffar T, Hussain R, Kamarul T. The Fabrication and Characterization of PCL/Rice husk derived bioactive glass-ceramic composite scaffolds. Journal of Nanomaterials 2014; 2014

[7]   Rezwan K, Chen QZ, Blaker JJ, Boccaccini AR. Biodegradable and bioactive porous polymer/inorganic composite scaffolds for bone tissue engineering. Biomaterials 2006; 27(18): 3413-31.
[http://dx.doi.org/10.1016/j.biomaterials.2006.01.039] [PMID: 16504284]

[8]   Okamoto M, John B. Synthetic biopolymer nanocomposites for tissue engineering scaffolds. Prog Polym Sci 2013; 38(10): 1487-503.
[http://dx.doi.org/10.1016/j.progpolymsci.2013.06.001]

[9]   Skrtic D, Antonucci JM, Eanes ED. Amorphous Calcium Phosphate-Based Bioactive Polymeric Composites for Mineralized Tissue Regeneration. J Res Natl Inst Stand Technol 2003; 108(3): 167-82.
[http://dx.doi.org/10.6028/jres.108.017] [PMID: 27413603]

[10]   Cheung HY, Lau KT, Lu TP, Hui D. A critical review on polymer-based bio-engineered materials for scaffold development. Compos, Part B Eng 2007; 38(3): 291-300.
[http://dx.doi.org/10.1016/j.compositesb.2006.06.014]

[11]   Van Vlierberghe S, Graulus GJ, Samal SK, Dubruel P. Porous hydrogel biomedical foam scaffolds for tissue repair. In: Netti, P, Ed. Biomedical foams for tissue engineering applications. 1st ed. Woodhead Publishing, 2014: p. 335.
[http://dx.doi.org/10.1533/9780857097033.2.335]

[12]   Alvarez K, Nakajima H. Metallic scaffolds for bone regeneration. Materials (Basel) 2009; 2(3): 790-832.
[http://dx.doi.org/10.3390/ma2030790]

[13]   Di Luca A, Van Blitterswijk C, Moroni L. The osteochondral interface as a gradient tissue: from development to the fabrication of gradient scaffolds for regenerative medicine. Birth Defects Res C Embryo Today 2015; 105(1): 34-52.

[http://dx.doi.org/10.1002/bdrc.21092] [PMID: 25777257]

[14] Dormer NH, Berkland CJ, Detamore MS. Emerging techniques in stratified designs and continuous gradients for tissue engineering of interfaces. Ann Biomed Eng 2010; 38(6): 2121-41.
[http://dx.doi.org/10.1007/s10439-010-0033-3] [PMID: 20411333]

[15] Fallahiarezoudar E, Ahmadipourroudposht M, Idris A, Mohd Yusof N. A review of: application of synthetic scaffold in tissue engineering heart valves. Mater Sci Eng C 2015; 48: 556-65.
[http://dx.doi.org/10.1016/j.msec.2014.12.016] [PMID: 25579957]

[16] Vacanti CA. Tribute to the Vacantis. J Cell Mol Med 2006; 10(1): 2-2.
[http://dx.doi.org/10.1111/j.1582-4934.2006.tb00284.x]

[17] Denry I, Kuhn LT. Design and characterization of calcium phosphate ceramic scaffolds for bone tissue engineering. Dent Mater 2015.
[PMID: 26423007]

[18] Neuss S, Apel C, Buttler P, *et al.* Assessment of stem cell/biomaterial combinations for stem cell-based tissue engineering. Biomaterials 2008; 29(3): 302-13.
[http://dx.doi.org/10.1016/j.biomaterials.2007.09.022] [PMID: 17935776]

[19] Zivkovic P, Petrovic V, Najman S, Stefanovic V. Stem cell-based dental tissue engineering. Sci World J 2010; 10: 901-16.
[http://dx.doi.org/10.1100/tsw.2010.81] [PMID: 20495769]

[20] Madaghiele. M and L Salvatore, Tailoring the pore structure of foam scaffolds for nerve regeneration. Biomedical Foams for Tissue Engineering Applications 2014; p. 101.

[21] Breunig JJ, Haydar TF, Rakic P. Neural stem cells: historical perspective and future prospects. Neuron 2011; 70(4): 614-25.
[http://dx.doi.org/10.1016/j.neuron.2011.05.005] [PMID: 21609820]

[22] Pittenger MF, Martin BJ. Mesenchymal stem cells and their potential as cardiac therapeutics. Circ Res 2004; 95(1): 9-20.
[http://dx.doi.org/10.1161/01.RES.0000135902.99383.6f] [PMID: 15242981]

[23] Segers VF, Lee RT. Stem-cell therapy for cardiac disease. Nature 2008; 451(7181): 937-42.
[http://dx.doi.org/10.1038/nature06800] [PMID: 18288183]

[24] Palakkan AA, Hay DC, Anil Kumar PR, Kumary TV, Ross JA. Liver tissue engineering and cell sources: issues and challenges. Liver Int 2013; 33(5): 666-76.
[http://dx.doi.org/10.1111/liv.12134] [PMID: 23490085]

[25] Shirakigawa N, Ijima H, Takei T. Decellularized liver as a practical scaffold with a vascular network template for liver tissue engineering. J Biosci Bioeng 2012; 114(5): 546-51.
[http://dx.doi.org/10.1016/j.jbiosc.2012.05.022] [PMID: 22717723]

[26] Du C, Narayanan K, Leong MF, Wan AC. Induced pluripotent stem cell-derived hepatocytes and endothelial cells in multi-component hydrogel fibers for liver tissue engineering. Biomaterials 2014; 35(23): 6006-14.
[http://dx.doi.org/10.1016/j.biomaterials.2014.04.011] [PMID: 24780169]

[27] Peloso A, Tamburrini R, Edgar L, *et al.* Extracellular matrix scaffolds as a platform for kidney regeneration. Eur J Pharmacol 2016; 790: 21-7.
[http://dx.doi.org/10.1016/j.ejphar.2016.07.038] [PMID: 27455902]

[28] Metcalfe AD, Ferguson MW. Tissue engineering of replacement skin: the crossroads of biomaterials, wound healing, embryonic development, stem cells and regeneration. J R Soc Interface 2007; 4(14): 413-37.
[http://dx.doi.org/10.1098/rsif.2006.0179] [PMID: 17251138]

[29] Mauney JR, Volloch V, Kaplan DL. Role of adult mesenchymal stem cells in bone tissue engineering applications: current status and future prospects. Tissue Eng 2005; 11(5-6): 787-802.

[http://dx.doi.org/10.1089/ten.2005.11.787] [PMID: 15998219]

[30]   Liu Y, Lim J, Teoh S-H. Review: development of clinically relevant scaffolds for vascularised bone tissue engineering. Biotechnol Adv 2013; 31(5): 688-705.
[http://dx.doi.org/10.1016/j.biotechadv.2012.10.003] [PMID: 23142624]

[31]   Shadjou N, Hasanzadeh M. Bone tissue engineering using silica-based mesoporous nanobiomaterials:Recent progress. Mater Sci Eng C 2015; 55: 401-9.
[http://dx.doi.org/10.1016/j.msec.2015.05.027] [PMID: 26117771]

[32]   Bose S, Roy M, Bandyopadhyay A. Recent advances in bone tissue engineering scaffolds. Trends Biotechnol 2012; 30(10): 546-54.
[http://dx.doi.org/10.1016/j.tibtech.2012.07.005] [PMID: 22939815]

[33]   Fu Q, Saiz E, Rahaman MN, Tomsia AP. Bioactive glass scaffolds for bone tissue engineering: state of the art and future perspectives. Mater Sci Eng C 2011; 31(7): 1245-56.
[http://dx.doi.org/10.1016/j.msec.2011.04.022] [PMID: 21912447]

[34]   Kolk A, Handschel J, Drescher W, *et al.* Current trends and future perspectives of bone substitute materials - from space holders to innovative biomaterials. J Craniomaxillofac Surg 2012; 40(8): 706-18.
[http://dx.doi.org/10.1016/j.jcms.2012.01.002] [PMID: 22297272]

[35]   Staton CA, Stribbling SM, Tazzyman S, Hughes R, Brown NJ, Lewis CE. Current methods for assaying angiogenesis *in vitro* and *in vivo*. Int J Exp Pathol 2004; 85(5): 233-48.
[http://dx.doi.org/10.1111/j.0959-9673.2004.00396.x] [PMID: 15379956]

[36]   Lanza R, Langer R, Vacanti JP. Principles of tissue engineering. Academic press 2011.

[37]   Harley BA, Yannas IV. *In vivo* synthesis of tissues and organs. In: Lanza R, Langer R, Vacanti JP, Eds. Principles of Tissue Engineering. Elsevier Inc. 2014; 325-55.

[38]   Ingber D. Mechanochemical control of cell fate switching Principles of Tissue Engineering. 2007.

[39]   Boehler RM, Graham JG, Shea LD. Tissue engineering tools for modulation of the immune response. Biotechniques 2011; 51(4): 239-240, 242, 244 passim.
[PMID: 21988690]

[40]   Franz S, Rammelt S, Scharnweber D, Simon JC. Immune responses to implants - a review of the implications for the design of immunomodulatory biomaterials. Biomaterials 2011; 32(28): 6692-709.
[http://dx.doi.org/10.1016/j.biomaterials.2011.05.078] [PMID: 21715002]

[41]   Janik H, Marzec M. A review: fabrication of porous polyurethane scaffolds. Mater Sci Eng C 2015; 48: 586-91.
[http://dx.doi.org/10.1016/j.msec.2014.12.037] [PMID: 25579961]

[42]   Henkel J, Woodruff MA, Epari DR, *et al.* Bone regeneration based on tissue engineering conceptions—a 21st century perspective. Bone Res 2013; 1(3): 216-48.
[http://dx.doi.org/10.4248/BR201303002] [PMID: 26273505]

[43]   Liu C, Czernuszka J. Development of biodegradable scaffolds for tissue engineering: a perspective on emerging technology. Mater Sci Technol 2007; 23(4): 379-91.
[http://dx.doi.org/10.1179/174328407X177027]

SUBJECT INDEX

www.ingramcontent.com/pod-product-compliance
Lightning Source LLC
Chambersburg PA
CBHW041725210326
41598CB00008B/782